Recombinant Lymphokines and Their Receptors

IMMUNOLOGY SERIES

1. Mechanisms in Allergy: Reagin-Mediated Hypersensitivity
   Edited by Lawrence Goodfriend, Alec Sehon and Robert P. Orange
2. Immunopathology: Methods and Techniques
   Edited by Theodore P. Zacharia and Sidney S. Breese, Jr.
3. Immunity and Cancer in Man: An Introduction
   Edited by Arnold E. Reif
4. *Bordetella pertussis:* Immunological and Other Biological Activities
   J.J. Munoz and R.K. Bergman
5. The Lymphocyte: Structure and Function (in two parts)
   Edited by John J. Marchalonis
6. Immunology of Receptors
   Edited by B. Cinader
7. Immediate Hypersensitivity: Modern Concepts and Development
   Edited by Michael K. Bach
8. Theoretical Immunology
   Edited by George I. Bell, Alan S. Perelson, and George H. Pimbley, Jr.
9. Immunodiagnosis of Cancer (in two parts)
   Edited by Ronald B. Herberman and K. Robert McIntire
10. Immunologically Mediated Renal Diseases: Criteria for Diagnosis and Treatment
    Edited by Robert T. McCluskey and Giuseppe A. Andres
11. Clinical Immunotherapy
    Edited by Albert F. LoBuglio
12. Mechanisms of Immunity to Virus-Induced Tumors
    Edited by John W. Blasecki
13. Manual of Macrophage Methodology: Collection, Characterization, and Function
    Edited by Herbert B. Herscowitz, Howard T. Holden, Joseph A. Bellanti, and Abdul Ghaffar
14. Suppressor Cells in Human Disease
    Edited by James S. Goodwin
15. Immunological Aspects of Aging
    Edited by Diego Segre and Lester Smith
16. Cellular and Molecular Mechanisms of Immunologic Tolerance
    Edited by Tomáš Hraba and Milan Hašek

17. Immune Regulation: Evolution and Biological Significance
Edited by Laurens N. Ruben and M. Eric Gershwin

18. Tumor Immunity in Prognosis: The Role of Mononuclear Cell Infiltration
Edited by Stephen Haskill

19. Immunopharmacology and the Regulation of Leukocyte Function
Edited by David R. Webb

20. Pathogenesis and Immunology of Treponemal Infection
Edited by Ronald F. Schell and Daniel M. Musher

21. Macrophage-Mediated Antibody-Dependent Cellular Cytotoxicity
Edited by Hillel S. Koren

22. Molecular Immunology: A Textbook
Edited by M. Zouhair Atassi, Carel J. van Oss, and Darryl R. Absolom

23. Monoclonal Antibodies and Cancer
Edited by George L. Wright, Jr.

24. Stress, Immunity, and Aging
Edited by Edwin L. Cooper

25. Immune Modulation Agents and Their Mechanisms
Edited by Richard L. Fenichel and Michael A. Chirigos

26. Mononuclear Phagocyte Biology
Edited by Alvin Volkman

27. The Lactoperoxidase System: Chemistry and Biological Significance
Edited by Kenneth M. Pruitt and Jorma O. Tenovuo

28. Introduction to Medical Immunology
Edited by Gabriel Virella, Jean-Michel Goust, H. Hugh Fudenberg, and Christian C. Patrick

29. Handbook of Food Allergies
Edited by James C. Breneman

30. Human Hybridomas: Diagnostic and Therapeutic Applications
Edited by Anthony J. Strelkauskas

31. Aging and the Immune Response: Cellular and Humoral Aspects
Edited by Edmond A. Goidl

32. Complications of Organ Transplantation
Edited by Luis H. Toledo-Pereyra

33. Monoclonal Antibody Production Techniques and Applications
Edited by Lawrence B. Schook

34. Fundamentals of Receptor Molecular Biology
Donald F. H. Wallach

35. Recombinant Lymphokines and Their Receptors
Edited by Steven Gillis

36. Immunology of the Male Reproductive Organs
Edited by Pierre Luigi Bigazzi

Additional Volumes in Preparation

Recombinant Lymphokines and Their Receptors

edited by
Steven Gillis
Immunex Corporation
Seattle, Washington

MARCEL DEKKER, INC. New York and Basel

Library of Congress Cataloging-in-Publication Data

Recombinant lymphokines and their receptors.

(Immunology series ; 35)
Includes bibliographies and index.
1. Lymphokines. 2. Lymphokines--Receptors.
3. Recombinant DNA. I. Gillis, Steven.
II. Series: Immunology series ; v. 35.
QR185.8.L93R43 1987 616.07'95 87-8856
ISBN 0-8247-7753-0

MARCEL DEKKER, INC.
270 Madison Avenue, New York, New York 10016

Current printing (last digit):
10 9 8 7 6 5 4 3 2 1

PRINTED IN THE UNITED STATES OF AMERICA

Series Introduction

It has been obvious for many years that the cells of the immune system communicate with one another on a continuing basis. How else could such an intricate system be kept in proper balance? And how could it respond to so many different stimuli in a stereotyped pattern? For a time, it appeared that most regulatory interactions required cell-to-cell contact. Gradually, however, evidence has accumulated that soluble products are also intricate members of the immunological community.

One by one, these soluble products have been isolated and their individual functions defined. The receptor(s) for each, and its target cell population, have been determined. The latest and potentially most exciting phase of investigation has begun with the production of some of these regulatory substances—the interleukins and colony-stimulating factors, for instance—by recombinant cDNA cloning. The availability of these substances in large quantities now opens new, exciting possibilities for treatment of infectious, immunological, and malignant diseases. In the present volume, Dr. Gillis and his collaborators have given us a comprehensive and authoritative glimpse of that future.

Noel R. Rose

Preface

Over the past 10 years, no other subspecialty within the field of immunology has enjoyed a more rapid pace of development than has the investigation of soluble mediators of immune response. In the mid-1970s, lymphokines were dismissed by most of the cognoscenti of cellular immunology as mere mythical molecules present in crude supernates of mitogen- or antigen-activated leukocytes. Indeed, at that point in time, not a single lymphokine had been purified to molecular homogeneity, and the isolation of a lymphokine cDNA was closer to fantasy than it was to reality. Now, in the mid-1980s, most, if not all, of the better characterized lymphokine systems have been laid open. Several important regulators of the immune response have been identified. As such, the genes encoding these hormones have been cloned and placed into bacterial and mammalian expression systems, affording the immunologist the opportunity not only to study the mechanism behind cell-mediated immune function, but also to begin to dissect the cytoplasmic elements behind immune hormone action. Finally, and perhaps most important, the generation of large quantities of recombinant immunoregulatory proteins has fostered their testing in various pathological conditions where clinicians have long theorized that perturbance of host immune function might be more beneficial to the outcome of the patient than mere antibiotic or chemotherapeutic treatment of the causative lesion.

Why has the molecular characterization of lymphokines, as hormones of the immune response, enjoyed such a rapid development in the past decade?

First, and perhaps foremost, investigators came to the common conclusion that, in order to understand how cells of the immune response spoke to one another, it would be necessary to conduct experiments on homogeneous and, in the best of circumstances, clonal populations of immunocytes—whether they be macrophages, B cells, or T cells of any particular effector lineage. The investigation of cell-mediated immune responses in vitro, at the clonal level, led to an appreciation that the soluble products of mixed populations of immunocytes could have marked effects on both the vigor and direction of a given immune response. The marriage of investigation at the clonal cell level, with previously documented effects of immunocyte culture supernates on in vitro assays of cell-mediated immune function, led to the development of the first truly reproducible in vitro assays for lymphokine function. Whether they were assays that measured the ability of a cloned T cell to proliferate, or whether they were assays that monitored immunoglobulin production at the level of a single B lymphocyte, in vitro assays of lymphokine function were the first early key to rapid progress in the area of research that dealt most closely with soluble mediators of immune function.

The attraction of biochemists to the field of immunology led to successful experimentation aiming at the biochemical characterization and purification of discrete molecules that functioned in the unambiguous assays mentioned above. In addition, the techniques of molecular biology, when focused on this narrow subspecialty of immunology, led to the rapid isolation and characterization of lymphokine genes.

Finally, the availability of large quantities of soluble immune response mediators, all of which function in vitro or in vivo at subnanomolar levels, allowed membrane biochemists to unlock the door leading to a glimpse of how lymphokines function at the cell surface, which in turn led to biochemical characterization of lymphokine receptor genes. Such rapid progress was fueled not only by the efforts of investigators trained in disciplines far afield from immunology (most notably biochemists and molecular biologists), but by an outpouring of resources in this particular area of scientific inquiry, both from funding agencies and from the private sector, as the field of biotechnology embraced immunology as a produce orchard where high-value-added pharmaceuticals might be ripe for the plucking. Thus, a number of immunoregulatory molecules have passed out of the realm of existence as mythological mediators in a culture supernate, to cloned gene products being tested in human clinical trials for their ability to augment or alter immune function.

It is hoped that the present volume will serve as a collective anthology describing experimentation that resulted in the successful molecular characterization of various lymphokines and their receptors. Unfortunately, as in most volumes, the following chapters represent only a still life of the field of immune regulation at a given point in time—unfortunate only in that the field has continued to move at its rapid pace and, thus, several of its most recent developments could not be included in this volume. Nevertheless, it is hoped that this volume will be of benefit, not only to investigators involved in dissection of immune function, but also to students of molecular biology, biochemistry, and, of course, immunology.

The first molecule that most investigators would agree could be characterized as a lymphokine is interferon. In his chapter, Sidney Pestka reviews experimentation which successfully allowed for the production of recombinant interferon—a molecule that has gone on through all phases of clinical testing and has become an approved therapeutic.

The next lymphokine to make the voyage from conjecture to cloning to the clinic is interleukin-2 (IL-2). Investigators from Cetus Corporation have reviewed in their chapter the cloning and expression of human IL-2. This molecule was originally, and perhaps more appropriately, known as T-cell growth factor and is of paramount importance for the proliferation of any antigen-stimulated effector T-cell clone. IL-2, because of its central role in the development of an immune response either in vitro or in vivo, continues to hold great promise as a therapeutic entity, most notably for the treatment of malignancy, either alone or in concert with adoptive immunotherapy or chemotherapy regimens. In recent days, IL-2 has also been shown to act on a wide variety of cell populations from B lymphocytes to monocytes to bone marrow precursors of varying types of hematopoietic cells. In keeping with these varied functions of IL-2, James Watson, and collaborators from the University of Auckland in New Zealand, explore in their chapter theories of the mechanism behind induction of IL-2 responsiveness in a wide variety of cell types. Finally, in a world where analogous gene products in different species can be uncovered after development of a single Southern blot, Paul Baker and Douglas Pat Cerretti describe the use of cross-species hybridization for the isolation of a bovine IL-2 cDNA.

As intimated above, the availability of large quantities ofpurified natural or recombinant lymphokines, made possible by the efforts of biochemists and molecular biologists, has allowed investigators of another discipline to become fascinated by the actions of immunoregulatory hormones. As such, membrane biochemists have turned their attention to the action of lymphokines at the cell surface. Teams of such investigators, who once again have embraced the power of biochemistry and molecular biology, have made great strides with respect to the biochemical and molecular characterization of lymphokine receptors, the most well characterized of which is the interleukin-2 receptor.

In their chapter, David Urdal and colleagues review Immunex Corporation's experimentation that led to isolation of human IL-2 cDNA and its expression in mammalian cells. As well, Kathleen McKereghan et al. chronicle an investigation that resulted in the successful molecular characterization of the murine IL-2 receptor. Although both investigations were successful in characterizing the gene that codes for an IL-2-binding protein, they fell somewhat short of solving what today remains a central question in the area of lymphokine research; namely, what is the molecular foundation for high-affinity binding of IL-2 to responsive cells? The cDNA clones isolated to date (those described by Urdal, McKereghan, and their co-workers) when transfected into many mammalian cells give rise to expression of a cell surface protein that mediates only low-affinity binding of IL-2 (an affinity several orders of magnitude below the high-affinity binding observed in antigen-activated T cells, or when receptor cDNAs are appropriately transfected into T cells). It is hoped that experimentation over the next 6–12 months will unlock the molecular mechanism behind high-affinity IL-2 binding and, more important, help to elucidate whether the complex molecular mechanism responsible for IL-2 receptor interactions will be a common one for other lymphokine-binding proteins.

Interleukin-1 (IL-1) can largely be thought of as the "original sin" lymphokine. Although at first technically outlawed as a lymphokine (as it was known to be produced most notably by macrophages and keratinocytes), IL-1 has now been found to be produced by a wide variety of B lymphocytes and cloned T-cell lines. Most interestingly, its functions appear to be as diverse as its cellular source. IL-1 is required for IL-2 production and is thus centrally involved in initiation of cell-mediated immune responses. It is capable of fueling B-lymphocyte proliferation as well. Furthermore, in addition to its effects on cells of the immune response, IL-1 has been shown to function as an endogenous pyrogen, to foster fibroblast proliferation, to stimulate prostaglandin and collagenase production by synovial cells, and to induce acute-phase protein synthesis by hepatocytes. As a result, scientists in the early 1980s questioned how a single molecule could possibly be responsible for so many of the functions attributed to IL-1. The answer was unearthed in 1985 through a series of studies which documented that, in fact, IL-1 activities were not mediated by a single protein, but could be attributed to the function of two remarkably distinct immunoregulatory molecules.

In one chapter, Andrew Webb and colleagues review the molecular characterization of human IL-1β, as it was unearthed from a cDNA library prepared from mRNA harvested from activated macrophages. In a second chapter, dealing with the molecular characterization of IL-1 genes, David Cosman et al. review the use of hybrid select translation as a means for unearthing the human IL-1α gene. Both chapters serve as appropriate examples of how molecular biology has been used to solve important questions of cell-mediated immunity.

As has been the case with IL-2, membrane biochemists have most recently turned their attention to IL-1 and have begun a variety of studies aimed at biochemical characterization of the IL-1 receptor. In his chapter, Steven Dower reviews these experiments and puts forth the now well-accepted conclusion that both interleukin-1s, α and β, although only 25% homologous at the amino acid level, appear to bind to the same high-affinity cell-surface receptor. How two such structurally diverse and yet biologically similar molecules can bind to the same cell-surface structure with the apparent same high affinity is a question that will hopefully be answered shortly by the molecular characterization of the IL-1 receptor.

In addition to controlling the proliferation and the vigor of immunocyte function, soluble products of immune cells also control hematopoiesis and, as such, the proliferation and differentiation of a wide variety of blood cells—from granulocytes to macrophages to pluripotent precursors of eosinophils, megakaryocytes, and normoblasts. An ever-growing list of such T-cell products have now been analyzed at the molecular level. A number of chapters detailing the results of such studies are contained in this volume.

Mosmann and colleagues review the efforts of investigators at DNAX, who successfully isolated the gene for murine interleukin-3 (IL-3), a molecule that controls proliferation and differentiation of early multipotent hematopoietic cells and gives rise in vitro to the generation of a wide variety of hematopoietic cell types, most notably basophils and mast cells.

Another chapter (by Belinda Avalos and colleagues) reviews the molecular isolation of a gene coding for human erythroid-potentiating activity, a molecule that enhances the development of erythroid cells in vitro and, interestingly, functions as an inhibitor of metaloproteinase activity.

Michael Cantrell and colleagues review the cloning, expression, and activity of human granulocyte macrophage colony-stimulating factor (GM-CSF), a product of T cells that directly controls the in vitro and in vivo proliferation of both granulocytes and macrophages.

Finally, Christine Martens and colleagues chronicle their experiments that have led to the isolation of a molecule which functions in allergic reactions by binding to immunoglobulin E and inhibiting histamine release by basophils.

One of the key areas where clinicians and biotechnicians hope to use recombinant lymphokines or their receptors as pharmaceutical products remains the treatment of malignancy. As such, a wide variety of lymphokines are being tested clinically in cancer patients because they are known to augment the function of cells capable of mediating destruction of malignant cells, whether they be T cells (following stimulation with IL-2) or macrophages and granulocytes (following activation with GM-CSF). However, two lymphokines have long been known to act directly to mediate tumor cell destruction. Late during the period of the mid-1980s both these molecules have fallen to the dissection of molecular biologists. Patrick Gray reviews the isolation of human lymphotoxin genes, and Diane Pennica et al. chronicle expression of tumor necrosis factors. Both chapters continue to emphasize the speed with which investigators (having been given an appropriate unambiguous assay for biological activity and a crude cellular source of that activity) can rapidly isolate and characterize genes that encode the protein(s) responsible for such activities.

As mentioned above, the field of the molecular characterization of lymphokines and their receptors continues to move at an almost frenzied pace. Thus, although this volume will serve as a reference for the elucidation of a variety of lymphokine genes, it cannot, by definition, provide a truly up-to-date accounting. Predictably, several more immune response modulators have now given way to analysis at the biochemical and molecular level. Genes for human IL-3, granulocyte colony-stimulating factor, and macrophage colony-stimulating factor have been cloned and expressed in heterologous hosts. As well, molecules that function to control B-lymphocyte growth and differentiation have recently been described in molecular terms. B-cell-stimulating factor-1 (BSF-1) and B-cell-stimulating factor-2 (BSF-2), the latter being synonymous with a subtype of human interferon-β, have recently been characterized and produced in quantities sufficient for contemplation of in vivo studies. At the cell surface level, the oncogene product, c-fms, is known to be the receptor for macrophage colony-stimulating factor, or CSF-1. High-affinity cell surface-binding proteins have also been identified for GM-CSF and for human and murine BSF-1. Given the rapid progress that has been made since this volume was written, it is safe to assume that the future for molecular characterization of recombinant lymphokines and their receptors remains a bright one.

Steven Gillis

Contributors

John S. Abrams Department of Immunology, DNAX Research Institute of Molecular and Cellular Biology, Palo Alto, California

Alan R. Alpert Department of Membrane Biochemistry, Immunex Corporation, Seattle, Washington

Dirk M. Anderson Department of Molecular Biology, Immunex Corporation, Seattle, Washington

Ken-ichi Arai Department of Molecular Biology, DNAX Research Institute of Molecular and Cellular Biology, Palo Alto, California

Naoko Arai Department of Molecular Biology, DNAX Research Institute of Molecular and Cellular Biology, Palo Alto, California

Philip E. Auron Department of Medicine, Harvard–M.I.T. Division of Health Sciences and Technology, Cambridge, Massachusetts; The New England Medical Center and Tufts University School of Medicine, Boston, Massachusetts

Belinda R. Avalos Division of Hematology-Oncology, Department of Medicine, UCLA School of Medicine, Los Angeles, California

Paul E. Baker Animal Health Laboratory, Immunex Corporation, Seattle, Washington

Martha W. Bond Department of Molecular Biology, DNAX Research Institute of Molecular and Cellular Biology, Palo Alto, California

Michael A. Cantrell Department of Molecular Biology, Immunex Corporation, Seattle, Washington

Douglas Pat Cerretti Department of Molecular Biology, Immunex Corporation, Seattle, Washington

Steven C. Clark Genetics Institute, Cambridge, Massachusetts

Paul J. Conlon Department of Cellular Immunology, Immunex Corporation, Seattle, Washington

David J. Cosman Department of Molecular Biology, Immunex Corporation, Seattle, Washington

Michael C. Deeley Department of Molecular Biology, Immunex Corporation, Seattle, Washington

Steven K. Dower Department of Membrane Biochemistry, Immunex Corporation, Seattle, Washington

Michael V. Doyle Department of Cell Biology, Cetus Corporation, Emeryville, California

Byron M. Gallis Department of Cellular Biochemistry, Immunex Corporation, Seattle, Washington

Judith C. Gasson Division of Hematology-Oncology, Department of Medicine, UCLA School of Medicine, Los Angeles, California

Steven Gillis Research and Development, Immunex Corporation, Seattle, Washington

David W. Golde Department of Medicine, UCLA School of Medicine, Los Angeles, California

Kenneth Grabstein Department of Cellular Immunology, Immunex Corporation, Seattle, Washington

Patrick W. Gray Department of Molecular Biology, Genentech, Inc., South San Francisco, California

Thomas P. Hopp Department of Protein Chemistry, Immunex Corporation, Seattle, Washington

Kimishige Ishizaka Subdepartment of Immunology, Johns Hopkins University School of Medicine, Baltimore, Maryland

Kirston Koths Department of Protein Chemistry, Cetus Corporation, Emeryville, California

Shirley R. Kronheim Department of Protein Chemistry, Immunex Corporation, Seattle, Washington

Frank D. Lee Department of Molecular Biology, DNAX Research Institute of Molecular and Cellular Biology, Palo Alto, California

Graham S. Le Gros Department of Immunobiology, School of Medicine, University of Auckland, Auckland, New Zealand

Andrew J. Lewis Department of Membrane Biochemistry, Immunex Corporation, Seattle, Washington

Randell T. Libby Department of Molecular Biology, Immunex Corporation, Seattle, Washington

David F. Mark Department of Molecular Biology, Cetus Corporation, Emeryville, California

Christine L. Martens Department of Immunology, DNAX Research Institute of Molecular and Cellular Biology, Palo Alto, California

Kathleen N. McKereghan Department of Molecular Biology, Immunex Corporation, Seattle, Washington

Atsushi Miyajima Department of Molecular Biology, DNAX Research Institute of Molecular and Cellular Biology, Palo Alto, California

Shoichiro Miyatake Department of Molecular Biology, DNAX Research Institute of Molecular and Cellular Biology, Palo Alto, California

Diane Y. Mochizuki Department of Cellular Biochemistry, Immunex Corporation, Seattle, Washington

Kevin W. Moore Department of Immunology, DNAX Research Institute of Molecular and Cellular Biology, Palo Alto, California

Bruce Mosley Department of Molecular Biology, Immunex Corporation, Seattle, Washington

Tim R. Mosmann Department of Immunology, DNAX Research Institute of Molecular and Cellular Biology, Palo Alto, California

Robert W. Overell Department of Molecular Biology, Immunex Corporation, Seattle, Washington

Michael A. Palladino, Jr. Department of Molecular Immunology, Genentech, Inc., South San Francisco, California

Linda S. Park Department of Membrane Biochemistry, Immunex Corporation, Seattle, Washington

Diane Pennica Department of Molecular Immunology, Genentech, Inc., South San Francisco, California

Sidney Pestka* Department of Biochemistry, Roche Institute of Molecular Biology, Roche Research Center, Nutley, New Jersey

Virginia L. Price Department of Molecular Biology, Immunex Corporation, Seattle, Washington

---

**Present affiliation*: Department of Molecular Genetics and Microbiology, UMDNJ--Robert Wood Johnson Medical School, Piscataway, New Jersey.

Donna M. Rennick Department of Immunology, DNAX Research Institute of Molecular and Cellular Biology, Palo Alto, California

Lanny J. Rosenwasser Department of Medicine, The New England Medical Center and Tufts University School of Medicine, Boston, Massachusetts

Jolanda Schreurs Department of Molecular Biology, DNAX Research Institute of Molecular and Cellular Biology, Palo Alto, California

M. Refaat Shalaby Department of Pharmacological Sciences, Genentech, Inc., South San Francisco, California

Craig A. Smith Department of Immunology, DNAX Research Institute of Molecular and Cellular Biology, Palo Alto, California

Yutaka Takebe Department of Molecular Biology, DNAX Research Institute of Molecular and Cellular Biology, Palo Alto, California

Robert J. Tushinski Department of Cellular Biochemistry, Immunex Corporation, Seattle, Washington

David L. Urdal Department of Membrane Biochemistry, Immunex Corporation, Seattle, Washington

James D. Watson Department of Immunobiology, School of Medicine, University of Auckland, Auckland, New Zealand

Andrew C. Webb Department of Biological Sciences, Wellesley College, Wellesley, Massachusetts

Takashi Yokota Department of Molecular Biology, DNAX Research Institute of Molecular and Cellular Biology, Palo Alto, California

Gerard Zurawski Department of Molecular Biology, DNAX Research Institute of Molecular and Cellular Biology, Palo Alto, California

Sandra M. Zurawski Department of Molecular Biology, DNAX Research Institute of Molecular and Cellular Biology, Palo Alto, California

Contents

Recombinant Lymphokines and Their Receptors

1

Human Interleukin-2

DAVID F. MARK, MICHAEL V. DOYLE, and KIRSTON KOTHS
Cetus Corporation, Emeryville, California

INTRODUCTION

Human interleukin-2 was first reported by Morgan et al. (1) as a T-cell growth factor (TCGF) found in mitogen-stimulated human lymphocyte-conditioned medium that supported the long-term proliferation of human T cells. Subsequently, it has been shown that a number of lymphokine activities, such as T–cell-replacing factor, costimulator, and killer cell helper factor shared similar characteristics with TCGF. These lymphokines are now characterized under a single name, interleukin-2 (IL-2) (2,3).

The biological effects of IL-2, although originally defined on the basis of the growth of T cells in culture, have expanded to include interactions with macrophages, B cells, natural killer (NK) and other cytotoxic cells, and immunotherapy of cancer and infectious diseases.

Human IL-2 is produced in very small quantities by helper T cells present in peripheral blood lymphocytes (PBL). However the development of high producer tumor cell lines, such as the human Jurkat leukemia line, the gibbon MLA 144 line, and the murine EL4 line, has facilitated the purification of several IL-2s to homogeneity and the determination of their protein sequence (4). Purified Jurkat-derived human IL-2 has a relative molecular weight of approximately 15,000 (4–6) and is glycosylated at a single location, the threonine residue at position 3 (5).

The complementary DNA (cDNA) for human IL-2 has been cloned from a number of human cell sources (7–10) and the gene for recombinant human

IL-2 (*IL2*) has been expressed in *Escherichia coli* and yeast, as well as in insect and mammalian tissue culture cells. In this report we will describe (a) the molecular cloning of the human IL-2 cDNA from the Jurkat human T-cell line and from human peripheral blood lymphocytes (PBL), (b) the expression of the IL-2 protein in *E. coli*, (c) the site-specific modification of the IL-2 gene, and (d) the purification and biological characterization in vivo and in vitro of recombinant IL-2.

MOLECULAR CLONING OF THE HUMAN INTERLEUKIN-2 COMPLEMENTARY DNA

Identification of a High Interleukin-2-Producing Jurkat Subclone

The Jurkat cell line (11) was passaged in Iscove's modified Dulbecco's medium supplemented with 15% fetal calf serum, penicillin, and streptomycin. Cell density was maintained between 2×10^5 and 2×10^6 cells/ml. Cloning of the Jurkat cell line was performed by limiting dilution. The cells were diluted to a concentration of 1-5 cells/ml and then dispensed into 96-well plastic microtiter plates in 200 μl aliquots. The plates were maintained in a humidified incubator containing 5% CO_2 at 37°C until the clones had expanded sufficiently to permit passaging. The clones were then tested for their ability to produce IL-2 upon induction with 10 ng/ml phorbol myristate acetate (PMA) and 3 μg/ml phytohemagglutinin (PHA). Those clones with high levels of production were subjected to a second cycle of subcloning. The Jurkat A5 subclone, isolated after the second cycle of subcloning, consistently produced up to 1000 times as much IL-2 as the parent line and therefore was expanded for use in RNA isolation.

Isolation of Messenger RNA from Induced Cells

Jurkat A5 Subclone

The Jurkat A5 line (2×10^6 cells/ml) was induced for production of IL-2 RNA for 8 hr, as described earlier. Cells were washed twice in phosphate-buffered saline (PBS) at 4°C and resuspended in 10 mM Tris (pH 8), containing 140 mM NaCl, 1.5 mM $MgCl_2$, and 10 mM vanadyl adenosine complex (12). The cellular membranes were lysed by the addition of NP-40 to 0.3% and the nuclei were removed by centrifugation at $1000 \times g$ for 10 min. The cytoplasmic fraction was extracted four times with equal volumes of phenol/chloroform (1:1). Total cytoplasmic RNA was then recovered by ethanol precipitation. Poly-A+ RNA was obtained by chromatography on oligo-dT cellulose (13), and concentrated by ethanol precipitation.

Human Peripheral Blood Lymphocytes

Human PBLs were purified from buffy coats by Ficoll-Hypaque centrifugation and induced for IL-2 production (4×10^6 cells/ml) by the addition of PMA (5 ng/ml) and concanavalin A (Con A) (10 μg/ml) for 48 hr. Total cytoplasmic RNA and poly-A+ mRNA were prepared as described for the Jurkat A5 subclone.

Fractionation of Jurkat and Peripheral Blood Lymphocyte Messenger RNA

Jurkat and PBL poly-A+ mRNA (250 μg) were separately fractionated on identical 5-20% sucrose gradients. The mRNAs were recovered from each gradient fraction by ethanol precipitation and dissolved in distilled water. Aliquots from each fraction were tested for IL-2 biological activity by injection into frog oocytes (14) and by subsequent testing of the oocyte incubation medium for IL-2 biological activity (15) on a murine IL-2-dependent cell line, HT-2 (16). Figure 1 shows the activity profiles of the sucrose gradients, plotted together for purposes of comparison. The mRNAs were pooled from two fractions of each gradient (13 and 14) with high IL-2 activity and used for the construction of cDNA banks.

Construction of Complementary DNA Banks

Complementary DNA was made from the Jurkat and PBL mRNA fractions that contained IL-2 activity (as determined by the IL-2 assay of injected oocytes) using oligo-dT priming of the poly-A tails and avian myeloblastosis virus (AMV) reverse transcriptase (17). The mRNAs were denatured by treatment with 10 mM methyl mercury at 22°C for 5 min and detoxified by the addition of 100 mM 2-mercaptoethanol (18). Single-stranded cDNAs were synthesized in the presence of 2 mM vanadyl adenosine complex as previously described (12). The second-strand cDNAs were synthesized according to the oligonucleotide-priming method described by Rougeon et al. (19). The cDNAs from both the PBL and Jurkat mRNAs were inserted into the Pst I site of the plasmid, pBR322, by the G-C tailing method (20) and were transformed into competent *E. coli* K12 strain MM294 to generate two cDNA banks.

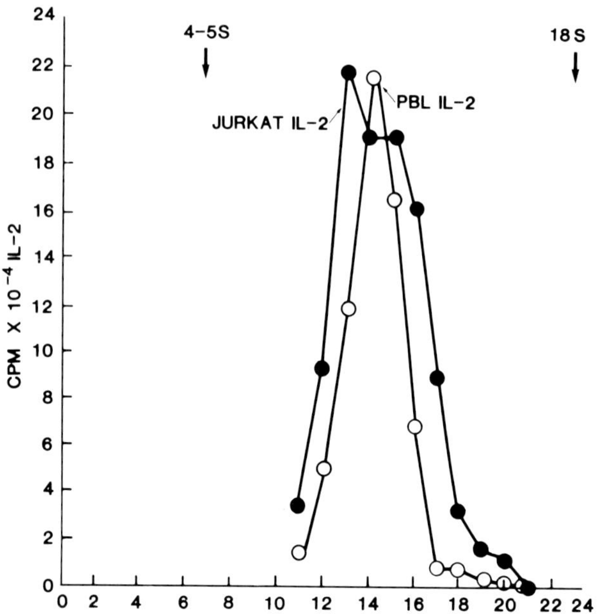

Figure 1 IL-2 activity profile from oocytes injected with mRNAs fractionated by sucrose gradient centrifugation.

Identification of Interleukin-2 Complementary DNA Clones

A 20-mer oligonucleotide probe, based on the nucleotide sequence near the middle of the IL-2 gene as described by Taniguchi et al. (7) was chemically synthesized. This probe, GTGGCCTTCTTGGGCATGTA, was labeled with ^{32}P and used to screen the Jurkat cDNA bank. From 10,000 clones screened by the method of filter hybridization (21), 21 clones hybridized to the probe. Six of the 21 were identified as full-length cDNA clones by restriction enzyme mapping. The nucleotide sequences of two full-length clones (clones 7 and 8) were determined and are shown in Fig. 2. Clone 7 differed from clone 8 by two single-base substitutions (at positions 77 and 504). These changes did not affect the predicted amino acid sequence of the mature protein. The PBL cDNA library (10,000 clones) was screened with a 490 base pair Rsa I/Stu I fragment isolated from the Jurkat clone 7 cDNA insert. A total of 24 clones hybridized to this probe and two

```
         1
                                                                         MET TYR ARG MET
CLONE7   TAT CAC TCT CTT TAA TCA CTA CTC ACA GTA ACC TCA ACT CCT GCC ACA ATG TAC AGG ATG
CLONE8   -------------------------------------------------------------------------------
CLONE26  -------------------------------------------------------------------------------
CLONE60  -------------------------------------------------------------------------------

         61
         GLN LEU LEU SER CYS THR ALA LEU SER LEU ALA LEU VAL·THR ASN SER ALA PRO THR SER
CLONE7   CAA CTC CTG TCT TGC ACT GCA CTA AGT CTT GCA CTT GTC ACA AAC AGT GCA CCT ACT TCA
CLONE8   ---------------------T---------------------------------------------------------
CLONE26  ---------------------T---------------------------------------------------------
CLONE60  ---------------------T---------------------------------------------------------
                            (ILE)
         121
         SER SER THR LYS LYS THR GLN LEU GLN LEU GLU HIS LEU LEU LEU ASP LEU GLN MET ILE
CLONE7   AGT TCT ACA AAG AAA ACA CAG CTA CAA CTG GAG CAT TTA CTG CTG GAT TTA CAG ATG ATT
CLONE8   -------------------------------------------------------------------------------
CLONE26  -----------------------------------------------------A-------------------------
CLONE60  -------------------------------------------------------------------------------

         181
         LEU ASN GLY ILE ASN ASN TYR LYS ASN PRO LYS LEU THR ARG MET LEU THR PHE LYS PHE
CLONE7   TTG AAT GGA ATT AAT AAT TAC AAG AAT CCC AAA CTC ACC AGG ATG CTC ACA TTT AAG TTT
CLONE8   -------------------------------------------------------------------------------
CLONE26  -------------------------------------------------------------------------------
CLONE60  -------------------------------------------------------------------------------

         241
         TYR MET PRO LYS LYS ALA THR GLU LEU LYS HIS LEU GLN CYS LEU GLU GLU GLU LEU LYS
CLONE7   TAC ATG CCC AAG AAG GCC ACA GAA CTG AAA CAT CTT CAG TGT CTA GAA GAA GAA CTC AAA
CLONE8   -------------------------------------------------------------------------------
CLONE26  -------------------------------------------------------------------------------
CLONE60  -------------------------------------------------------------------------------

         301
         PRO LEU GLU GLU VAL LEU ASN LEU ALA GLN SER LYS ASN PHE HIS LEU ARG PRO ARG ASP
CLONE7   CCT CTG GAG GAA GTG CTA AAT TTA GCT CAA AGC AAA AAC TTT CAC TTA AGA CCC AGG GAC
CLONE8   -------------------------------------------------------------------------------
CLONE26  -------------------------------------------------------------------------------
CLONE60  -------------------------------------------------------------------------------

         361
         LEU ILE SER ASN ILE ASN VAL ILE VAL LEU GLU LEU LYS GLY SER GLU THR THR PHE MET
CLONE7   TTA ATC AGC AAT ATC AAC GTA ATA GTT CTG GAA CTA AAG GGA TCT GAA ACA ACA TTC ATG
CLONE8   -------------------------------------------------------------------------------
CLONE26  -------------------------------------------------------------------------------
CLONE60  -------------------------------------------------------------------------------

         421
         CYS GLU TYR ALA ASP GLU THR ALA THR ILE VAL GLU PHE LEU ASN ARG TRP ILE THR PHE
CLONE7   TGT GAA TAT GCT GAT GAG ACA GCA ACC ATT GTA GAA TTT CTG AAC AGA TGG ATT ACC TTT
CLONE8   -------------------------------------------------------------------------------
CLONE26  -------------------------------------------------------------------------------
CLONE60  -------------------------------------------------------------------------------

         481
         CYS GLN SER ILE ILE SER THR LEU THR ***
CLONE7   TGT CAA AGC ATC ATC TCA ACA CTG ACT TGA TAA TTA AGT GCT TCC CAC TTA AAA CAT ATC
CLONE8   ------------------------------A------------------------------------------------
CLONE26  ------------------------------A------------------------------------------------
CLONE60  ------------------------------A------------------------------------------------

         541
CLONE7   AGG CCT TCT ATT TAT TTA AAT ATT TAA ATT TTA TAT TTA TTG TTG AAT GTA TGG TTT GCT
CLONE8   -------------------------------------------------------------------------------
CLONE26  -------------------------------------------------------------------------------
CLONE60  -------------------------------------------------------------------------------

         601
CLONE7   ACC TAT TGT AAC TAT TAT TCT TAA TCT TAA AAC TAT AAA TAT GGA TCT TTT ATG ATT CTT
CLONE8   -------------------------------------------------------------------------------
CLONE26  -------------------------------------------------------------------------------
CLONE60  -------------------------------------------------------------------------------

         661
CLONE7   TTT GTA AGC CCT AGG GGC TCT AAA ATG GTT TCA CTT ATT TAT CCC AAA ATA TTT ATT ATT
CLONE8   -------------------------------------------------------------------------------
CLONE26  -------------------------------------------------------------------------------
CLONE60  -------------------------------------------------------------------------------

         721
CLONE7   ATG TTG AAT GTT AAA TAT AGT ATC TAT GTA GAT TGG TTA GTA AAA CTA TTT AAT AAA TTT
CLONE8   -------------------------------------------------------------------------------
CLONE26  -------------------------------------------------------------------------------
CLONE60  -------------------------------------------------------------------------------

         781
CLONE7   GAT AAA TAT AAC AAA AAA AA
CLONE8   --------------------------
CLONE26  --------------------------
CLONE60  --------------------------
```

Figure 2 Nucleotide sequences of human IL-2 cDNA clones. Clones 7 and 8 were isolated from a Jurkat-derived cDNA library, and clones 26 and 60 were from a PBL-derived cDNA library.

full-length cDNA clones (clone 26 and clone 60) were completely sequenced and compared with the Jurkat-derived IL-2 clones (Fig. 2). Clone 60 was found to be identical to the Jurkat clone 8 and clone 26 was shown to have a single base change at position 161.

EXPRESSION OF RECOMBINANT HUMAN INTERLEUKIN-2 IN *ESCHERICHIA COLI*

Human IL-2 was expressed in *E. coli* under the control of the *trp* promoter (22–24), using the scheme described in Fig. 3. The resulting IL-2 expression plasmid, pLW1, encoded an IL-2 lacking the NH_2-terminal alanine (des-Ala-1 IL-2). When *E. coli* harboring pLW1 was grown in the absence of tryptophan to induce the *trp* promoter and the total cell extract analyzed on sodium dodecyl sulfate polyacrylamide gels (SDS-PAGE), a new protein, of approximately 15,000 Da, was induced (Fig. 4, lane 3). The induced IL-2 protein represented approximately 5% of the total cellular protein, and the total cell extract contained about 10^5 units of IL-2 biological activity per milliliter.

SITE-SPECIFIC MUTAGENESIS OF THE INTERLEUKIN-2 COMPLEMENTARY DNA

Substitution of the Cysteine Residues

The presence of three cysteine residues in the IL-2 protein permits the formation of three different disulfide bridges upon controlled oxidation of the reduced protein in vitro. To investigate the disulfide bond structure of IL-2 and to identify the cysteine residues responsible for the disulfide bridge found in the biologically active protein, we selectively modified each of the three cysteines of IL-2 to serine residues by site-specific mutagenesis of the IL-2 cDNA (25,26). Following oligonucleotide-directed mutagenesis of the cDNA in single-stranded M13 phage, the three mutants were individually subcloned into an expression vector under the control of the *E. coli trp* promoter. Extracts of cells containing the plasmids pLW42 (Ser-58), pLW44 (Ser-105), and pLW46 (Ser-125) were assayed for IL-2 activity on the murine HT-2 cell line. The results are shown in Table 1. Compared with the parent, pLW21, two of the mutants, pLW42 (Ser-58) and pLW44 (Ser-105) were essentially inactive, while pLW46 (Ser-125) exhibited full biological activity. When these extracts were analyzed on an

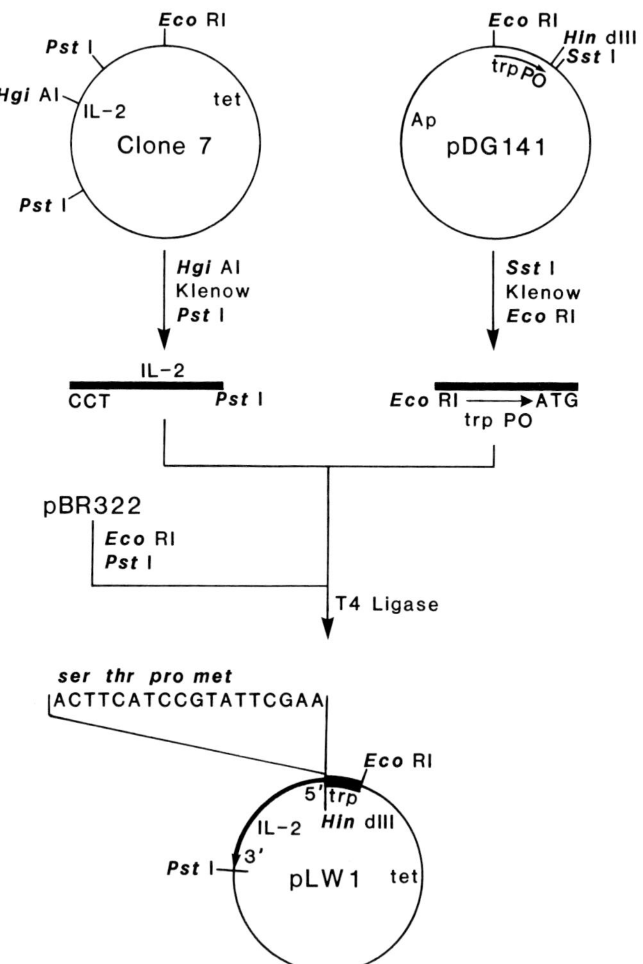

Figure 3 Scheme for the expression of des-Ala-1 IL-2 (*Source*: Ref. 9. Copyright 1984 by the AAAS.)

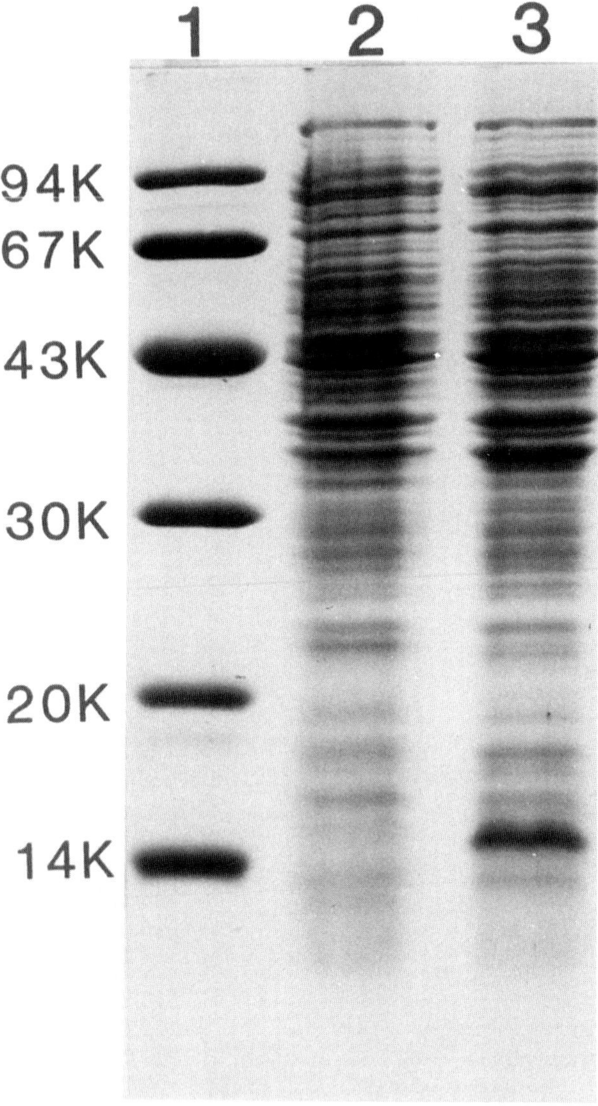

Figure 4 Polyacrylamide gel electrophoresis of IL-2 produced in *E. coli*. The *E. coli* containing pLW1 was grown in minimal medium in the absence of tryptophan to derepress the *trp* promoter, and total cell extracts were analyzed on a 15% SDS-PAGE stained with Coomassie blue. Lane 1, molecular weight markers; lane 2, extract of *E. coli* containing the plasmid vector without the IL-2 cDNA; lane 3, extract of *E. coli* containing pLW1.

Table 1 Biological Activities of Serine-Substituted IL-2s

Extracts[a]	IL-2 activity (U/ml)
pIL2-7 (negative control)	<69
pLW21 (positive control)	9.0×10^5
pLW42	4.4×10^3
pLW44	1.7×10^4
pLW46	1.2×10^6

[a]Normalized for IL-2 polypeptide content.

SDS-PAGE, all four had a 15-kDa band, characteristic of IL-2, of similar intensity (data not shown), suggesting that the differences seen in the biological activity were not the result of different levels of expression of the IL-2 protein. The specific activities of highly purified parental and Ser-125 IL-2s were subsequently shown to be identical.

These results indicate that cysteines at position 58 and 105 are involved in a disulfide bridge necessary for maintaining a biologically active conformation, while cysteine-125 is not involved in disulfide bridge formation and is not necessary for biological activity. Similar conclusions were reached by Robb et al., based on biochemical studies of native Jurkat IL-2 (5).

Modification of Methionine-104 to Alanine-104

Some proteins contain methionine residues that are particularly sensitive to oxidation to methionine sulfoxide, and this may contribute to microheterogeneity of the purified protein. On the basis of biochemical analysis of purified recombinant IL-2 (see the following discussion), we suspected that a specific methionine in IL-2 was particularly susceptible to oxidation. To prove that methionine-104 was responsible for this microheterogeneity and to determine if it was required for IL-2 biological activity, we substituted an alanine residue at position 104 using the site-specific mutagenesis technique. As described in the following section, the purified protein derived from mutant plasmid pSY3001 (des-Ala-1, Ala-104, Ser-125) had the same specific biological activity as IL-2 derived from the parental plasmid pLW45 (des-Ala-1, Ser-125).

PURIFICATION OF RECOMBINANT INTERLEUKIN-2 AND DISULFIDE BOND FORMATION

Recombinant human IL-2 (IL-2) is produced in *E. coli* in a fully reduced, insoluble state which causes it to accumulate as inclusion bodies within the cells. Typical published procedures for purifying such IL-2 begin by solubilizing the protein using denaturants such as guanidinium hydrochloride (27,28). These protocols also take advantage of the unusually hydrophobic behavior of the solubilized IL-2 on reverse-phase high-performance liquid chromatography (RP-HPLC) to achieve a high degree of purity in the finished product.

We have found that accurate formation of the native disulfide bond of IL-2 is an important step in obtaining a monocomponent preparation with full activity. Before initiating disulfide bond formation in vitro, we isolated and purified the reduced recombinant IL-2 by taking advantage of its insolubility. The purification protocol (summarized in Table 2) involves (a) extraction of the soluble contaminants from the insoluble IL-2 contained in the *E. coli* cell debris, (b) solubilization of the IL-2 with detergent, (c) partial purification using molecular sieve chromatography, (d) oxidation to form the correct disulfide bond, and (e) purification to homogeneity by RP-HPLC.

Escherichia coli MM294 cells containing the cloned IL-2 were induced, washed, and resuspended in 50 mM Tris, 1 mM EDTA (pH 8.1–8.5). The high pH aided in selective extraction of *E. coli* proteins in the subsequent steps. The cells were sonicated or homogenized and the homogenate was centrifuged to collect the cell debris, which contained most of the IL-2. The debris was resuspended in 60 ml of the Tris/EDTA mixture at room temperature, and over a 5-min period an equal volume of 8 M urea in Tris/EDTA buffer was added to the suspension with rapid stirring to yield a final urea concentration of 4 M. The resulting mixture was stirred for 15–30 min at room temperature and centrifuged at 12,000 × *g* for 15 min at room temperature to remove soluble contaminants. The pellet, which contained most of the IL-2, was then resuspended in 50 mM sodium phosphate (pH 6.8), 1 mM EDTA, 10 mM dithiothreitol (DTT) at 20°C and solubilized by addition of SDS to 2% with vigorous mixing. The resuspension was centrifuged at 12,000 × *g* for 10 min at room temperature, and the insoluble material was discarded. The cleared supernatant was 35–60% pure IL-2 at this point. The solution was then heated to 40°C for 15 min to make certain that all of the IL-2 was fully reduced, and the protein was loaded onto a Sephacryl-200 or Sephadex G-100 column run in 50 mM

Table 2 Recombinant IL-2 Purification Protocol Summary

	Volume (ml)	Total protein (mg)	Total activity (U)	Specific activity (U/mg)	Recovery (%)	Fold purification (X)
Cell lysate[a] (from 20 g wet cells)	200	690	8.0×10^{7}	1.2×10^{5}	100	
Cell debris[a]	60	324	5.3×10^{7}	1.6×10^{5}	66	1.3
SDS-solubilized, urea-extracted pellet	8.8	77	7.3×10^{7}	9.5×10^{5}	91	8
S-200 pool (following S-S formation)	11	19	6.4×10^{7}[b]	3.5×10^{6}[b]	80[b]	29[b]
RP-HPLC pool	7.6	11.4	6.2×10^{7}[b]	5.4×10^{6}[b]	77[b]	45[b]

[a]An aliquot was solubilized in 0.1% SDS, 10 mM DTT at 37°C for 15 min before determination of protein concentration and bioactivity relative to the BRMP International IL-2 standard.
[b]These numbers reflect an apparent two-fold increase in specific activity following the disulfide bond formation step in the protocol.

sodium phosphate (pH 6.8), 1 mM EDTA, 1 mM DTT, 1% (w/v) SDS. Interleukin-2 was located by SDS-PAGE analysis of the resulting fractions, and those containing the 15.5-kDa IL-2 were pooled and concentrated to 5–10 ml using an Amicon YM5 ultrafilter. The preparation was 70–90% pure, and the recovery was about 40% at this point.

To form the disulfide bond in IL-2, the peak fractions from this column were treated as follows: DTT was added to the preparation to a concentration of 2.5 mM, and the sample was heated to 60°C for 10 min to ensure full reduction. Reducing agent was removed using a Sephadex G-25 column equilibrated in 50 mM sodium phosphate buffer (pH 7.0) containing 0.1% SDS. The protein peak was pooled and diluted to 0.25 mg/ml in the column buffer. Disulfide bond formation was initiated by addition of $CuCl_2$ to a concentration of 50 μM at 25°C. The extent of the reaction was measured by assaying residual free sulfhydryl groups or by RP-HPLC, which is capable of resolving disulfide-bonded and reduced proteins (29). At the end of the reaction (typically 30–60 min), EDTA was added to a concentration of 10 mM to chelate free copper ions. One-tenth volume of 100% acetonitrile/5% trifluoroacetic acid (TFA) was added, and the disulfide-bonded IL-2 was then separated from remaining *E. coli* protein and endotoxin by preparative RP-HPLC in acetonitrile/0.1% TFA. Interleukin-2 was recovered in 60% acetonitrile, following gradient elution at 2 ml/min using 10 to 30% acetonitrile for 5 min and 30 to 60% acetonitrile in 45 min. The peak of IL-2 was pooled, and the total protein recovered was determined by absorption at 280 nm. At this point the protein was formulated as follows: mannitol was added to pooled HPLC fractions to a concentration of 1.5%, and SDS was added to 0.03%. The sample was lyophilized overnight and resuspended in 50 mM sodium phosphate (pH 6.8) in water for injection (WFI). The final concentrations of SDS and mannitol were 0.1 and 5%, respectively, and the solubilized protein was stable for at least 2 months at 4°C.

These methods for the purification of IL-2 from *E. coli* and reformation of the disulfide bond worked equally well for both of the IL-2s described in the previous section. Figure 5 shows an SDS-PAGE analysis of these two purified IL-2s, which differ in only one amino acid. When analyzed under nonreducing conditions (lane 4), the final product was over 98% pure, and it contained less than 2% protein migrating in the position expected for IL-2 dimers (which can form when disulfide bonds are generated intermolecularly). If necessary, residual IL-2 oligomers can be removed by molecular sieve chromatography following the IL-2 disulfide

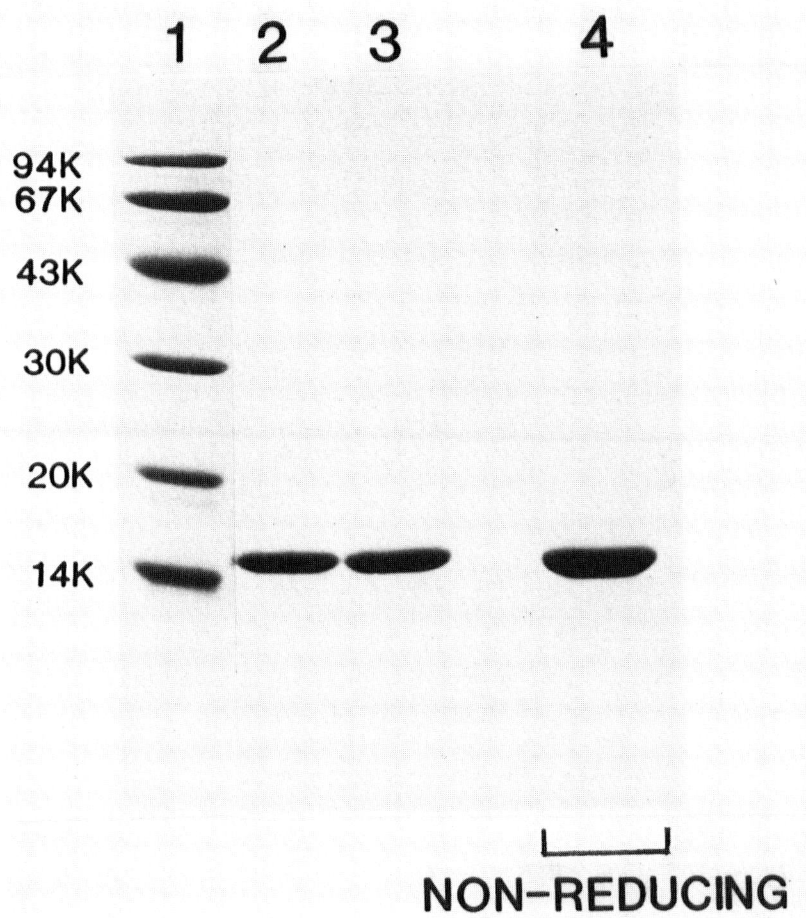

Figure 5 SDS-PAGE analysis of purified, disulfide-bonded IL-2s. Proteins were reduced (lanes 1–3) and run on a 14% acrylamide gel and visualized by Coomassie staining: lane 1, molecular weight standards; lane 2, des-Ala-1, Ala-104, Ser-125 IL-2; lane 3, des-Ala-1, Ser-125 IL-2; lane 4, des-Ala-1, Ala-104, Ser-125 IL-2 (nonreducing conditions).

bond formation step. The RP-HPLC step was very effective at removing residual *E. coli* contaminants and endotoxins.

The specific bioactivity of the purified IL-2 was determined to be 5–10 × 10^6 units/mg, based on the standardized HT-2 cell proliferation assay (15,16) and on protein content measured by the method of Lowry et al. (30). This value agreed well with the specific activity obtained for native Jurkat IL-2 purified to homogeneity and assayed in parallel.

CHARACTERIZATION OF RECOMBINANT INTERLEUKIN-2 WITH IMPROVED PROPERTIES

An Interleukin-2 with Directed Disulfide Bond Formation

When the reaction to form disulfide bonds was carried out on a reduced IL-2 containing all three of the cysteines present in the native molecule, a uniform product was not obtained. Using the conditions described in the previous section, approximately 85% of the product appeared to have the correct disulfide linkage and was fully active in the HT-2 cell proliferation assay (Fig. 6A). However 15% of the material was biologically inactive, eluted earlier on RP-HPLC, and represented the two other possible isomers of IL-2 that contain incorrect disulfide linkages (31).

This interpretation was confirmed when the disulfide bond was reformed in des-Ala-1, Ser-125 IL-2. Because this form of IL-2 lacked the cysteine at residue 125, it was expected that only the active form of the molecule (with a disulfide between the remaining two cysteines) would be generated. The RP-HPLC analysis of this reaction product shows that it contains only the desired form of IL-2 and no inactive isomers (Fig. 6B). The single amino acid change at position 125 affects the RP-HPLC elution position (compare Figs. 6A and B), but the specific bioactivity of the molecule is unchanged.

When the cysteine at position 125 was replaced with alanine instead of serine, no inactive isomers were formed, and the purified, disulfide-containing product had the normal specific bioactivity of IL-2 (data not shown). Thus site-directed mutagenesis of cysteines has been successfully used [as it had previously with recombinant β-interferon production, Mark et al. (22)] to simplify the production and increase the yield of the active form of the product. By replacing a cysteine that participates in unwanted side reactions, we have "directed" the disulfide bond formation reaction to produce only the desired form of IL-2.

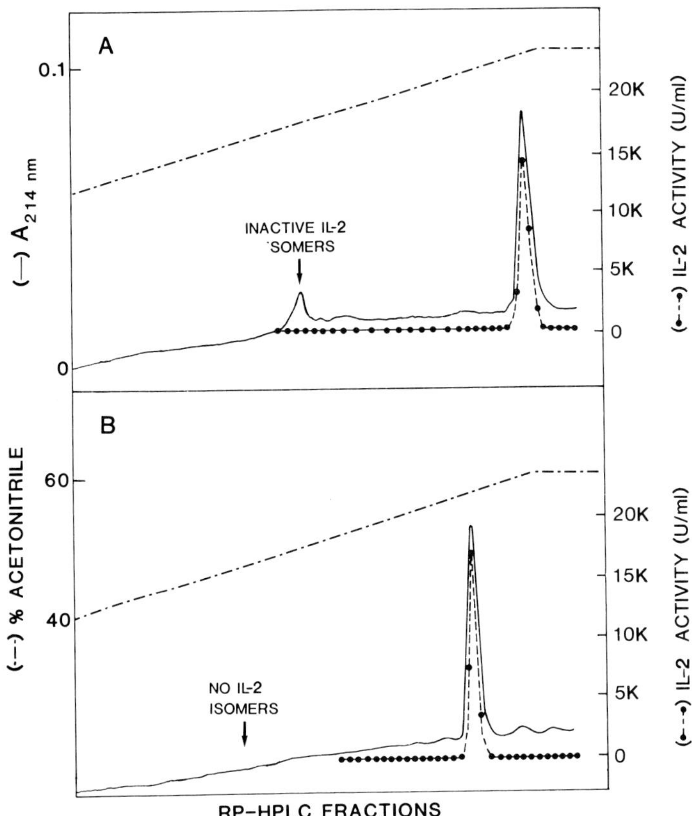

Figure 6 An RP-HPLC analysis of two IL-2s with different disulfide-bonding characteristics. Des-Ala-1 IL-2 and des-Ala-1, Ser-125 IL-2 proteins were purified and treated to reform disulfide bonds as described in the text. An equivalent amount of each protein was analyzed by RP-HPLC on a 5 μm C4 Vydac column, using a gradient of acetonitrile in 0.1% trifluoroacetic acid as the mobile phase. Fractions were immediately diluted into tissue culture medium and assayed in duplicate for cell proliferation activity: panel A, des-Ala-1 IL-2; panel B, des-Ala-1, Ser-125 IL-2.

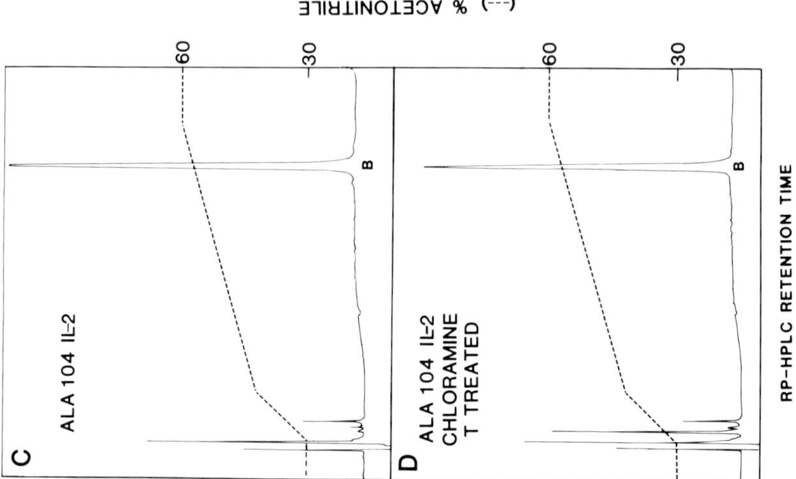
(---) % ACETONITRILE
60
30
C
ALA 104 IL-2
B
D
ALA 104 IL-2
CHLORAMINE
T TREATED
B
RP-HPLC RETENTION TIME

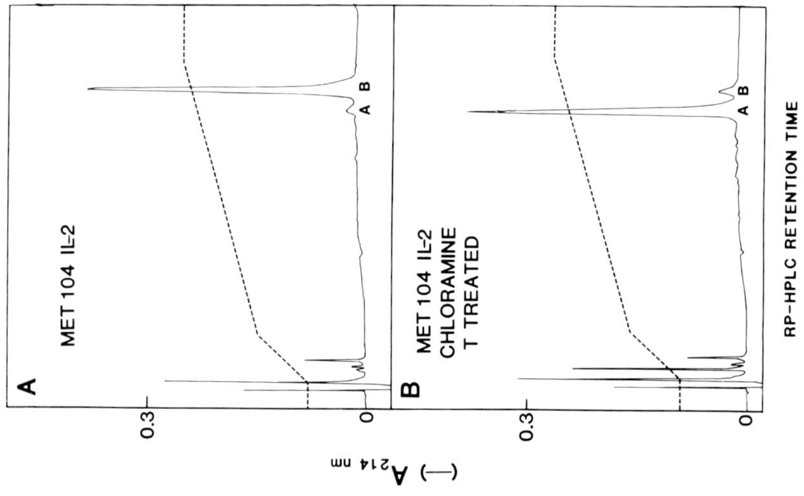
(—) A214 nm
0.3
0
A
MET 104 IL-2
A B
B
MET 104 IL-2
CHLORAMINE
T TREATED
A B
RP-HPLC RETENTION TIME

An Interleukin-2 with Resistance to Undesirable Oxidation

When the disulfide bond in purified, reduced des-Ala-1, Ser-125 IL-2 was reformed and the protein was subjected to analytical RP-HPLC, the results shown in Fig. 7A were obtained. The major IL-2-containing peak (peak B) was preceded by a much smaller peak (peak A). The peak-A material was shown by biological assay and chemical characterization to be active, full-length IL-2, but it contained a methionine that had been oxidized to methionine sulfoxide.

This conclusion was supported by an experiment in which the entire sample was oxidized with chloramine T, which is known to preferentially oxidize methionines (32). Figure 7B shows the RP-HPLC profile of the same IL-2 preparation after chloramine T oxidation. Essentially all of the peak-B protein in Fig. 7A was converted to the peak-A position by chloramine T oxidation. Similar results were obtained in an analogous experiment in which 30 mM hydrogen peroxide was used in place of chloramine T as the oxidizing agent (data not shown).

The exact location of the oxidation-sensitive methionine(s) in IL-2 was determined by exposure to cyanogen bromide (which cleaves protein sequences at methionine, but not at methionine sulfoxide residues). Peaks A and B were purified by RP-HPLC, cleaved with cyanogen bromide, and the resulting mixture of peptides was sequenced by Edman degradation. Several amino acids were recovered at each cycle, corresponding to the sequences of the predicted CNBr fragments. Where methionine sulfoxide was present and cleavage did not occur, amino acids corresponding to the missing peptide were absent. Analysis of the results obtained showed that

---

Figure 7 An RP-HPLC characterization of oxidation-sensitive (Met-104) and oxidation-resistant (Ala-104) forms of IL-2. The IL-2 was purified and treated to reform the disulfide bond as described in the text. The RP-HPLC of the two IL-2s was carried out as in Fig. 6: panel A, des-Ala-1, Ser-125 IL-2 (Met-104 IL-2); panel C, des-Ala-1, Ala-104, Ser-125 IL-2 (Ala-104 IL-2).

Equal amounts of these two samples were chemically treated to oxidize methionines, using chloramine T (five-fold molar excess in 25 mM Tris pH 8.0, 0.1% SDS for 15 min at 25°C). The RP-HPLC analyses are shown in panel B (des-Ala-1, Ser-125 IL-2) and panel D (des-Ala-1, Ala-104, Ser-125 IL-2).

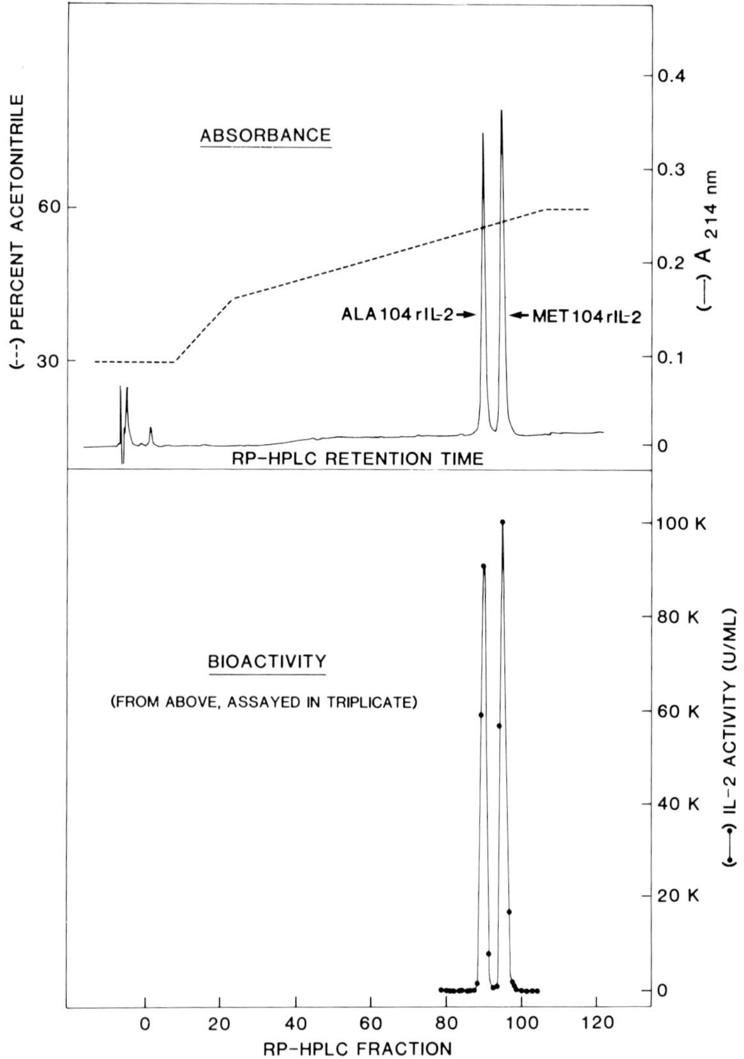

Figure 8 Comparison of the retention times and specific activities of two altered IL-2s following RP-HPLC. Equivalent amounts of purified, disulfide-containing des-Ala-1, Ser-125 IL-2 and des-Ala-1, Ala-104, Ser-125 IL-2 were mixed and subjected to RP-HPLC (upper panel). Fractions were diluted into tissue culture medium and assayed for bioactivity in triplicate (lower panel).

all methionines in peak B IL-2 were unmodified, but in peak A, only the methionine residue at position 104 of each molecule had been oxidized. The same conclusion was obtained using the techniques of tryptic mapping and amino acid analysis to identify the modified methionine (31).

To eliminate the oxidation-sensitivity of IL-2 at methionine-104, we used site-directed mutagenesis to produce an IL-2 containing alanine at residue 104. This new form of IL-2 was purified in the standard fashion and analyzed by RP-HPLC (Fig. 7C). A single, symmetrical peak was obtained, showing that the peak-A material that was generated in similarly purified "parental" IL-2 had been eliminated. Figure 7D shows the results of chloramine T treatment of this preparation, conducted exactly as described for the parental IL-2. As expected, no change in the RP-HPLC pattern was seen for des-Ala-1, Ala-104, Ser-125 IL-2, indicating that this IL-2 lacks the methionine residue preferentially susceptible to oxidation by chloramine T. Interestingly, mouse IL-2 (which is 65% homologous to human IL-2) has glutamic acid instead of methionine at the residue corresponding to position 104 of human IL-2 (33). This supports the observation that methionine-104 is not required for IL-2 activity.

The RP-HPLC retention time of the oxidation-resistant IL-2 differs slightly from that of the parental protein, as has been observed for other IL-2s with single amino acid substitutions (31). This fact has allowed us to mix the oxidation-resistant IL-2 (des-Ala-1, Ala-104, Ser-125) and the parental protein (des-Ala-1, Ser-125) and still resolve them on RP-HPLC (Fig. 8, top). Equivalent bioactivities are observed for the two IL-2s in the T-cell proliferation assay of fractions containing equivalent amounts of protein (Fig 8, bottom). Both altered forms of IL-2 also efficiently activated NK cells. The creation of an oxidation-resistant, monocomponent IL-2 through the introduction of two step-wise amino acid changes has apparently been accomplished without deleterious effects on bioactivity. Thus protein engineering can be used to facilitate production of more homogeneous proteins by eliminating microheterogeneity and by creating products more resistant to changes during storage.

BIOLOGICAL CHARACTERIZATION OF RECOMBINANT INTERLEUKIN-2

The cloning and expression in *E. coli* of the gene for human IL-2 has provided an exciting and significant tool for studying the biology of this immunomodulatory lymphokine. Over the past few years the availability of large quantities of homogeneously pure IL-2 has offered the opportunity to unambiguously determine some of its in vitro and in vivo properties. This work has included experiments confirming a variety of known or suspected properties of native IL-2 that previously might have been attributed to contaminating lymphokines or cytokines in the preparation. In addition, extensive in vivo investigations in humans, mice, and other animal species are now possible. The following discussion will briefly summarize the published biological activities of IL-2 produced in *E. coli*, with particular emphasis on the des-Ala-1, Ser-125 mutein.

Effects on T Cells and Natural Killer Cells

The hallmark of the biological activities of IL-2 has been the ability to maintain the proliferation of populations of activated T cells. Recombinant IL-2 supports the growth, in vitro, of both murine and human long-term lines of T cells. The specific activities (units/mg) of des-Ala-1, Ser-125 IL-2 and of native IL-2 purified from both human peripheral blood mononuclear cells (PBMC) and the Jurkat cell line were the same when measured in a short-term (18-hr), [^{3}H] thymidine incorporation assay (15) using the HT-2 cell line (16). Compared to the human IL-2 reference standard supplied by the Biological Response Modifiers Program of the NCI-FCRF, the specific activities were 5–10 $\times$ 10^6 units/mg protein. The long-term growth in culture of IL-2-dependent cell lines was also maintained equally well by des-Ala-1, Ser-125 IL-2 and native IL-2 (34).

A variety of cytolytic cell activities are affected by IL-2. Allocytotoxic T-cell activity was enhanced both in vitro and in vivo by treatment with des-Ala-1 IL-2 (9). Also, natural killer cell and lymphokine activated killer (LAK) cell activities were increased by exposure of PBMC, in vitro, to des-Ala-1, Ser-125 IL-2 (34–36). Recombinant des-Ala-1, Ser-125 IL-2 and native IL-2 were equivalent in their enhancement of NK cell cytolytic activity (37).

Native IL-2 and des-Ala-1, Ser-125 IL-2 were demonstrated to be equally effective in their direct, dose-dependent, mitogenic effects on PBMC populations and their induction of interferon gamma (34). Ettinghausen et al. (38) have recently demonstrated that in vivo, des-Ala-1, Ser-125 IL-2 caused a dose-dependent proliferation of T cells in mice. They also showed that lymphocytes from certain organs of des-Ala-1, Ser-125 IL–2-treated mice, such as the mesenteric lymph nodes and lungs, were activated to lyse a fresh murine sarcoma target cell.

Interleukin-2 interacts with T cells through attachment to a specific high-affinity receptor (Tac antigen) on activated cells (39–41). The mechanism(s) by which this receptor/IL-2 complex produces effects upon the cellular metabolism, including an up-regulation of the receptor itself (42), is unclear. Work by Farrar and Humes (43) has indicated that the lipoxygenase enzyme pathway of arachidonic acid metabolism may be involved.

Effects on B Cells

Recent work has produced evidence for the presence of a functional IL-2 receptor on cells of the B lineage in humans (44). Des-Ala-1, Ser-125 IL-2 has been demonstrated to induce the proliferation of purified human B cells activated by anti-IgM (45) and to enhance the secretion of IgG and IgM by *Staphylococcus aureus* Cowan I bacteria (SAC)-activated, purified B cells (46). Ralph et al. (47) have shown that high levels of IL-2, including des-Ala-1, Ser-125 IL-2, induce IgM and IgG secretion by SAC-stimulated, purified human B cells as well as by certain Epstein-Barr virus (EBV)-infected B cell lines. This response was not sensitive to inhibition by anti-Tac antibody and possibly functioned through a low-affinity Tac receptor or through a presently undescribed receptor. This result is in contrast to the previously mentioned publications (44–46) that indicated that IL-2 works on B cells through a classic high-affinity Tac receptor. Tomita et al. (48) have used des-Ala-1, Ser-125 IL-2 to induce the differentiation to IgM secretion of HTLV-1-infected B cells in the absence of a proliferative increase through interaction with the Tac receptor. In addition, Murray et al. (49) have examined the lymphokine requirements for IgA and IgM production by B cells in response to the thymus-independent antigen, dextran. They found a differential enhancement of the production of the two immunoglobulin classes by combinations of des-Ala-1, Ser-125 IL-2 and recombinant murine interferon gamma. In summary, while these and other experiments demonstrate an effect of des-Ala-1, Ser-125 IL-2 on B cells, both as a growth factor (BCGF) and as a differentiation factor (BCDF), more information is required to understand the mechanism(s) and significance of these activities.

Pharmacokinetics of ^{35}S-Labeled Recombinant Interleukin-2

Pharmacokinetic studies on purified native and des-Ala-1, Ser-125 IL-2 have generally been limited to experiments that measured the disappearance of bioactivity in serum samples over time following injection of IL-2 into mice (50–52) or humans (53). As expected for a protein of such small size, IL-2 was cleared relatively rapidly, and kidney filtration was implicated as a major route of clearance (50).

We have labeled des-Ala-1, Ser-125 IL-2 in vivo in *E. coli*, using [^{35}S] sulfate, to follow the fate of the IL-2 protein independent of its bioactivity (52). When this radioactive IL-2 was injected intravenously, the rate of clearance of bioactivity from serum was indeed rapid. However it appeared to be significantly more rapid than the rate of clearance of radioactivity (Fig. 9). We do not attribute this to the presence of IL-2 inhibitors, which have been reported to exist in serum (54,55) but rather to proteolysis of the IL-2 (which could inactivate the molecule without decreasing the radioactive signal).

When sequential serum samples from a single animal from this study were immediately sized by molecular sieve HPLC, labeled peptides with relative molecular weights less than IL-2 were seen to accumulate within 20 min (Fig. 10). The profile in Fig. 10 also suggests that a substantial portion of IL-2 has formed a 350 kDa complex, apparently with a component in mouse serum. The rate of clearance of the complexed IL-2 appeared to be slower than that of the free IL-2. The identity of this IL–2-binding component is unknown, but it seems to be present at very low concentrations, because injection of larger amounts of IL-2 shows an increase in the proportion of free IL-2, which has an apparent relative molecular weight of 17,000. When the same labeled IL-2 is mixed with fresh human serum in vitro and sized by HPLC, a similar complex is observed, but it has a smaller apparent relative molecular weight, 150,000 (K. Koths et al., in preparation). The distribution of ^{35}S recovered in various organs of the mouse following injection of labeled IL-2 indicated that the kidney and liver were involved in removal of IL-2 from the circulation (52).

In Vivo Activities

Major progress in the investigation of the in vivo function(s) and utility of IL-2 has resulted from the availability of sufficient quantities of pure material. The capacity of des-Ala-1, Ser-125 IL-2 to affect the antibody-forming response to a protein antigen under the control of *Ir* genes was studied by Kawamura et al. (56). They showed that des-Ala-1, Ser-125 IL-2 could rescue the low responsiveness of BIO.BR mice to sperm whale myoglobin. The kinetics of production and the levels of antimyoglobin

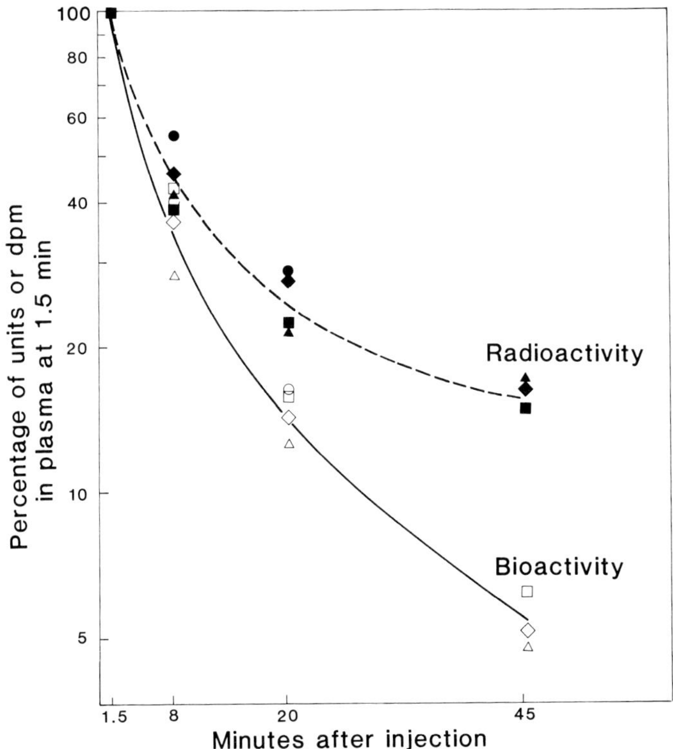

Figure 9 Pharmacokinetics of ^{35}S-labeled IL-2 injected iv into mice. The ^{35}S-labeled des-Ala-1, Ser-125 IL-2 was produced by in vivo labeling with $^{35}SO_4$ in *E. coli* as described (52). The purified, disulfide-containing product was fully active and had a specific radioactivity of about 5×10^6 cpm/μg. To determine plasma clearance rates, 80 μl of [^{35}S]IL-2 (1 μg) was injected into the tail vein and 100 μl samples were removed retro-orbitally at the indicated times. Plasma was immediately prepared, an aliquot was assayed for radioactivity, and an aliquot was diluted in duplicate for bioassay. (Reprinted with permission of Academic Press.)

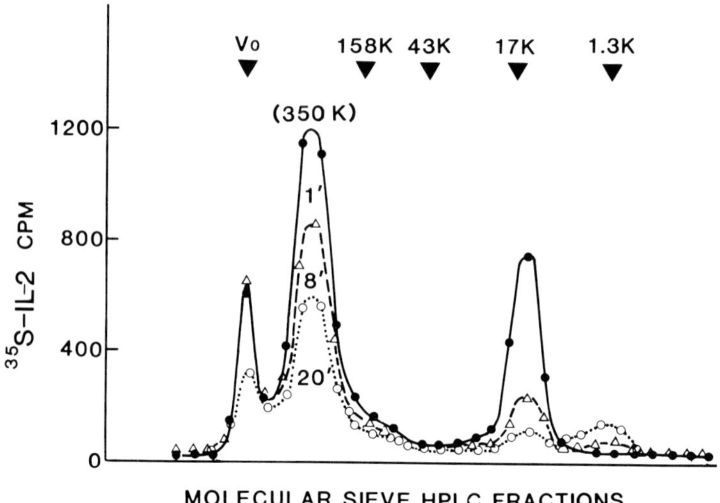

Figure 10 Molecular weight of [^{35}S] IL-2 in mouse plasma, following iv injection. Plasma samples were prepared from retroorbital blood samples taken at 1.5, 8, and 20 min from one of the animals described in Fig. 9. The apparent native molecular weight of the [^{35}S] IL-2 was determined within 5–30 min of sample collection, using molecular sieve HPLC (TSK-250) run in 10 mM phosphate (pH 7.4) containing 150 mM NaCl. (*Source*: Ref. 52. Reprinted with permission of Academic Press.)

antibodies in the low-responder mice were restored to those of the congenic, high-responder strain in a dose-dependent manner by administration of des-Ala-1, Ser-125 IL-2 together with the antigen. Thoman and Weigle (57) have used des-Ala-1, Ser-125 IL-2 administration in vivo to reconstitute the levels of spleen cell-mediated lympholysis against the allogeneic P815 cell line in aged mice (24–30 months old). Both primary and secondary responses were increased to levels equivalent to those seen in young mice (3–5 months old).

The field of parasitology offers a potentially rewarding area for investigation of the effects of IL-2 on in vivo immune responses. *Trypanosoma cruzi*, the causative agent of Chagas' disease, produces a nonspecific suppression of the immunological responsiveness of acutely infected animals. Choromanski and Kuhn (58) have demonstrated that recombinant IL-2 administration in vivo increased the response of infected animals to both *T. cruzi* antigens and to sheep red blood cells (SRBC). In addition, there was evidence of a prolonged survival in the IL-2-treated mice. In a recent study, Sharma et al. (59) concluded that des-Ala-1, Ser-125 IL-2 administration could reduce the mortality in mice infected with the intracellular parasite *Toxoplasma gondii*. These initial studies provide an encouraging basis for the examination of the effects of IL-2 administration on the therapy for parasitic infections.

In vitro experimentation has encouraged continued investigations of in vivo application of des-Ala-1, Ser-125 IL-2 in human infectious disease settings. Haregewoin and coworkers (60) demonstrated the ability of des-Ala-1, Ser-125 IL-2 to reverse the T-cell unresponsiveness of leprosy patients to *Mycobacterium leprae* antigens. At the moment, these results remain controversial because of the reported inability of Mohagheghpour et al. to demonstrate the same effects (61). Des-Ala-1, Ser-125 IL-2 also has been shown to partially reconstitute the mitogen- and alloantigen-induced proliferation of and to enhance the activity of the natural killer cells in PBMC populations from patients with acquired immune deficiency syndrome (AIDS) (62).

Veterinary Applications

The broad cross-species reactivity of human IL-2 was demonstrated in the early work of Ruscetti and Gallo (63). More recently, native IL-2 and des-Ala-1, Ser-125 IL-2 were shown to be equally active in maintaining the long-term growth of mitogen-activated PBMC populations from several nonmurine, animal species (34). Table 3 summarizes the activities of purified or partially purified IL-2s from various sources on cells isolated from a variety of animals. A more detailed examination of the response of bovine and porcine PBMC to des-Ala-1, Ser-125 IL-2 also showed a direct, dose-dependent mitogenic effect and the induction of cytolytic cell activities, as previously shown to occur with human PBMC (64).

An in vivo study of the use of des-Ala-1, Ser-125 IL-2 in an infectious disease model of pneumonia in pigs has indicated one of the potential veterinary uses of IL-2. Preliminary experiemnts performed in collaboration with Dr. G. Anderson at the University of Nebraska have demonstrated that des-Ala-1, Ser-125 IL-2 administration in combination with injection of a bacterin provided significantly increased protection of young pigs against a lethal challenge with *Haemophilus pleuropneumoniae* compared with the bacterin alone. Encouraging results regarding the ability of des-Ala-1, Ser-125 IL-2 to minimize the morbidity and mortality associated with respiratory distress syndrome (shipping fever) in cattle have also been obtained (data not shown).

Table 3 Cross-Species Reactivities of IL-2

Source of IL-2	Source of cells tested for response[a]										
	Human	Monkey	Cow	Horse	Pig	Rabbit	Dog	Sheep	Chicken	Rat	Mouse
Human[b]	+	+	+	+	+	+		+		+	+
Monkey	+	+									+
Cow			+								+
Horse				+							
Pig	–				+			+			+
Rabbit	–					+					+
Dog							+				
Sheep					–			+			
Chicken									+		
Rat[c]	–	–	–	–						+	+
Mouse	–	–					+			–	+

[a]Ability to cause T cells to proliferate. A blank means not tested.
[b]Human IL-2 also causes responses on cat and guinea pig cells.
[c]Rat IL-2 also shows no activity on cat or guinea pig cells.
Source: Data from Ref. 34, 63, 64, and 70–77.

Cancer Immunotherapy

The ability of IL-2 to control growth of various tumors in experimental animal systems has recently been tested. In low dosages, IL-2 alone controlled growth of tumors when injected near the tumor site (J. Vaage, personal communication). At much higher concentrations, systemic administration was also efficacious (65). In experiments that we have carried out with Dr. W. Laird at Cetus Corporation, IL-2 alone (administered intraperitoneally once a day for 5 days) completely inhibited growth of Meth A tumors in mice. The dose-response curve for des-Ala-1, Ser-125 IL-2 in this system is shown in Fig. 11.

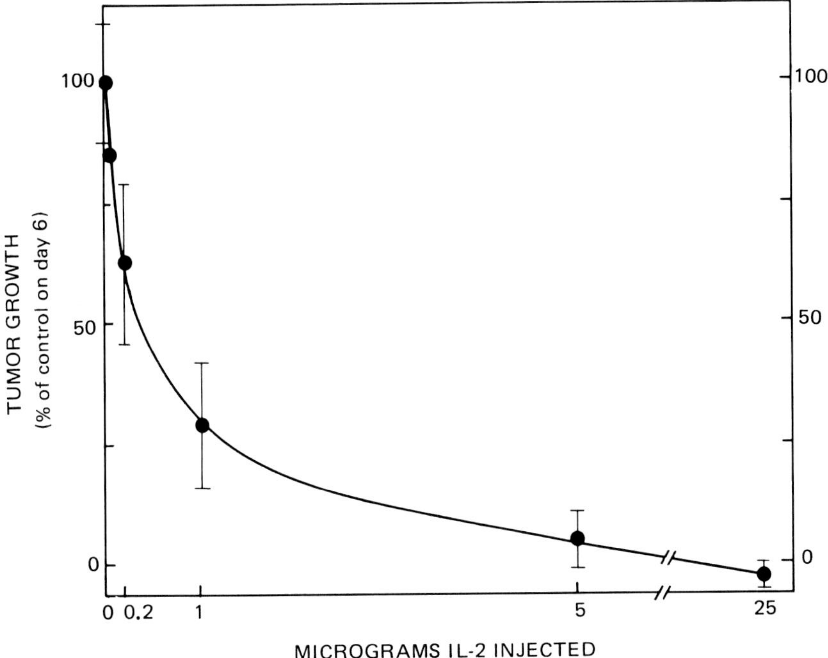

Figure 11 Effect of increasing amounts of des-Ala-1, Ser-125 IL-2 on tumor growth in mice. Groups of four mice containing 7-day-old subcutaneous methylcholanthrine-induced sarcomas of equivalent size (30 mm^3) were injected with various amounts of IL-2 in 100 μl (ip once a day for 5 days). Tumor volumes were measured 6 days after the beginning of treatment and expressed as percentage of control on day 6 (323 ± 36 mm^3).

Rosenberg and others have shown that des-Ala-1, Ser-125 IL-2 alone or in combination with adoptive transfer of LAK cells can cause the regression of a variety of established tumor cell metastases in mice (65–68). These promising results have led to phase I and phase II clinical studies of LAK cell administration in conjunction with des-Ala-1, Ser-125 IL-2 in human cancer patients. Preliminary results from these trials have been published (69) and provide encouragement for the use of such an approach for the treatment of a number of different cancers.

Future Prospects

The spectrum of biological activities and the specific activity of des-Ala-1, Ser-125 IL-2 have been shown to be equal to those of native IL-2. The application of des-Ala-1, Ser-125 IL-2 in both humans and animals for prophylactic and therapeutic purposes in infectious disease, cancer, and parasitic disease settings now appears promising. Given the short half-life of IL-2 following in vivo administration, development of more efficacious forms of the molecule using chemical modification or slow-release delivery mechanisms may be required to facilitate medical applications. Immunomodulation with IL-2 offers opportunities for important advances in our understanding of the mechanism(s) of immune responses and in our ability to use that knowledge for improving the quality of life in certain human and animal disease states.

REFERENCES

1. Morgan, D. A., Ruscetti, F. W., and Gallo, R. C. (1976). *Science 193*: 1007.
2. Watson, J. and Mochizuki, D. (1980). *Immunol. Rev. 51*:257.
3. Aarden, L. A. et al. (1979). *J. Immunol. 123*:2928.
4. Robb, R. J., Kunty, R. M., and Chowdhry, V. (1983). *Proc. Natl. Acad. Sci. USA 80*:5990.
5. Robb, R. J., Kunty, R. M., Panico, M., Morris, H. R., and Chowdhry, V. (1984). *Proc. Natl. Acad. Sci. USA 81*:6486.
6. Henderson, L. E., Hewetson, J. F., Hopkins, R. F., III, Sowder, R. C., Neubauer, R. H., and Rabin, H. (1983). *J. Immunol. 131*:810.
7. Taniguchi, T., Matsui, H., Fujita, T., Takaoka, C., Kashima, N., Yoshimoto, R., and Hamuro, J. (1983). *Nature 302*:305.
8. Devos, R., Plaetinck, G., Cheroutre, H., Simmons, G., Degrave, W., Tavernier, J., Remaut, E., and Fiers, W. (1983). *Nucleic Acids Res. 11*: 4307.

9. Rosenberg, S. A., Grimm, E. A., McGrogan, M., Doyle, M., Kawasaki, E., Koths, K., and Mark, D. F. (1984). *Science 223*:1412.
10. Clark, S. C., Arya, S. K., Wong-Staal, F., Matsumoto-Kobayashi, M., Kay, R. M., Kaufman, R. J., Brown, E. L., Shoemaker, C., Copeland, T., Oroszlan, S., Smith, K., Sarngadharan, M. G., Lindner, S. G., and Gallo, R. C. (1984). *Proc. Natl. Acad. Sci. USA 81*:2543.
11. Kaplan, J., Tilton, J., and Peterson, W. D. (1976). *Am. J. Hematol. 1*: 219.
12. Berger, S. L. and Birkenmeier, C. S. (1979). *Biochemistry 18*:5143.
13. Aviv, J. and Leder, P. (1972). *Proc. Natl. Acad. Sci. USA 69*:1408.
14. Gurdon, J. B., Lane, C. D., Woodland, H. R., and Marbaix, G. (1971). *Nature 233*:177.
15. Gillis, S., Fern, M. M., Ou, W., and Smith, K. A. (1978). *J. Immunol. 120*:2027.
16. Watson, J. (1979). *J. Exp. Med. 150*:1510.
17. Wickens, M. P., Buell, G. N., and Schimke, R. T. (1978). *J. Biol. Chem. 253*:2483.
18. Payvar, F. and Schimke, R. T. (1979). *J. Biol. Chem. 254*:7636.
19. Rougeon, F., Kounilsky, P., and Mach, B. (1975). *Nucleic Acids Res. 2*:2365.
20. Deng, G. and Wu, R. (1981). *Nucleic Acids Res. 9*:4173.
21. Grunstein, M. and Hogness, D. (1975). *Proc. Natl. Acad. Sci. USA 72*: 3961.
22. Mark, D. F., Lu, S. D., Creasey, A. A., Yamamoto, R., and Lin, L. S. (1984). *Proc. Natl. Acad. Sci. USA 81*:5662.
23. Weck, P. K., Apperson, S., Stebbing, N., Gray, P. W., Leung, D., Shepard, H. M., and Goeddel, D. V. (1981). *Nucleic Acids Res. 9*:6153.
24. Goeddel, D. V., Shepard, H. M., Yelverton, E., Leung, D., and Crea, R. (1980). *Nucleic Acids Res. 8*:4057.
25. Wang, A., Lu, S. D., and Mark, D. F. (1984). *Science 224*:1431.
26. Wang, A., Lu, S. D., and Mark, D. F. (1985). *Cellular and Molecular Biology of Lymphokines.* Edited by C. Sorg and A. Schimpl. Academic Press, New York, p. 641.
27. Liang, S., Allet, B., Rose, K., Hirschi, M., Liang, C., and Thatcher, D. (1985). *Biochem. J. 229*:429.
28. Kato, K., Yamada, T., Kawahara, K., Onda, H., Asano, T., Sugino, H., and Kakinuma, A. (1985). *Biochem. Biophys. Res. Commun. 130*:692.
29. Perry, L. J. and Wetzel, R. (1984). *Science 226*:555.
30. Lowry, O. H., Rosebrough, N., Farr, A., and Randall, R. (1951). *J. Biol. Chem. 193*:265.
31. Kunitani, M., Hirtzer, P., Johnson, D., Halenbeck, R., Boosman, A., and Koths, K. (1986). *J. Chromatog. 359*:391.

32. Schechter, Y., Burstein, Y., and Patchornik, A. (1975). *Biochemistry 14*:4497.
33. Fiers, W., Degrave, W., Devos, R., Plaetinck, G., Cheroutre, H., Tavernier, J., Simons, G., and Remaut, E. (1985). *Cellular and Molecular Biology of Lymphokines.* Edited by C. Sorg and A. Schimpl. Academic Press, New York, p. 595.
34. Doyle, M. V., Lee, M. T., and Fong, S. (1985). *J. Biol. Resp. Mod. 4*:96.
35. Lanier, L. L., Benike, C. J., Philips, J. H., and Engleman, E. G. (1985). *J. Immunol. 134*:794.
36. Grimm, E. A. and Rosenberg, S. A. (1984). *Lymphokines 9*:279.
37. Ralph, P., Nakoinz, I., Doyle, M., Lee, M. T., Jeong, G., Halenbeck, R., Mark, D. F., and Koths, K. (1986). *Immune Reg. by Charact. Poly., UCLA Symposium 41.*
38. Ettinghausen, S. E., Lipford, E. H., III, Mule, J. J., and Rosenberg, S. A. (1985). *J. Immunol. 135*:1488.
39. Robb, R. J., Munck, A., and Smith, K. A. (1981). *J. Exp. Med. 154*: 1455.
40. Cantrell, D. A. and Smith, K. A. (1984). *Science 224*:1312.
41. Leonard, W. J., Depper, J. M., Robb, R. J. Waldmann, T. A., and Greene, W. C. (1983). *Proc. Nat. Acad. Sci. USA 80*:6957.
42. Smith, K. A. and Cantrell, D. A. (1985). *Proc. Natl. Acad. Sci. USA 82*:864.
43. Farrar, W. A. and Humes, J. L. (1985). *J. Immunol. 135*:1153.
44. Waldmann, T. A., Goldman, C. K., Robb, R. J., Depper, J. M., Leonard, W. J., Sharron, S. O., Bongiovanni, K. F., Kopsmeyer, S. J., and Greene, W. C. (1984). *J. Exp. Med. 160*:1450.
45. Mittler, R., Rao, P., Olini, G., Westberg, E., Newman, W., Hoffmann, M., and Goldstein, G. (1985). *J. Immunol. 134*:2393.
46. Muraguchi, A., Kehrl, J. H., Lango, D. L., Volkman, D. J., Smith, K. A., and Fauci, A. S. (1985). *J. Exp. Med. 161*:181.
47. Ralph, P., Jeong, G., Welte, K., Mertelsmann, R., Rabin, H., Henderson, L. E., Sonja, L. M., Boone, T. C., and Robb, R. J. (1984). *J. Immunol. 133*:2442.
48. Tomita, S., Ambrus, J. L., Jr., Volkman, D. L., Longo, D. L., Mitsuja, H., Reitz, M. S., Jr., and Fauci, A. S. (1985). *J. Exp. Med. 162*:393.
49. Murray, P. D., Swain, S. L., and Kagnoff, M. P. (1985). *J. Immunol. 135*:4015.
50. Donahue, J. and Rosenberg, S. (1983). *J. Immunol. 130*:2203.
51. Chang, A., Hyatt, C., and Rosenberg, S. (1984). *J. Biol. Resp. Mod. 3*: 561.
52. Koths, K. and Halenbeck, R. (1985). *Cellular and Molecular Biology of Lymphokines.* Edited by C. Sorg and A. Schimpl. Academic Press, New York, p. 779.

53. Lotze, M., Frana, L., Sharrow, S., Robb, R., and Rosenberg, S. (1985). *J. Immunol. 134*:157.
54. Male, D., Lelchuk, R., Curry, S., Pryce, G., and Playfair, J. (1985). *Immunology 56*:119.
55. Hooton, J., Riendeau, D., and Paetkau, V. (1985). *Cell Immunol. 95*: 311.
56. Kawamura, H., Rosenberg, S. A., and Berzofsky, J. A. (1985). *J. Exp. Med. 162*:381.
57. Thoman, M. L. and Weigle, W. O. (1985). *J. Immunol. 134*:949.
58. Choromanski, L. and Kuhn, R. E. (1985). *Infect. Immun. 50*:354.
59. Sharma, S. D., Hofflin, J. M., and Remington, J. S. (1985). *J. Immunol. 135*:4160.
60. Haregewoin, A., Mustafa, A. S., Helle, I., Waters, M. F. R., Leiker, D. L., and Godal, T. (1984). *Immunol. Rev. 80*:77.
61. Mohagheghpour, N., Gelber, R. H., Larrick, J. W., Sasaki, D. T., Brennan, P. J., and Engelman, E. G. (1985). *J. Immunol. 135*:1443.
62. Lifson, J. D., Mark, D. F., Benike, C. J., Koths, K., and Engelman, E. G. (1984). *Lancet 1*:698.
63. Ruscetti, F. W. and Gallo, R. C. (1981). *Blood 57*:379.
64. Fong, S. and Doyle, M. V. (1986). *Vet. Immunol. Immunopathol. 11*:91.
65. Mule, J. J., Shu, S., and Rosenberg, S. A. (1985). *J. Immunol. 135*:646.
66. Rosenberg, S. A., Mule, J. J., Spiess, P. J., Reichart, C. M., and Schwarz, S. L. (1985). *J. Exp. Med. 161*:1169.
67. Lafreniere, R. and Rosenberg, S. A. (1985). *Cancer Res. 45*:3735.
68. Mazumder, A. (1985). *Lymphokine Res. 4*:215.
69. Rosenberg, S. A., Lotze, M. T., Muul, L. M., Leitman, S., Chang, A. E., Ettinghausen, S. E., Matory, Y. L., Skibben, J. M., Shiloni, E., Vetto, J. T., Seip, C. A., Simpson, C., and Reichert, C. M. (1985). *N. Engl. J. Med. 313*:1485.
70. Redelman, D. and Bussett, E. (1983). *J. Immunol. Meth. 56*:359.
71. Daemen, A. J. J. M., Buurman, W. A., Linden, C. J. V. D., Groenewegen, G., and Kootstra, G. (1983). *Vet. Immunol. Immunopathol. 5*:247.
73. English, L. S., Binns, R. M., and License, S. T. (1985). *Vet. Immunol. Immunopathol. 9*:59.
74. Rabin, H., Hopkins, R. F., III, Ruscetti, F. W., Neubauer, R. H., Brown, R. L., and Kawakami, T. G. (1981). *J. Immunol. 127*:1852.
75. Magnuson, N., Perryman, L., Wyatt, C., Ishizaka, T., Mason, P., Namen, A., Banks, K., and Magnuson, J. (1984). *J. Immunol. 133*:2518.
76. Schnetzler, M., Oommen, A., Nowak, J., and Franklin, R. (1983). *Eur. J. Immunol. 13*:560.
77. Miller-Edge, M. and Splitter, G. A. (1984). *Vet. Immunol. Immunopathol. 7*:119.

2

Induction of Growth Responsiveness to Interleukin-2

Evidence for Intracellular Control Mechanisms Shared with Interleukin-3

JAMES D. WATSON and GRAHAM S. LE GROS
School of Medicine, University of Auckland, Auckland, New Zealand

LINDA S. PARK
Immunex Corporation, Seattle, Washington

INTRODUCTION

The activation of helper T lymphocytes by antigen or mitogen leads to the synthesis and secretion of a number of lymphokines, some of which act as growth factors for select cell types within hemopoietic and lymphoid lineages. The genes encoding growth-promoting lymphokines in these cells appear to be coordinately regulated (1). Since the molecular cloning of human interleukin-2 (IL-2) (2), there have been rapid advances in the understanding of the structure of murine (3,4) and human IL-2, murine interleukin-3 (IL-3) (5,6), and murine (7) and human (8-10) colony-stimulating factors (CSF). Despite extensive biological and molecular analysis, a human analogue of murine IL-3 has not been found. Each of these lymphokines are single polypeptides, with a molecular weight (M_r) of 14,000-18,000, and each found as a glycolysated series of molecules when secreted by cells (11,12). As IL-2, IL-3 and granulocyte-macrophage (GM)-CSF are coordinately synthesized by murine helper T cells and function as growth regulators for cells that share a common ancestory in the hemopoietic system, it is surprising that these lymphokines share no major amino acid homology (2–10) and are encoded as single genomic copies. The murine and human cell surface receptors for IL-2 have now been isolated (11) and cloned (13–15), but the receptors for IL-3 and GM-CSF have yet to be purified (16,17).

The uniqueness of lymphokines in the study of growth control lies in the establishment of lymphokine-dependent cell lines. Bone marrow or lymphoid cell populations, cultured in the presence of IL-2 (18,19) or IL-3 (19,20), have lead to the development of continuous cell lines that maintain a strict requirement for the appropriate lymphokine for continued growth. There are now a large number of IL–2-dependent T-cell lines, IL–3-dependent bone marrow-derived cells of diverse myeloid lineages, and several GM–CSF-dependent monocytic cell lines (20–25). These cells are apparently "immortal" in the sense that their growth potential is not limited unless deprived of lymphokine, and rarely exhibit transformation to a lymphokine-independent state of growth. There are now reports of retroviruses that have been used to infect and transform several lymphokine-dependent cell lines to a lymphokine-independent growth state (25–28). These retroviruses contain either the v-*abl*, v-*raf*/*myc* or the v-*myc* (25–28) oncogenes, implying that the products of select oncogenes are associated with the biochemical pathways activated by lymphokines involved in growth control.

It has been a general finding that IL-2 is a specific growth regulator for thymus-derived lymphocytes (18,19,23). Although IL-3 differs in having specificity for a number of myeloid lineages found in bone marrow (20,22), it is interesting that IL-3 was originally described as a growth regulator for an immature population of thymocyte progenitors (29,30). We discuss here the relationship of IL–3-dependent bone marrow cells to the pathway of T-cell development. Our recent observation has been that a number of IL–3-dependent cell lines can be induced to undergo phenotypic switching to an IL–2-dependent growth state (31). The expression of IL–2-specific receptors appears to occur when IL-2 is added to the culture medium supporting growth of a number of IL–3-dependent cell lines (32). We raise a number of issues that relate to the intracellular control mechanisms involved in growth regulation by lymphokines (29). In particular, although IL-2 and IL-3 show little homology in structure and interact with separate cell surface receptors, the intracellular biochemical pathways activated as a result of cells binding each of these lymphokines appear closely related.

This also has been recently suggested as a result of the observation that both IL-2 and IL-3 induce the rapid translocation of protein kinase C from the cytosol to the plasma membrane, an event thought to be associated with a transmembrane signaling mechanism (33,34).

MATERIALS AND METHODS

Murine Factor-Dependent Cell Lines

The FD.C/1 and FD.C/2 cell lines were developed from the FDC-P2 IL–3-dependent cell line originally derived by Dexter et al. (20) from long-term culture of DBA/2J mouse bone marrow. The derivation of these variant factor-dependent cell lines is detailed elsewhere (31). The FD.C/1 cell line is a cloned line maintained in culture medium containing 10% horse serum and 5% WEHI–3-conditioned medium. The FD.C/2 cell line is a cloned line maintained in culture medium containing 5% fetal calf serum and 7% concanavalin A (Con A)-stimulated rat spleen-conditioned medium (31). The 32D cl-23 cell line was derived from C3H/HeJ mouse strain bone marrow culture (21). These cells were cultured in either the RPMI 1640 medium just described, containing 7% Con A-stimulated rat spleen-conditioned medium and termed here, 32D/IL-2, or in RPMI containing 5% WEHI-3 conditioned medium, termed 32D/IL-3. The KP3 cell line was derived from long-term culture of CBA/N bone marrow cells in IL-3. These cells are cultured as for 32D cl-23 cells, either in IL–3- or IL–2-supplemented medium and are referred to as KP3/IL-3 or KP3/IL-2 cells respectively.

Recombinant Lymphokines

Recombinant murine IL-3, human IL-2, and murine granulocyte-macrophage colony-stimulating factors were gifts from Immunex Corporation, Seattle. The expression of cDNA encoding these lymphokines and subsequent biochemical purification are described elsewhere (10,12).

Cell Surface Binding

Recombinant human IL-2 (35) and purified murine IL-3 from WEHI-3 cells (11) were radiolabeled as previously described with the Enzymobead reagent (Biorad) (16,35). The specific activities of radiolabeled IL-2 and IL-3 were in the range of 10^{15} cpm/mmole.

RESULTS

Phenotypic Switching of Lymphokine-Dependent Growth States

The rationale underlying experiments that led to the discovery of lymphokine switching was originally directed toward a search for a human analogue of IL-3. As molecular cloning of human IL-2 (2) and murine GM-CSF (7) rapidly lead to the development of gene probes for the isolation of cDNA encoding murine IL-2 (3,4) and human GM-CSF (9,10), it has been surprising to us that probes developed from the cloning of murine IL-3 (5,6) have so far failed to identify a gene(s) or CDNA encoding human IL-3. As murine IL-3 is a product of murine T lymphocytes (1,11), we decided to examine conditioned media derived from human T lymphocytes for factor(s) that might be revealed by the growth-stimulation of murine IL-3-dependent cell lines. By comparison, as human IL-2 is known to stimulate the growth of murine T cells, we reasoned human IL-3 might also stimulate the growth of murine IL-3-dependent cell lines.

Interleukin-2 Stimulates Growth of Interleukin-3-Dependent Cell Lines

Initially, the culturing of IL-3-dependent FD.C/1 cells in medium supplemented with human tonsil conditioned medium (CM) led to the observation that growth of FD.C/1 cells was readily stimulated (Fig. 1A) (31). The FD.C/1 cells were then cultured continuously in culture medium in the presence of human tonsil CM. At regular stages throughout a 1-month period, FD.C/1 cells were harvested and washed, and the proliferative response of the cells to various lymphokines determined. Initially, the FD.C/1 cells responded maximally to purified murine IL-3, showed partial responses to human tonsil CM, but no response to purified murine IL-2. After 14-days growth in medium containing tonsil CM, cells responded similarly to both murine IL-3 and tonsil CM and showed a partial response to murine IL-2. By 28-days culture, the cells showed a marked decrease in responsiveness to murine IL-3, but responded well to tonsil CM, and were becoming increasingly responsive to murine IL-2. At this stage, the cells were cloned twice in culture medium supplemented with tonsil CM. The resulting cloned cell lines (designated FD.C/2 cells) were all equally responsive to human IL-2 and murine IL-2 and showed a low response to murine IL-3 (Fig. 1B).

We have examined the culture conditions that could be used to develop IL-2-responsive cell lines from FD.C/1 cells. The culture of FD.C/1 cells

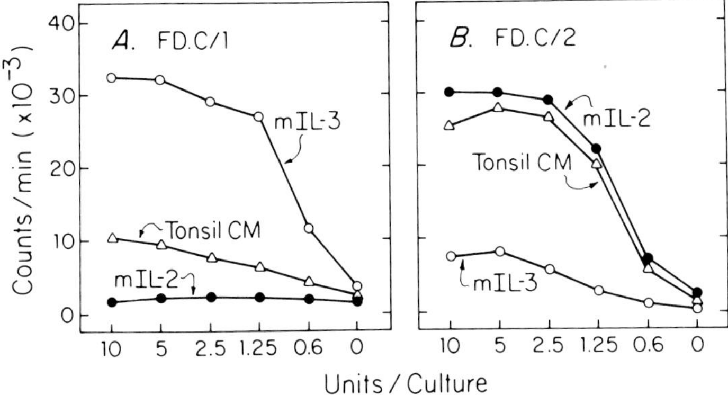

Figure 1 Long-term culture of FD.C/1 cells with tonsil CM. The FD.C/1 cells were maintained in complete culture medium containing 10% human tonsil CM. (A) At day 0 of culture, the cells were tested for their proliferative response to human tonsil CM, murine IL-2, and murine IL-3. (B) The growth responsiveness of the cell line FD.C/2 to murine IL-2 and IL-3, as well as tonsil CM. The concentration of IL-2 activity (units/ml) in tonsil CM was determined using an IL–2-independent T-cell line.

in medium supplemented with either human tonsil CM or recombinant human IL-2 reproducibly results in the growth of FD.C/2 cell lines (31). Once established, FD.C/2 cells grow equally in medium supplemented with human, murine, or rat IL-2. The FD.C/1 to FD.C/2 transformation process can be followed by counting the total number of viable cells. Initially, 90% of FD.C/1 cells remain viable for 48 hr in the presence of tonsil CM or recombinant human IL-2. After 7-days culture in human IL–2-conditioned medium, 1% of FD.C/1 cells remain viable. These surviving cells continue to grow, are readily cloned, and become FD.C/2. The spontaneous emergence of lymphokine-independent cells has rarely been observed. Thus IL-2 is all that is required to induce IL–2-responsive cells in this IL–3-dependent cell line.

Two other bone marrow-derived, IL–3-dependent cell lines, 32D cl-23 and KP3, have been examined for growth responses to IL-2. Unlike the FD.C/1 cell lines where a small number of cells initially appear to respond and grow (31), 32D cl-23 and KP3 cells can be more readily switched from IL–3-dependent to IL–2-dependent growth. The 32D cl-23 cells growing in IL-3 (termed 32D/IL-3) when cultured in IL–2-supplemented medium, showed a decrease in growth rate (Fig. 2A) that lasted approximately 4 days when cells appeared to adapt to the presence of IL-2 and then grow at a rate indistinguishable from that observed in IL–3-dependent growth conditions (Fig. 3A). The 32D/IL-2 cells respond virtually identically to the presence of either IL-2 or IL-3 (Fig. 3A). A similar response of KP3/IL-3 cells to IL-3 or IL-2 (Fig. 2B), or KP3/IL-2 cells to IL-2 and IL-3 (Fig. 3B) was observed. It was apparent that 32D cl-23 and KP3 cells growing in IL-3, when cultured in the presence of IL-2, have undergone a period of growth adaptation to the IL-2; however these cells growing in IL-2 were then able to be passaged into IL–3-supplemented medium without an apparent change in growth rate. Thus IL–3-dependent growth pathways were maintained in cells growing in IL-2, whereas the IL–2-dependent growth state appeared to be associated with some change in expression of these pathways. This may reflect a change in the number of cell surface receptors for IL-2 required to support growth in the presence of IL-2. Alternatively, the intracellular pathway through which the IL-2 receptor is linked to growth processes may differ in some way from those used by the IL-3 receptor and require an induction period before cell division can proceed normally.

Cell Surface Antigens

It was of interest to analyze a range of cell surface antigens expressed by FD.C/1, 32D cl-23, and KP3 cells growing in IL-3 and IL-2. These data have been summarized in Table 1. All cells were sIg^-, weakly Thy-1^+, and express the Fc receptors detected by the 2.4G2 monoclonal antibody (36). In addition, although FD.C/1, FD.C/2, 32D/IL-3, and 32D/IL-2 were L3T4^-, KP3/IL-3 and KP3/IL-2 cells were L3T4^+. All cells are Lyt-1^- and Lyt-2^- (Table 1). The Thy-1^+, L3T4^-, Ly2^- phenotype of the FD.C/1, FD.C/2, and 32D cell lines is similar to that exhibited by a subpopulation of murine embryonic thymocytes (37,38) that appears to give rise to the thymocyte population of adults. There is an interesting difference in the KP3 cell line. While FD.C/1, FD.C/2, 32D/IL-3, and 32D/IL-2 cells were J11D^+, $B220^+$, and MAC-1^-, KP3/IL-3 and KP3/IL-2 cells were J11D^-, $B220^-$, and MAC-1^+ (see Table 1). J11D is an antigen expressed on immature T cells, B cells, and various hemopoietic progenitors (43), although the monoclonal antibody RA3-2C2 recognizes the B220 antigen common to early B- and T-cell lineages (40). MAC-1 is often found on early T cells (44). The implication of these data is that while FD.C/1, FD.C/2, 32D/IL-3, and 32D/IL-2 cells express antigens common to hemopoietic progenitors and

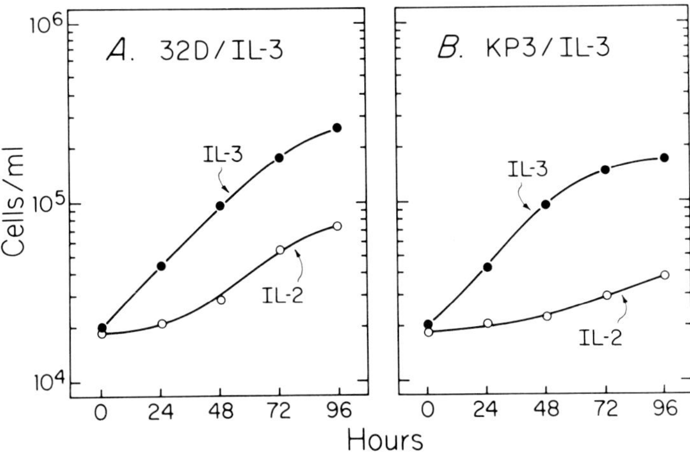

Figure 2 Growth of 32D c/23 and KP3 cell lines maintained in IL–3-supplemented growth medium in the presence of IL-2. (A) 32D/IL-3 and (B) KP3/IL-3 cells were harvested and seeded at 2×10^4 cells/ml in medium supplemented either with 600 units/ml murine recombinant IL-3, or with 300 units/ml human recombinant IL-2. At 24, 48, 72, and 96 hr, cells were harvested from cultures and viable cell numbers determined.

early lymphoid lineages, the lack of B220 and J11D antigens on KP3/IL-3 and KP3/IL-2 cell lines may reflect a cell that is found further along an immature T-cell pathway of development (37–45).

In general, the cell surface antigens detected under IL-3 growth conditions were identical with those seen when cells are switched to an IL–2-dependent growth state. There was one difference that might have been expected. The IL-2 receptor, detected by binding of the 7D4 (44,45) monoclonal antibody (see Table 1), was weakly expressed on FD.C/1 cells, 32D/IL-3, and KP3/IL-3 cells and increased markedly when cells were cultured in the presence of IL-2. This finding was reflected in the binding studies discussed later (Table 2).

Expression of Interleukin-2- and Interleukin-3-Specific Binding Sites

The number of binding sites for IL-2 and IL-3 on the cells in different growth states and the affinity with which each lymphokine is bound have

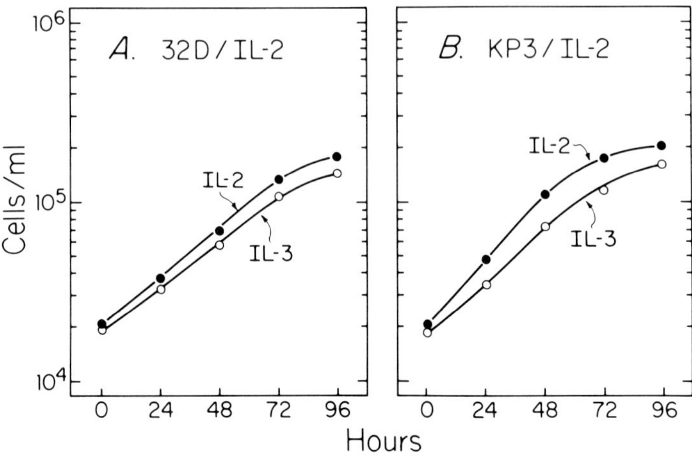

Figure 3 Growth of 32D c/23 and KP3 cell lines maintained in IL–2-supplemented growth medium in the presence of IL-3. (A) 32D/IL-2 and (B) KP3/IL-2 cells were harvested and seeded at 2×10^4 cells/ml in medium supplemented either with 600 units/ml murine recombinant IL-3, or with 300 units/ml human recombinant IL-2. At 24, 48, 72, and 96 hr, cells were harvested from cultures and viable cell numbers determined.

been determined by the binding of radiolabeled lymphokines to each cell type (16,35). Using ^{125}I-labeled IL-3, all cells (FD.C/1, FD.C/2, 32D/IL-3, 32D/IL-2, KP3/IL-3, KP2/IL-2) exhibited a small number (200–2000) of binding sites per cell (Table 2). Two separate issues were of particular interest. First, only high-affinity binding sites for IL-3 appeared to be present on cells, exhibiting a K_a of 10^9–10^{10} M^{-1}. Second, the number of binding sites on FD.C/1, FD.C/2, 32D, and KP3 cells appeared constant on cells growing in medium supplemented with either IL-3 or with IL-2, implying that the IL-3-specific receptor on the cell surface was constitutively expressed on the cell surface of these cell lines.

The specific binding of ^{125}I-labeled IL-2 to these same cell lines showed interesting differences. Two classes of receptor, distinguished by the affinity with which they bind IL-2, were detected on FD.C/1, FD.C/2, 32D/IL-3, 32D/IL-2, and KP3/IL-2 (Table 3). This observation has been described as a general characteristic of IL-2 receptor binding (46,47). For the KP3/IL-3 cells, we have been able to measure only one class of IL-2-binding receptor with an apparent low affinity (see Table 3). The K_a of

Table 1 Expression of Cell Surface Antigens by Lymphokine-Dependent Cell Lines

Antigen	FD.C/1	FD.C/2	32D/IL-3	32D/IL-2	KP3/IL-3	KP3/IL-2
sIg	–	–	–	–	–	–
Thy-1	–/+	–/+	–/+	–/+	++	++
J11D	++	++	++	++	–	–
B220	++	++	++	++	–	–
L3T4	–	–	–	–	+	+
Lyt-1	–	–	–	–	–	–
Lyt-2	–	–	–	–	–	–
2.4G2	+	+	+	+	+	+
MAC-1	–	–	–	–	–	–
7D4	+	++	+	++	+	++

Cells were stained with a fluorescent anti-Ig reagent made in our laboratory (31). The anti-thy 1 was from clone T24-31.7 (39), anti-B220 from clone RA3-2C2 (40, L3T4 from clone GK1.5 (41), Lyt-1 and Lyt-2 from clones 53-7.3 and 53-6.7, respectively (42). The monoclonal antibodies J11D (43), MAC-1 (44), 2.4G2 (36), and 7D4 (45) were gifts from Dr. P. Conlon, Immunex Corporation, Seattle, Washington.

Table 2 ^{125}I-Labeled IL-3 Binding to Lymphokine-Dependent Cell Lines

Cell line	K_a	Sites/cell
FD.C/1	$2.4 \pm 1.2 \times 10^{10}$	690 ± 700
FD.C/2	$8.1 \pm 2.9 \times 10^{10}$	1260 ± 420
32D/IL-3	$2.0 \pm 1.5 \times 10^{10}$	550 ± 380
32D/IL-2	$1.5 \pm 0.7 \times 10^{10}$	640 ± 440
KP3/IL-3	$3.8 \pm 2.6 \times 10^{10}$	990 ± 760
KP3/IL-2	$1.2 \pm 0.8 \times 10^{10}$	1020 ± 270

Binding experiments were performed as described elsewhere (16). The data represents the mean of two to four experiments with each cell line.

Table 3 ^{125}I-Labeled IL-2 Binding to Lymphokine-Dependent Cell Lines

	High-affinity		Low-affinity: Molecules bound/cell at 3.5×10^{-9} M
Cell line	K_a	Sites/cell	Sites/cell
FD.C/1	$3.7 \pm 1.6 \times 10^9$	750 ± 290	2150 ± 600
FD.C/2	$1.3 \pm 0.1 \times 10^9$	6270 ± 550	$12{,}500 \pm 1500$
32D/IL-3	$1.5 \pm 0.6 \times 10^9$	1895 ± 645	6500 ± 1500
32D/IL-2	$7.3 \pm 0.5 \times 10^8$	9160 ± 600	$14{,}000 \pm 2000$
KP3/IL-3	ND[a]	ND	$12{,}500 \pm 2000$
KP3/IL-2	$1.66 \pm 0.94 \times 10^9$	2400 ± 600	$16{,}000 \pm 4000$

Binding experiments were performed as described elsewhere (14). The data represent the mean data from two to four experiments performed with each cell line.
The number of low-affinity binding sites were generally 10- to 20-fold higher than the high-affinity sites measured, with a K_a of approximately 1×10^7.
[a]ND = high-affinity binding sites not detected.

the low-affinity binding sites measured for IL-2 was in the range of 10^8 M^{-1}, while the K_a of high-affinity measured sites was 10^9–10^{10} M^{-1} (see Table 3). The number of IL-2-binding sites was also lower on cell lines growing in the presence of IL-3, but it increased when cells were switched to IL-2-dependent growth conditions. As recombinant IL-2 was all that was required for growth, it appeared that IL-2 functioned as an inducer for the synthesis and expression of IL-2 receptors. The high-affinity binding sites for IL-2 exhibited on FD.C/1, FD.C/2, 32D/IL-3, 32D/IL-2, and KP3/IL-2 cells were accurately measured and showed an increase of five- to 10-fold in numbers when cells were changed from IL-3- to IL-2-dependent growth conditions. However the low-affinity binding sites could only be estimated using ^{125}I-labeled IL-2 binding to cells because the conditions used were not saturating. However these numbers were approximately 10-fold higher per cell than were high-affinity binding sites. The failure to detect high-affinity binding sites for IL-2 on KP3/IL-3 cells may have reflected that such sites were present in extremely low numbers on these cells (<100) representing the limitation of measurement, rather than a complete absence of such sites on KP3/IL-3 cells (see Table 3).

DISCUSSION

Ontogeny of Lymphokine-Dependent Cells

One of the hallmarks of thymocytes and peripheral T cells is that under the appropriate conditions of stimulation, the induction of IL-2 receptor RNA closely followed by expression of receptors on the cell surface, occurs in response to the presence of antigen and IL-2. In fetal thymus development one of the earliest cell subpopulations described exhibits a phenotype of Thy-1$^+$, L3T4$^-$, Lyt-1$^-$, and Lyt-2$^-$, but these cells are IL-2 receptor-positive (37,38,47). As fetal development proceeds these cells appear to give rise to the thymocyte population that characterizes the adult thymus (37), being Thy-1$^+$, L3T4$^+$, but IL-2-R$^-$. In light of these reports, our finding that certain bone marrow-derived IL-3-dependent cell lines can be converted to an IL-2-dependent growth state can be interpreted along two general lines: First, as originally described (22,29,30), some IL-3-dependent cell lines may represent progenitors of cells destined to mature through the thymus. The FD.C/1, 32D cl-23, and KP3 may represent progenitor cells responsive to IL-3 but that have yet to be committed to differentiation events normally seen in immature cells in the T lymphocyte lineage. These cells express very small numbers of receptors for IL-2 but are capable of response to IL-2 by the induction of increased synthesis of these receptors. Intracellular pathways activated by IL-2 receptor binding are either induced coordinately with the receptor or shared by those previously linked to the IL-3 receptor signal system. As the expression of major cell surface antigens associated with the T-cell lineage does not change in the switch to IL-2 growth dependence in these cell lines, it is likely that other events are required to continue the process of differentiation in the T-cell lineage.

A second explanation is that a number of progenitor cells in the bone marrow may constitutively express receptors for a number of growth regulators including IL-2 and IL-3. Growth is regulated by the availability of a specific lymphokine in a particular microenvironment (49). The intracellular biochemical pathways that control cell division may be common to all hematopoietic cell types. The "entry" into this common pathway may occur through similar or slightly different entry sites. A small number of different lymphokine-specific receptors may be expressed on cells in different lineages. The sequence in which receptors are used, thus influencing how cells develop, may normally be a function of the microenvironment that cells proceed through during development. In cell culture, it may be possible to induce the expression of high levels of a particular lymphokine-specific receptor. The switching of FD.C/1, 32D cl-23, or KP3 cells from an IL-3- to an IL-2-dependent growth state may merely reflect this process.

The Interleukin-2 Receptor

The molecular cloning of the human and murine IL-2 receptor has now been achieved (13-15). It is an unusually small size for a receptor molecule, consisting of a single polypeptide of 251 amino acids. Transfection of cells with the cDNA encoding this polypeptide has shown that its expression is sufficient to confer IL-2-binding ability upon non-T-cell populations (50). A comparison of the human and murine receptor polypeptides has shown that the two most highly conserved regions are the 21 amino acid transmembrane domain and the 13 amino acid cytoplasmic domain. Presumably, these highly conserved regions are associated with important functional properties. Two forms of the IL-2 receptor are found on activated T cells and are distinguished by the affinity with which they bind IL-2 (46,47). Approximately 5-10% of the receptors bind IL-2 with a K_a of $>1 \times 10^9$ M^{-1} and the remaining receptors with a K_a of 1×10^7 M^{-1}.

The problem of determining how IL-2 receptor binding leads to a biochemical response is unknown. Current thinking is based on similar observations with other growth receptors, such as those for insulin (51), epidermal growth factor (51,53), and platelet-derived growth factor (54) where it is believed that the high-affinity receptors are active in signal delivery. The interaction of IL-2 with its receptor does not result in the phosphorylation of the receptor, although the sequence of amino acids surrounding serine at position 247 resembles a concensus protein kinase C phosphorylation site (13–15). This serine on the small cytoplasmic domain, can be phosphorylated in response to phorbol myristate; however there is no evidence this phosphorylation is necessary for receptor function (55). If high-affinity sites are associated with function, it is possible there may be a receptor-specific subunit that confers upon the IL-2 receptor the ability to bind IL-2 with high affinity. Because the cytoplasmic domain of the receptor is very short, it is possible it could be associated with a subunit protein that functions as a signal-transducing unit. Alternatively, the transmembrane domain, highly conserved between mouse and human, may have a role other than a stretch of hydrophobic amino acids spanning the lipid bilayer. This domain could interact with proteins in the membrane that function as the transducing elements involved in signal delivery.

Although the structure of the IL-3 receptor is not yet known, it may share size characteristics and functional properties in common with the IL-2 receptor. The physiological characteristics of switching cells from an IL-3- to IL-2-dependent growth state may be possible only if these two growth regulators act similarly. Cells remain lymphokine-dependent for growth and do not undergo marked morphological changes. The 32D/IL-2 and KP3/IL-2 cells can be readily converted back to an IL-3-dependent growth state, again suggesting the lymphokines are acting similarly. If the IL-3 receptor is similar in size to the IL-2 receptor, the cytoplasmic domain of the IL-3 receptor may also be small and need a signal-transducing mechanism like that discussed for the IL-2 receptor. It would be of great interest to know whether or not these two receptors share a common transducing system for signal delivery.

Transducing Mechanisms for Interleukin-2 and Interleukin-3 Receptors

There are several observations that suggest some differences in the basic signal/transduction mechanism for IL-2 and IL-3. First, only high-affinity binding sites for IL-3 have been detected (see Table 2). Second, these IL-3-binding sites do not vary markedly in number on cells utilizing IL-2 or IL-3 for growth (see Table 3). Third, while conversion of cells from an IL-3- to an IL-2-dependent growth state requires an adaptational period for growth to continue normally, the reciprocal conversion of these cells from an IL-2- to an IL-3-dependent growth state occurs without a substantial change in cell division time (see Figs. 2,3). Thus cells growing in the presence of IL-2 appear to continue constitutively synthesizing the necessary cellular components that allow the cells to respond to IL-3. However these cells growing in IL-3 appear to induce a cellular constituent(s) when placed in IL-2 growth medium before IL-2-dependent growth continues at a similar cell division rate. This induction involves the increased expression of the IL-2 receptor. As IL-2-specific low-affinity binding sites are always in excess of high-affinity sites on these cells, and the high-affinity sites increase in response to IL-2, transducing elements may not be present in sufficient quantities in IL-3-dependent cells and may also require synthesis during this induction period to convert the low-affinity binding sites to high-affinity binding sites.

Recent reports that Abelson murine leukemia virus (25,28) and recombinant retroviruses expressing v-*myc* oncogenes (26,27) can abrogate the dependence of select cell lines for IL-2 or IL-3 have led to the suggestion that the cellular products of these genes function in the intracellular pathways normally regulated by ligand receptor binding. It is interesting that the epidermal growth factor (EGF) receptor has an intracellular tyrosine kinase domain (56), and that the insulin receptor is closely associated with a tyrosine kinase activity in the membrane (57). Because v-*abl* encodes a tyrosine kinase activity (58), it is tempting to speculate that the IL-2 and IL-3 receptors are closely associated with proteins that possess similar enzymatic activity. What is striking concerning the high-affinity IL-2- and IL-3-specific receptors, is their presence in very small numbers on growth-responsive cells. This may also reflect the situation with respect to the numbers of intracellular transducing elements for these receptors. Tyrosine kinases are present in small numbers in cells and remain attractive candidates for such transducing functions. The use of oncogenes, particularly those encoding tyrosine kinase, transfected into IL-2- and IL-3-dependent cells may play a major role in the elucidation of intracellular biochemical pathways that regulate growth. The more we learn of how different hematopoietic and lymphoid cell lineages respond to IL-2 and IL-3, the more similarities rather than differences in modes of action appear to emerge.

ACKNOWLEDGMENTS

This work was supported by the Auckland Medical Research Foundation, the Medical Research Council of New Zealand, the Welcome Trust, London, and the Auckland Division, Cancer Society of New Zealand Inc.

REFERENCES

1. Watson, J. D. (1983). Biology and biochemistry of T cell-derived lymphokines. I. The coordinate synthesis of interleukin 2 and colony-stimulating factors in a murine T cell lymphoma. *J. Immunol. 131*:293-296.
2. Tanaguchi, T., Matsui, H., Fujita, T., Takaoka, C., Kashima, N., Yosimoto, R., and Hamuro, J. (1983). Structure and expression of a cloned cDNA for human interleukin 2. *Nature 302*:305-310.
3. Kashima, N., Nishi-Takaoka, C., Fujita, T., Taki, S., Yamada, G., Hamuro, J., and Taniguchi, T. (1985). Unique structure of murine interleukin 2 as deduced from cloned cDNAs. *Nature 313*:403-404.
4. Yokata, T., Arai, N., Lee, F., Rennick, D., Mosmann, T., and Arai, K. (1985). Use of a cDNA expression vector for isolation of mouse interleukin 2 cDNA clones: Expression of T cell growth factor activity after transfection of monkey cells. *Proc. Natl. Acad. Sci. USA 82*:68-72.
5. Fung, M. C., Hapel, A. J., Ymer, S., Cohen, D. R., Johnson, R. M., Campbell, H. D., and Young, I. G. (1984). Molecular cloning of cDNA for murine interleukin-3. *Nature 307*:233-235.
6. Yokata, T., Lee, F., Rennick, D., Hall, C., Arai, N., Mosmann, T., Nabel, G., Cantor, H., and Arai, K.-I. (1984). Isolation and characterization of a mouse cDNA clone that expresses mast cell growth factor activity in monkey cells. *Proc. Natl. Acad. Sci. USA 81*:1070-1073.
7. Gough, N. M., Gough, J., Metcalf, D., Kelso, A., Grail, D. Nicola, N. A., Burgess, A. W., and Dunn, A. R. (1984). Molecular cloning of granulocyte-macrophage colony stimulating factor. *Nature 309*:763-765.
8. Wong, G. G., Witek, J. S., Temple, P. A., Wilkens, K. M. et al. (1985). Human GM-CSF: Molecular cloning of the complementary DNA and purification of the natural and recombinant proteins. *Science 228*: 810-813.
9. Lee, F., Yokota, T., Otsuka, T., Gemmell, L., Larson, N., Luh, J. et al. (1985). Isolation of cDNA for a human granulocyte-macrophage colony-stimulating factor by functional expression in mammalian cells. *Proc. Natl. Acad. Sci. USA 82*:4360-4364.
10. Cantrell, M. A., Anderson, D., Cerretti, D. P., Price, V. et al. (1985). Cloning, sequence and expression of a human granulocyte-macrophage colony stimulating factor. *Proc. Natl. Acad. Sci. USA 82*:6250-6254.

11. Prestidge, R. L., Watson, J. D., Urdal, D. L., Mochizuki, D., Conlon, P., and Gillis, S. (1984). Biochemical comparison of murine colony stimulating factors secreted by a T cell lymphoma and a myelomonocytic leukaemia. *J. Immunol. 133*:293–298.
12. Watson, J. D., Mochizuki, D. Y., and Gillis, S. (1983). Molecular characterisation of interleukin 2. *Fed. Proc. 42*:2747–2752.
13. Urdal, D. L., March, C. J., Gillis, S., Larsen, A., and Dower, S. K. (1984). Purification and characterisation of the receptor for interleukin 2 from activated human T lymphocytes and from a human T cell lymphoma line. *Proc. Natl. Acad. Sci. USA 81*:6481–6485.
14. Cosman, D., Cerretti, D. P., Larsen, A., Park, L., March, C., Dower, S., Gillis, S., and Urdal, D. (1984). Cloning, sequence and expression of human interleukin 2 receptor. *Nature 312*:768–771.
15. Miller, J., Malek, T. R., Leonard, W. J., Green, W. C., Shevach, E. M., and Germain, R. N. (1985). Nucleotide sequence and expression of a mouse interleukin 2 receptor cDNA. *J. Immunol. 134*:4212–4217.
16. Park, L. S., Friend, D., Gillis, S., and Urdal, D. L. (1986). Characterization of the cell surface receptor for a multi-lineage colony-stimulating factor (CSF-2). *J. Biol. Chem. 261*:205–210.
17. Gasson, J. C., Kaufman, S. E., Weishert, R. H., Tomonaga, M., and Golde, D. W. (1986). High affinity binding of granulocyte-macrophage colony-stimulating factors to normal and leukemic human myeloid cells. *Proc. Natl. Acad. Sci. USA 83*:669–673.
18. Gillis, S. and Smith, K. S. (1977). Long term culture of tumour-specific cytoxic T cells. *Nature 268*:154–156.
19. Watson, J. (1979). Continuous proliferation of murine antigen-specific helper T lymphocytes in culture. *J. Exp. Med. 150*:1510–1519.
20. Dexter, T. M., Garland, J., Scott, D., Scolnick, E., and Metcalf, D. (1980). Growth of factor-dependent hematopoietic precursor cell lines. *J. Exp. Med. 152*:1036–1045.
21. Greenberger, J. L. et al. (1983). Interleukin 3-dependent hematopoietic progenitor cell lines. *Fed. Proc. 42*:2762–2766.
22. Ihle, J. N., Keller, J., Henderson, L., Klein, F., and Palaszynski, E. (1982). Procedures for the purification of interleukin 3 to homogeneity. *J. Immunol. 129*:2431–2438.
23. Gillis, S. and Watson, J. D. (1981). Interleukin 2-dependent culture of cytolytic T cell lines. *Immunol. Rev. 54*:81–109.
24. Hapel, A. J., Warren, H. S., and Hume, D. A. (1984). Different colony-stimulating factors are detected by the "interleukin-3" dependent cell lines, FDC-Pl and 32D cl-23. *Blood 64*:786–792.
25. Cook, W. D., Metcalf, D., Nicola, N. A., Burgess, A. W., and Walker, F. (1985). Malignant transformation of a growth factor-dependent myeloid cell line by Abelson virus without evidence of an autocrine mechanism. *Cell 41*:677–683.

26. Blasi, E., Mathieson, B. J., Varesio, L., Cleveland, J. L., Borchert, P. A., and Rapp, U. R. (1985). Selective immortalisation of murine macrophages from fresh bone marrow by a raf/myc recombinant murine retrovirus. *Nature 318*:667–670.
27. Rapp, U. R., Cleveland, J. L., Brightman, K., Scott, A., and Ihle, J. N. (1985). Abrogation of IL3 and IL2 dependence by recombinant murine retroviruses expressing v-*myc* oncogenes. *Nature 317*:434–437.
28. Pierce, J. H., Di Fiore, P. P., Aaronson, S. A., Potter, M., Pumphrey, J., Scott, A., and Ihle, J. N. (1985). Neoplastic transformation of mast cells by Abelson-MuLV: Abrogation of IL3 dependence by a nonautocrine mechanism. *Cell 41*:685–693.
29. Ihle, J. N., Pepersack, L., and Rebar, L. (1981). Regulation of T cell differentiation: In vitro induction of 20-β-hydroxysteroid dehydrogenase in splenic lymphocytes is mediated by a unique lymphokine. *J. Immunol. 126*:2184–2189.
30. Ihle, N., Keller, J., Greenberger, J. S., Henderson, L., Yetter, R. A., and Morse, H. C. (1982). Phenotypic characteristics of cell lines requiring IL3 for growth. *J. Immunol. 129*:1377–1384.
31. Le Gros, G. S., Gillis, S., and Watson, J. D. (1985). Induction of IL2 responsiveness in a murine IL3-dependent cell line. *J. Immunol. 135*: 4009–4013.
32. Koyasu, S., Yodoi, J., Nikaido, T., Tagaya, Y., Tanaguchi, Y., Honjo, T., and Yahara, I. (1986). Expression of interleukin 2 receptors on interleukin 3-dependent cell lines. *J. Immunol. 136*:984–987.
33. Farrar, W. L. and Anderson, W. B. (1985). Interleukin-2 stimulates association of protein kinase C with plasma membrane. *Nature 315*: 233–235.
34. Farrar, W. L., Thomas, P. T., and Anderson, W. B. (1985). Altered cytosol/membrane enzyme redistribution on interleukin-3 activation of protein kinase C. *Nature 315*:235–237.
35. Cosman, D., Cerretti, D. P., Larson, A., Park, L., March, C., Dower, S., Gillis, S., and Urdal, D. (1984). Cloning, sequence and expression of human interleukin-2 receptor. *Nature 312*:768–770.
36. Lamers, M. C., Heckford, S. E. ,and Kickles, H. B. (1982). Monoclonal anti-Fc IgG receptor antibodies trigger B lymphocyte function. *Nature 298*:178–180.
37. Raulet, D. H. (1985). Experiment and function of interleukin 2 receptors on immature thymocytes. *Nature 314*:101–103.
38. Kingston, R., Jenkinson, E. J., and Owens, J. J. T. (1985). A single stem cell can recognise an embryonic thymus, producing phenotypically distinct T cell populations. *Nature 317*:811–813.
39. Dennert, G., Hyman, R., Lesley, J., and Trowbridge, I. S. (1980). Effects of cytotoxic monoclonal antibody specific for T200 glycoprotein on functional lymphoid cell populations. *Cell. Immunol. 53*:350–356.

40. Coffman, R. L. (1982). Surface antigen expression and immunoglobulin gene arrangement during mouse pre-B cell development. *Immunology 69*:5–23.
41. Dyalynas, D. P., Quan, Z. S., Wall, K. A., Pierres, A., Quintans, J., Loken, M. R., Pierres, M., and Fitch, F. W. (1983). Characterization of the murine T cell surface molecule, designated L3T4, identified by the monoclonal antibody GK1.5: Similarity of L3T4 to the human Leu3/T4 molecule. *J. Immunol. 131*:2445–2452.
42. Ledbetter, J. A. and Herzenberg, L. A. (1979). Xenogeneic monoclonal antibodies to mouse lymphoid differentiation antigens. *Immunol. Rev. 47*:63–84.
43. Bruce, J., Symington, F. W., McKearn, T. J., and Sprent, J. (1981). A monoclonal antibody discriminating between subsets of T and B cells. *J. Immunol. 127*:2496–2501.
44. Springer, T., Galfre, G., Secher, D., and Milstein, C. (1978). Monoclonal xenogenic antibodies to mouse leukocyte antigens: Identification of macrophage specific and other differentiation antigens. *Curr. Top. Microbiol. Immunol. 81*:45–62.
45. Malek, T. R., Robb, R. J., and Shevach, E. M. (1983). Identification and initial characterization of a rat monoclonal antibody reactive with the murine interleukin 2 receptor-ligand complex. *Proc. Natl. Acad. Sci. USA 80*:5694–5698.
46. Robb, R. J., Greene, W. C., and Rusk, C. M. (1984). Low and high affinity cellular receptors for interleukin 2. Implications for the level of Tac antigen. *J. Exp. Med. 160*:1126–1134.
47. Lowenthal, J. W., Corthesy, P., Tougne, C., Lees, R., MacDonald, H. R., and Nabholz, M. (1985). High and low affinity IL2 receptors: Analysis by IL2 dissociation rate and reactivity with monoclonal anti-receptor antibody, Pc61. *J. Immunol. 135*:3988–3993.
48. Ceredig, R., Lowenthal, J. W., Nabholz, M., and MacDonald, H. R. (1985). Expression of interleukin 2 receptors as a differentiation marker on intrathymic stem cells. *Nature 314*:98–99.
49. Dexter, T. M., Whetton, A. D., Spooncer, E., Heyworth, C., and Simmons, P. (1985). The role of stromal cells and growth factors in haemopoiesis and modulation of their effects by the *src* oncogene. *J. Cell. Physiol. 3*:1–10.
50. Hatakeyama, M., Minamoto, S., Uchiyama, T., Hardy, R. R., Yamada, G., and Tanaguchi, T. (1985). Reconstitution of functional receptor for human interleukin 2 in mouse cells. *Nature 318*:467–470.
51. Corin, R. E. and Donner, D. B. (1982). Insulin receptors convert to a higher affinity state subsequent to hormone binding. *J. Biol. Chem. 257*:104–109.

52. King, A. C. and Cuatrecasas, P. (1982). Resolution of high and low affinity epidermal grow factor receptors. *J. Biol. Chem. 257*:3053–3056.
53. Shoyab, M., De Larco, J. E., and Todaro, G. J. (1979). Biologically active phorbol esters specifically alter affinity of epidermal growth factor membrane receptors. *Nature 219*:387–389.
54. Williams, L. T., Tremble, P. M., Lavin, M. F., and Sunday, M. E. (1984). Platelet-derived growth factor receptors from a high affinity state in membrane preparations. Kinetics and affinity cross-linking studies. *J. Biol. Chem. 259*:5287–5289.
55. Gallis, B., Lewis, A., Wignall, J., Alpert, A., Mochizuki, D. Y., Cosman, D., Hopp, T., and Urdall, D. (1986). Phosphorylation of the human interleukin 2 receptor and a synthetic peptide identical to its C-terminal cytoplasmic domain. *J. Biol. Chem. 261*:5075–5080.
56. Giugni, T. D., James, L. D., Haigler, H. T. (1985). Epidermal growth factor stimulates tyrosine phosphorylation of specific proteins in permeabilised human fibroblasts. *J. Biol. Chem. 260*:15081–15090.
57. White, M. F., Maron, F., and Kahn, C. R. (1985). Insulin rapidly stimulates tyrosine phosphorylation of a M-185,000 protein in intact cells. *Nature 318*:183–185.
58. Wang, J. Y. J. and Baltimore, D. (1985). Localisation of tyrosine kinase-coding region in v-*abl* oncogene by the expression of v-*abl*-encoded proteins in bacteria. *J. Biol. Chem. 260*:64–69.

3
Bovine Interleukin-2

PAUL E. BAKER and DOUGLAS PAT CERRETTI
Immunex Corporation, Seattle, Washington

INTRODUCTION

There are numerous reasons to study lymphokines in animal species other than man. From an academic point, knowledge of lymphokines in lower animals may reveal insight into the evolution of immune responses. In addition, relevance in diseases not affecting man may add to our understanding of defense mechanisms. Moreover, these studies may lead to novel applications. For example, to date most research dealing with interleukin-2 (IL-2) applications has focused on cancer therapy. Yet, a large body of information suggests that IL-2 might find beneficial use in communicable diseases.

Domestic animals suffer from a wide variety of protozoan, bacterial, and viral diseases. For economic reasons, communicable diseases of cattle have been studied more than others. Nonetheless, both beef and dairy cattle remain vulnerable to hundreds of infectious agents, costing farmers and ranchers billions of dollars every year. For example, the most debilitating and common disease of dairy cattle is mastitis. *Staphylococcus* sp. and *Streptococcus agalactia* are the most prominent causative agents, although enteric bacteria may occasionally be involved. Onset of the disease typically occurs early during the "dry period," when cessation of milking allows bacteria ready access to the teat cisternae. Macrophages predominate in normal mammary secretions, while neutrophils are the most common cell of mastitic udders. Both are capable of phagocytizing opsonized bacteria via binding immunoglobulin through Fc receptors. Immunity in the teat end is considered the first line of defense against pathogenic bacteria. Both B and T cells infiltrate the stroma during acute mastitis (1), suggesting a prominent role for lymphocytes. Given the direct effect of IL-2 on T cells, and thereby its indirect effect on B cells, it is likely that IL-2-directed lymphocyte proliferation may prove effective in augmenting pathogen-specific immunity.

Thus in cattle there exists not only an opportunity to expand our understanding of immune mechanisms but also a potential application of this knowledge to solving practical problems.

GENERATION OF BOVINE INTERLEUKIN-2-DEPENDENT BOVINE T-CELL LINES

Human IL-2 will induce replication of bovine T cells (2). However therapeutic or prophylactic administration of human IL-2 to cattle, especially dairy cattle where it may be utilized over several years, is likely to bring about an immune response to the molecule. Therefore administration of bovine IL-2 to cattle would be greatly preferred. Attempts to characterize bovine IL-2 have been hampered because the lymphokine is, to some extent, species-restricted. Because bovine IL-2 has no effect on the murine T cells used for human and murine studies, the development of a bovine IL-2-responsive T-cell line was considered a necessity.

Unfortunately, identification of bovine T cells was not a simple task. Numerous investigators had reported that those bovine lymphocytes that formed rosettes with sheep red blood cells (SRBC) were of the T-cell lineage (3,4). Others claimed that bovine T cells responded to lectins such as concanavalin A (Con A) and phytohemagglutinin (PHA) (5,6), known to induce blastogenesis of murine and human T cells. Finally, monoclonal antibodies (MAb) reactive with bovine leukocytes and specific leukocyte subsets had also been purported (7).

Rather than defining bovine T cells based on staining patterns, responses to lectins, or the like, we chose to use a physiological marker, antigen-specific cytotoxicity. Peripheral blood leukocytes (PBL) from two young Hereford steers were isolated and used throughout this study. The PBL from one animal were inactivated with mitomycin C and used as stimulators in one-way mixed leukocyte cultures (MLC) to generate alloantigen-specific cytotoxic T cells. It had been previously shown that generation of cytotoxic T cells in murine and human allogeneic MLC peaked on days 5 and 7, respectively, of culture (8,9). When responding leukocytes were harvested from MLC and used as effectors in 4-hr ^{51}Cr-release cytotoxicity assays, we found highly inconsistent results (Table 1). On the other hand, if we cultured the MLC for 15 days before lymphocyte-mediated cytolysis (LMC) assays, we found that highly cytotoxic, alloantigen-specific responder cells could be generated (Fig. 1). Effector cells thus generated demonstrated approximately 50% cytolysis against allogeneic target cells at an effector/target ratio (E/T) of 144:1, while providing only moderate killing of autologous or third-party ^{51}Cr-labeled targets. In addition, there was a distinct E/T dose response of cytolysis.

We found that if responder cells from primary allogeneic MLC were harvested 15 days after culture and restimulated with the same mitomycin C-inactivated allogeneic stimulator cells for an additional 5 days, even better alloantigen-specific cytotoxicity resulted (Fig. 2). This effector cell population showed approximately 97% lysis of the allogeneic target cell at the highest E/T tested. The effectors also exhibited alloantigen specificity as seen by the minimal cytotoxic activity against the autologous and third-party target cells. Additionally, there was a strict dose-dependent relationship between the E/T and percentage specific lysis of the allogeneic target.

Alloantigen-specific cytotoxic leukocytes from a secondary MLC were placed into medium containing 500 pg/ml human recombinant IL-2 (rIL-2). Eighteen days after the initiation of culture, these cells (termed BT2) were examined for proliferative responsiveness to various sources of IL-2 or lectin. As determined by [^{3}H]thymidine incorporation, BT2 displayed

Table 1 Maximum Percentage Cytolysis (% Cyto) of Target Cells Observed at the Highest Effector/Target Cell Ratio (E/T) on Day 5 of a Primary Bovine Mixed Leukocyte Culture

	Effector cells versus:					
	Allogeneic target cells		Autologous target cells		Third-party target cells	
Exp.	E/T	% Cyto	E/T	% Cyto	E/T	% Cyto
1	161	20	168	10	165	9
2	110	54	129	20	105	4
3	98	5	107	0	101	1

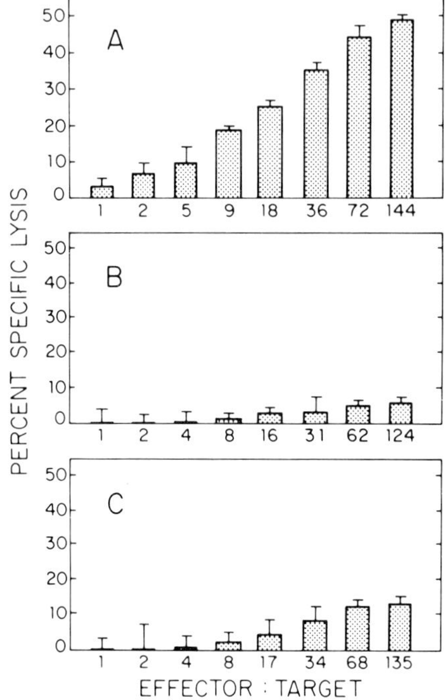

Figure 1 Responding cells were harvested from a primary mixed bovine leukocyte culture on day 15 and tested in a 4-hr ^{51}Cr-release assay against (A) allogeneic lymphoblasts, (B) autologous lymphoblasts, and (C) third-party lymphoblasts. Bars represent the percentage standard deviation of triplicate cultures (*Source*: From Picha, K. and Baker, P. E. (1986). *Immunology* 57:131–136. With permission).

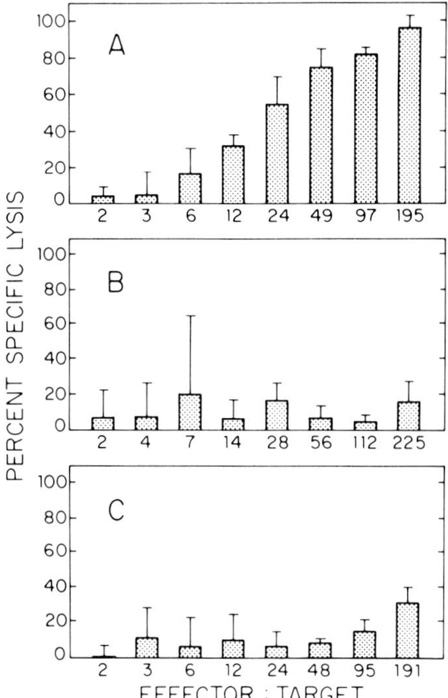

Figure 2 Responding cells were harvested 5 days after restimulation of a long-term primary mixed bovine leukocyte culture with allogeneic leukocytes, and lytic activity determined in a 4-hr ^{51}Cr-release assay against (A) allogeneic lymphoblasts, (B) autologous lymphoblasts, and (C) third-party lymphoblasts. Bars represent the percentage standard deviation of triplicate cultures (*Source*: From Picha, K. and Baker, P. E. (1986). *Immunology* *57*:131–136. With permission).

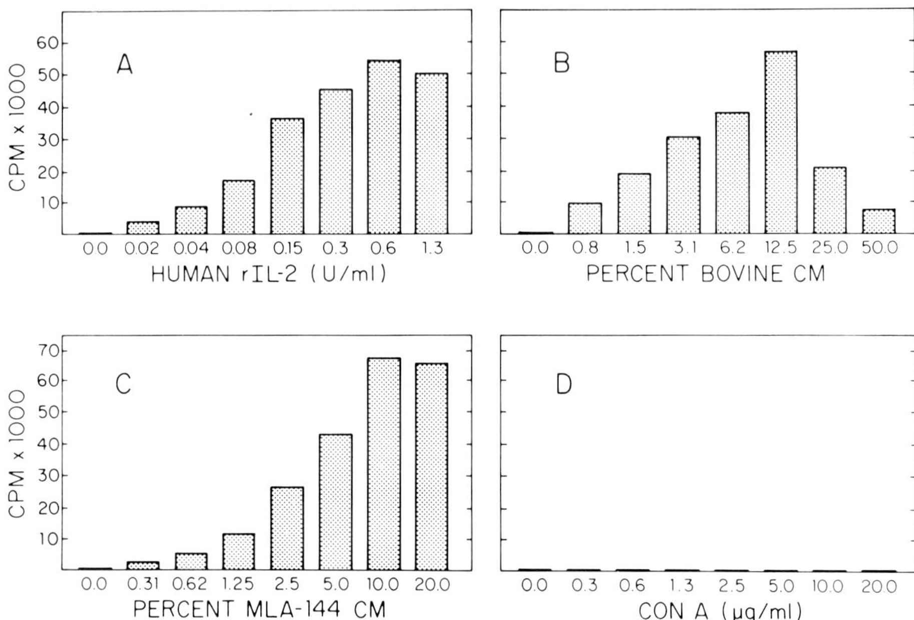

Figure 3 BT2 cells were examined 18 days after initiation of culture for proliferation via [^{3}H] thymidine incorporation in response to increasing $\log_2$ dilutions of (A) human recombinant IL-2, (B) bovine lymph node-conditioned medium, (C) MLA-144-conditioned medium, and (D) Con A (*Source*: From Picha, K. and Baker, P. E. (1986). *Immunology 57*:131–136. With permission).

exquisite sensitivity to human, simian, and bovine IL-2, but not to lectin alone (Fig. 3).

Four weeks after having been placed into IL-2-containing medium, BT2 cells were again assayed for lytic activity against autologous and allogeneic lymphoblasts in a 4-hr LMC assay. The BT2 effectors demonstrated 55% specific cytolysis against the allogeneic target cells at an E/T of 100:1, while simultaneously showing less than 3% cytotoxicity at the same E/T against autologous lymphoblasts (Fig. 4). Moreover, there was a strict relationship between the E/T and the percentage cytotoxicity against allogeneic targets and none against autologous lymphoblasts.

In an effort to determine the effect of extended culturing of BT2 cells on antigen-specific cytolysis, a similar LMC assay was performed 10 weeks after the initiation of culture. Autologous, allogeneic, and third-party

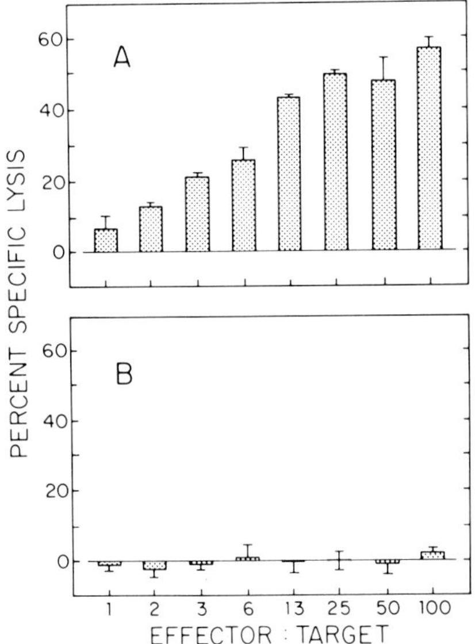

Figure 4 BT2 cells were examined 4 weeks after initiation of culture in a 4-hr ^{51}Cr-release assay for specific cytolysis against (A) allogeneic lymphoblasts and (B) autologous lymphoblasts. Bars represent the percentage standard deviation of triplicate cultures (*Source*: From Picha, K. and Baker, P. E. (1986). *Immunology* 57:131–136. With permission).

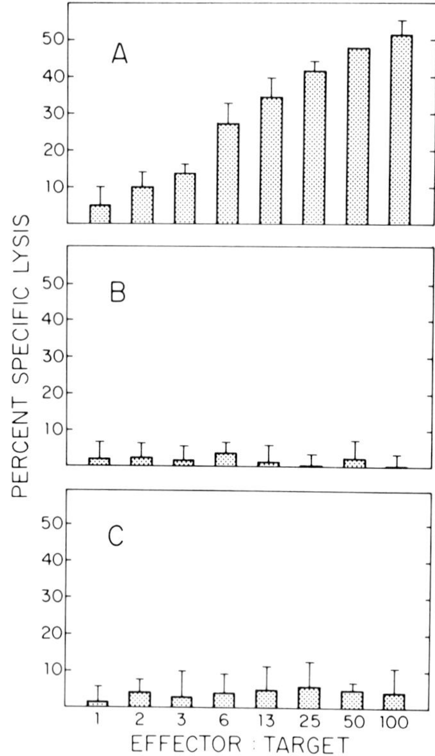

Figure 5 Ten weeks after initiation of culture, BT2 cells were examined for lytic activity in a 4-hr ^{51}Cr assay against (A) allogeneic lymphoblasts, (B) autologous lymphoblasts, and (C) third-party lymphoblasts. Bars represent the percentage standard deviation of triplicate cultures (*Source*: From Picha, K. and Baker, P. E. (1986). *Immunology* 57:131–136. With permission).

cytolyses were examined (Fig. 5). Again BT2 cells manifested over 50% cytolysis against allogeneic lymphoblasts, and none against autologous cells at an E/T of 100:1. Similarly, there was no significant lysis of third-party targets.

QUANTIFICATION OF BOVINE INTERLEUKIN-2: THE BOVINE INTERLEUKIN-2 ASSAY

The availability of a bovine IL-2-dependent bovine T-cell line, BT2, made it possible to quantify bovine IL-2 in conditioned medium. Moreover, this cell line was to prove crucial in cloning and optimizing expression of the lymphokine. For the purpose of quantification, we utilized the method that Gillis and associates (10) had previously described for assaying murine IL-2, with the following modifications. First, the bovine IL-2-dependent cytotoxic T-cell line, BT2, was used as indicator cells. Second, the cell concentration was doubled to 8×10^4/ml and the cells were cultured for 48 hr (instead of 24 hr) before the addition of [^{3}H] thymidine. Finally, because we found BT2 to grow adequately in a 20% solution of conditioned medium from the primate T-cell line MLA-144, containing primate IL-2, we utilized it as a 1 unit/ml IL-2 standard.

CLONING BOVINE INTERLEUKIN-2

Construction and Analysis of a Bovine Complimentary DNA Library

Before our attempts to clone bovine IL-2 from a cDNA library, the nucleic acid sequence for both murine (11) and human (12) IL-2 had been determined and were found to be remarkably homogeneous. This observation, and the fact that human rIL-2 would induce BT2 cells to divide in culture, led us to examine the possibility of utilizing a human cDNA probe to isolate its analogue from a bovine cDNA library.

Polyadenylated mRNA was isolated from bovine lymph node cells stimulated for 17 hr with Con A (7.5 μg/ml). Procedures for RNA purification and cDNA library construction were identical with those described previously (13). Small-scale plasmid DNA preparations from pools of 2.5×10^3 transformants, representing approximately 3.5×10^4 total transformants, were digested with Pst1, electrophoresed on 0.8% agarose gels, blotted onto nitrocellulose filters, and hybridized with a human cDNA probe (^{32}P-labeled by nick-translation) corresponding to nucleotides

52–759 of the published sequence. After hybridization, filters were washed extensively. Positive pools, as assessed by autoradiography, containing the largest hybridizing cDNAs were subdivided, and the process was repeated on pools of 500 transformants. Positive pools were then used in colony filter hybridization experiments to identify transformants that hybridized strongly with the probe.

Screening of a bovine cDNA library with a ^{32}P-labeled DNA fragment encoding human IL-2 resulted in several positive clones. One of these, pBIL2-4, was selected for further analysis. A partial restriction endonuclease map and DNA sequence is shown in Fig. 6. pBIL2-4 contained a cDNA insert of 775 base pairs (bp) including a stretch of adenylate residues corresponding to the poly-A tail of mRNA. These adenylate residues were preceded by the polyadenylation/maturation signal, AATAAA (14). The sequence also had an open-reading frame of 155 amino acids, starting with an initiator Met codon at nucleotide 18 and ending with a termination codon at nucleotide 485. This protein would have a predicted relative molecular weight of 17,555. Comparison of the amino acid sequence with that of human IL-2 (12) indicated that the amino-terminal residue of mature bovine IL-2 was Ala-21. The mature protein would be composed of 135 amino acids and have a predicted relative molecular weight of 15,452. The 5′ end of the open-reading frame encoded a region of 20 amino acids with many characteristics expected of a signal peptide for secreted proteins (15).

Expression of Bovine Recombinant Interleukin-2 in *Escherichia coli*

An *E. coli* expression vector was constructed by inserting a blunt-ended (by T4 polymerase) HgiAl/Pst1 fragment (encoding amino acids 22 to 135) from pBIL2-4 into pLNhumIL-2 with a synthetic oligonucleotide to provide an *E. coli* ribosomal-binding site, translational initiation site, and a codon for amino acid 21 (Fig. 7). The nucleotide sequences used for the ribosome-binding site were based on sequences used to give high-level expression of human rIL-2 in *E. coli* (16,17). pLNhumIL-2 was constructed by inserting a DNA fragment encoding human IL-2 into Hpal-digested pPL-lambda (Pharmacia) with a synthetic oligonucleotide. pPL-lambda contained the lambda P_L promoter on a pBR322-derived vector. The resulting recombinant plasmid, designated pLNBovIL-2, was transformed into *E. coli* strain RRl containing the plasmid pRK248cIts that has a gene encoding a thermolabile repressor of the P_L promoter. During the

[PstI] HgiAI XbaI [PstI]

(A)x

100bp

(A)

```
                                                     5'--CCTCAACTCCTGCCACA    17

Met Tyr Lys Ile Gln Leu Leu Ser Cys Ile Ala Leu Thr Leu Ala Leu Val Ala Asn Gly    20
ATG TAC AAG ATA CAA CTC TTG TCT TGC ATT GCA CTA ACT CTT GCA CTC GTT GCA AAC GGT    77
 *
Ala Pro Thr Ser Ser Ser Thr Gly Asn Thr Met Lys Glu Val Lys Ser Leu Leu Leu Asp    40
GCA CCT ACT TCA AGC TCT ACG GGG AAC ACA ATG AAA GAA GTG AAG TCA TTG CTG CTG GAT   137

Leu Gln Leu Leu Leu Glu Lys Val Lys Asn Pro Glu Asn Leu Lys Leu Ser Arg Met His    60
TTA CAG TTG CTT TTG GAG AAA GTT AAA AAT CCT GAG AAC CTC AAG CTC TCC AGG ATG CAT   197
                                     ▲
Thr Phe Asp Phe Tyr Val Pro Lys Val Asn Ala Thr Glu Leu Lys His Leu Lys Cys Leu    80
ACA TTT GAC TTT TAC GTG CCC AAG GTT AAC GCT ACA GAA TTG AAA CAT CTT AAG TGT TTA   257

Leu Glu Glu Leu Lys Leu Leu Glu Glu Val Leu Asn Leu Ala Pro Ser Lys Asn Leu Asn   100
CTA GAA GAA CTC AAA CTT CTA GAG GAA GTG CTA AAT TTA GCT CCA AGC AAA AAC CTG AAC   317

Pro Arg Glu Ile Lys Asp Ser Met Asp Asn Ile Lys Arg Ile Val Leu Glu Leu Gln Gly   120
CCC AGA GAG ATC AAG GAT TCA ATG GAC AAT ATC AAG AGA ATC GTT TTG GAA CTA CAG GGA   377

Ser Glu Thr Arg Phe Thr Cys Glu Tyr Asp Asp Ala Thr Val Asn Ala Val Glu Phe Leu   140
TCT GAA ACA AGA TTC ACA TGT GAA TAT GAT GAT GCA ACA GTA AAC GCT GTA GAA TTT CTG   437

Asn Lys Trp Ile Thr Phe Cys Gln Ser Ile Tyr Ser Thr Met Thr End                   155
AAC AAA TGG ATT ACC TTT TGT CAA AGC ATC TAC TCA ACA ATG ACT TGA TCACTAAGTGCCTCT   500

CATTTTAAACTATCAGGCTTTCTATTTATTTAAATATTTAAAATTTATATTTATTTTTTGATATATGTTTTCCTACCTT   579

TTGTAACTGTTAGTCTTAAGATGATAAATATGGATCTTTTAAGATTCTTTTTGTAAGCCCTACGGGCTTAAAAATTCAG   658

TTAAATTATTTATCCTGAAGTATTTATTTGTATATTGAATTTTTAAATATAATGTCTATGCAGGTCATTGACTAAAATT   737

ATTTAATAAAGTTGATGAATAAAAAACAAAAAAAAAAAA--3'                                        776
```

(B)

Figure 6 Restriction map and nucleotide sequence of bovine IL-2 cDNA. (A) Partial restriction map of the cDNA insert in pBIL2-4. Coding sequences are boxed. The open boxes represent the coding region for mature protein. The PstI sites in brackets were generated by the cloning procedure. (B) Nucleotide sequence and predicted amino acid sequence of bovine IL-2. The predicted amino terminus of mature bovine IL-2 is marked with a star (Ala-21). The triangle represents a possible *N*-linked glycosylation site and the 3′ polyadenylation/maturation signal is underlined (*Source*: From Cerretti, D. P. et al. (1986). *Proc. Natl. Acad. Sci. USA 83*:3223–3227. With permission).

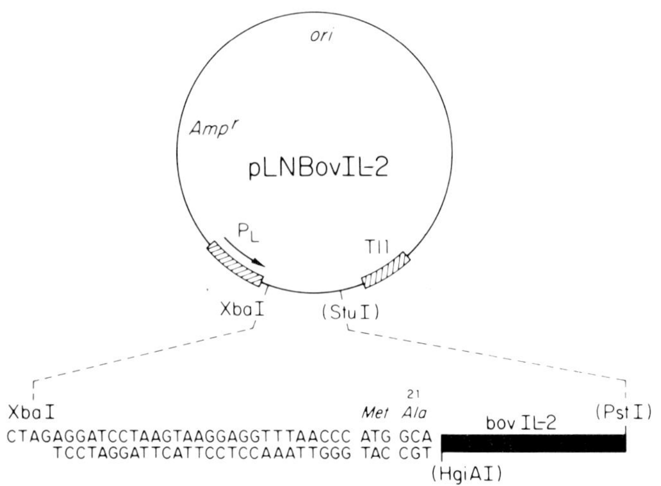

Figure 7 Structure of the *E. coli* expression plasmid pLNBovIL-2. The plasmid contains sequences derived from pBR322 containing the origin of replication (*ori*) and ampicillin resistance gene (Amp^r). The hatched boxes represent regions containing the lambda P_L promoter used to direct transcription of IL-2 and the transcriptional terminator, T11. The synthetic oligonucleotide containing a ribosome-binding site, an initiator Met codon and a codon for Ala-21 is shown fused to the coding region of bovine IL-2 (solid box) (*Source*: From Cerretti, D. P. et al. (1986). *Proc. Natl. Acad. Sci. USA 83*:3223–3227. With permission).

construction of pLNBovIL-2, human IL-2 DNA was deleted. Expression of bovine rIL-2 in *E. coli* and sample preparation were done as previously described (13).

After initial growth at 30°C, *E. coli* containing this plasmid, as well as one containing a control plasmid lacking bovine IL-2 sequences, were induced by raising the temperature to 42°C. Aliquots were taken at various times and total *E. coli* proteins were analyzed by sodium dodecyl sulfate polyacryamide gel electrophoresis (SDS-PAGE) (Fig. 8). A major new protein band (arrow), that was presumably bovine IL-2, continued to accumulate for up to 20 hr. An apparent relative molecular weight of 15,250 for this protein was in good agreement with the predicted relative molecular weight of 15,452 as deduced from the DNA sequence. Densitometer scanning of silver-stained gels of total *E. coli* protein from an induced

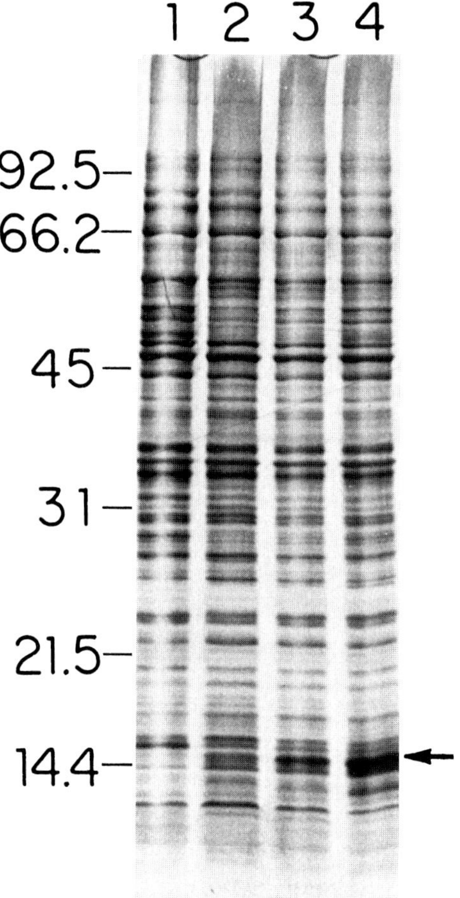

Figure 8 Induction of bovine IL-2 synthesis in *E. coli.* Aliquots of *E. coli* cultures were centrifuged and prepared for SDS-PAGE at the times after induction listed as follows: Lane 1, RR1(pRK248cIts) with a control plasmid containing P_L lacking bovine IL-2 sequences, 20 hr; lane 2, RR1(pRK248cIts) (pLNBovIL-2), 1.5 hr; lane 3, RR1(pRK248cIts) (pLNBovIL-2), 4 hr; lane 4, RR1(pRK248cIts) (pLNBovIL-2), 20 hr. The positions of protein molecular weight markers (in kilodaltons) are indicated at the far left. Arrow indicates position of recombinant bovine IL-2 (*Source*: From Cerretti, D. P. et al. (1986). *Proc. Natl. Acad. Sci. USA 83*:3223–3227. With permission).

culture (see Fig. 8, lane 4) indicated that bovine IL-2 represented about 10% of the cellular protein. Cultures that were induced for 20 hr (see Fig. 8, lane 4) were simultaneously assayed on BT2 cells for biological activity and were found to produce 2.8×10^6 units/ml. Control plasmids, lacking IL-2 sequences (see Fig. 8, lane 1), yielded no biological activity (<0.1 units/ml).

Analysis of Messenger RNA

Polyadenylated mRNA was isolated from Con A-stimulated and unstimulated lymph node cells as described previously for cDNA library construction. Samples were then electrophoresed in agarose gels containing formaldehyde, transferred to nylon membranes, and hybridized with a ^{32}P-labeled RNA probe transcribed with SP6 polymerase. The [^{32}P] RNA probe was synthesized from a 500 base pair Rsal/Dral fragment (isolated from pBIL2-4) that was inserted into pGem1 (Promega Biotec). Hybridization and washing of blots was as described (18).

A single RNA species of approximately 1100 nucleotide bases was detected in lymph node cells stimulated with Con A but not in unstimulated lymph node cells (Fig. 9). The size of bovine IL-2 mRNA was similar to the size of human and murine IL-2 mRNA (19,20).

Analysis of the Amino Acid Sequence

Analysis of the amino acid sequence, as deduced from the nucleotide sequence, revealed that mature bovine IL-2 would be composed of 135 amino acids and have a predicted relative molecular weight of 15,450. This was compared with the estimated relative molecular weight of 14,400–25,000 of bovine IL-2 isolated from lymph node cells. The heterogeneity in molecular weight has been attributed to variable degrees of glycosylation (21). The predicted amino acid sequence of bovine IL-2 aligned with the predicted amino acid sequences of human (12) and murine (11) IL-2 is shown in Fig. 10. The bovine analogue is more homologous to the human (approximately 69%) than to the murine (approximately 50%) sequence and this homology is dispersed throughout. However one region, the amino-terminal of mature IL-2 (see Fig. 10, star) has seven identical amino acids in all three proteins. In addition, the positions of all three cysteinyl (Cys) residues (see Fig. 10, arrows) are conserved, including the two cysteinyl residues (see Fig. 10, heavy arrows) thought to be involved in the formation of an active conformation (12). Bovine IL-2, like the human analogue,

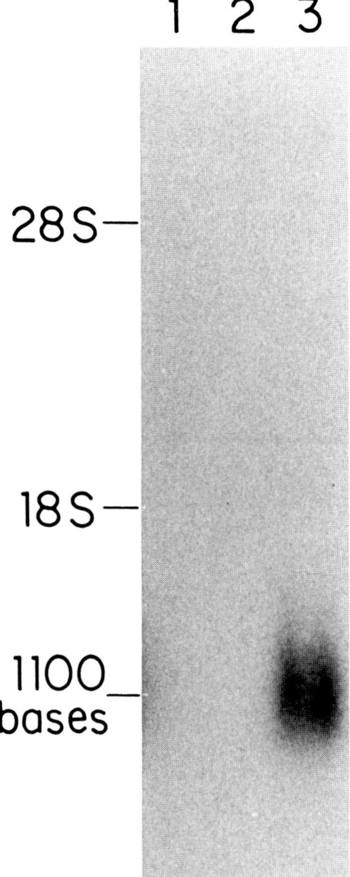

Figure 9 Autoradiographs of Northern blots of IL-2 mRNA. Hybridization of IL-2 probe to blots from lymph node cells. Lanes: 1, 4 μg polyadenylated RNA from unstimulated cells; 2, 4 μg polyadenylated RNA from unstimulated cells cultured for 17 hr; 3, 4 μg polyadenylated RNA from stimulated cells cultured for 17 hr with Con A. The position of 18S and 28S rRNA bands are indicated (*Source*: From Cerretti, D. P. et al. (1986). *Proc. Natl. Acad. Sci. USA 83*:3223–3227. With permission).

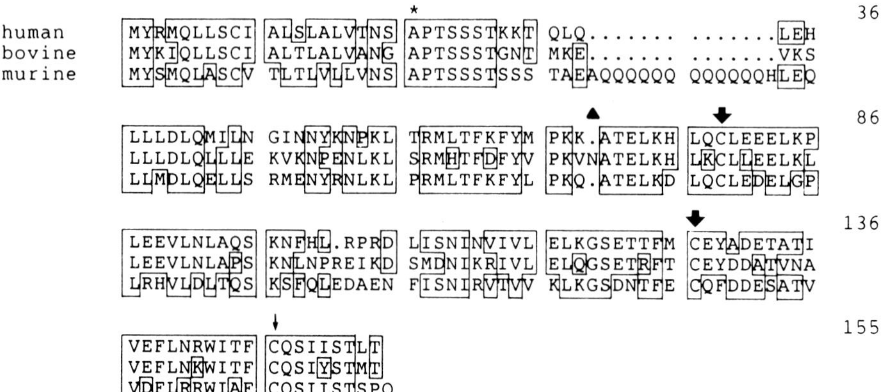

Figure 10 Alignment of human, bovine, and murine IL-2 amino acid sequences as deduced from their DNA sequences. Numbering, starting at the initiator Met, is for bovine IL-2. Boxed residues indicate homology at two or more residues. The star represents the predicted amino-terminus of mature IL-2. Arrows identify the conserved cysteine residues and the triangle indicates the position of the possible *N*-linked glycosylation site in bovine IL-2 (*Source*: From Cerretti, D. P. et al. (1986). *Proc. Natl. Acad. Sci. USA 83*:3223–3227. With permission).

lacked the unusual stretch of 12 glutaminyl (Gln) residues present in the murine polypeptide, but was unique in that it had one potential *N*-linked glycosylation site (Fig. 10, triangle). This was due to an insertion of an asparaginyl (Asn) residue at position 70 that is absent in the human and murine analogues.

Analysis of Genomic DNA

To determine the number of IL–2-related genes in cattle, a ^{32}P-labeled bovine IL-2 probe was hybridized to Southern blots of genomic DNA (isolated from PBL) digested with three different restriction endonucleases. Digestion with BamHI, EcoRI, and HindIII resulted in one (9.8 kb), two (5.8 kb, 5.0 kb), and three (5.0 kb, 3.3 kb, 1.9 kb) bands respectively (Fig. 11). These results suggested that the gene for bovine IL-2 probably exists as a single copy, as was predicted for human IL-2 (12,22,23).

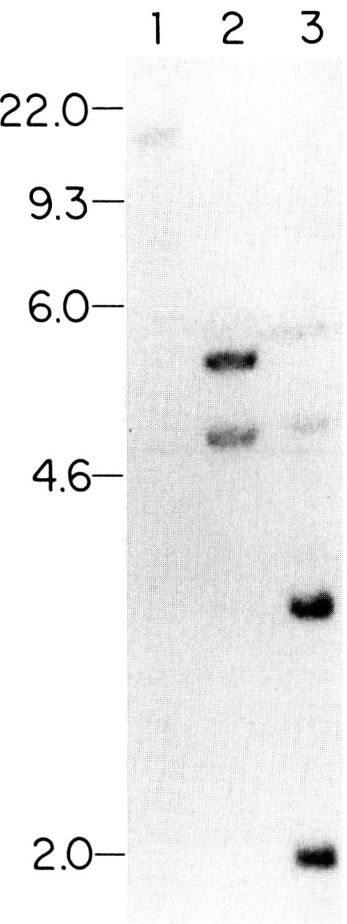

Figure 11 Autoradiograph of hybridizations with IL-2 cDNA probe to Southern blots of bovine genomic DNA. Genomic DNA (10 μg) was digested with BamHI (lane 1), EcoR1 (lane 2), and HindIII (lane 3), electrophoresed in a 0.7% agarose gel, blotted, and hybridized at high stringency to nick-translated ^{32}P-labeled IL-2 cDNA. The molecular weight markers (in kilobase pairs) are from HindIII-digested bacteriophage lambda DNA (*Source*: From Cerretti, D. P. et al. (1986). *Proc. Natl. Acad. Sci. USA 83*:3223–3227. With permission).

OPTIMIZATION OF BOVINE INTERLEUKIN-2 EXPRESSION AND PURIFICATION

Synthesis of Recombinant Interleukin-2 in Yeast

Synthesis and secretion of foreign proteins in *Saccharomyces cervisiae* can be an effective means of obtaining easily purified material, because yeasts secrete few proteins of their own. The well-characterized secretion pathway of the yeast alpha-factor has allowed this signal sequence to be exploited to direct secretion and proper processing of foreign proteins (24,25). To this end, we used a yeast expression vector, pNB2, that included (a) pBR322 sequences for selection and replication in *E. coli*, (b) the *TRP1* gene and 2μ origin of replication for selection and replication in *S. cerevisiae*, and (c) the yeast alcohol dehydrogenase 2 (*ADH2*) promoter followed by the alpha-factor leader sequence to allow foreign protein expression and secretion from yeast (24,25). A bovine IL-2 cDNA fragment from the HgiA1 site (blunt ended with T4 polymerase) at alanine-21 to an Ssp1 site (modified to a NcoI site with linkers) in the 3′ noncoding region was fused in-frame to the alpha-factor leader by means of a synthetic oligonucleotide that regenerated the last five amino acids of the alpha-factor leader and the Ala codon at position 1 of mature bovine IL-2. Ligation reactions and restriction enzyme digests were carried out by standard procedures (26). The yeast expression plasmid is depicted in Fig. 12.

This expression plasmid was transformed into a diploid yeast, strain XV2181 [*trp*-1, *leu*-2], selecting for Trp$^+$ transformants. Cultures to be assayed for biological activity were grown in 20–50 ml of YPD medium (1% yeast extract, 2% peptone, 1% glucose) at 30°C to a cell density of 1–5 $\times$ 10^8 cells/ml. Cells were then removed by centrifugation and the medium was filtered through a 0.45 μm cellulose acetate filter. Analysis of this material on BT2 cells indicated that the yeast containing the bovine IL-2 plasmid secreted approximately 1.26 $\times$ 10^6 units/ml. Large-scale fermentations were done in a 10 L New Brunswick Microferm fermentor. Cells were removed from the medium using a Millipore Pellicon filtration system.

Purification of Bovine Recombinant Interleukin-2

Given previous success at using reversed-phase high-performance liquid chromatography (RP-HPLC) for the final step in the purification of natural

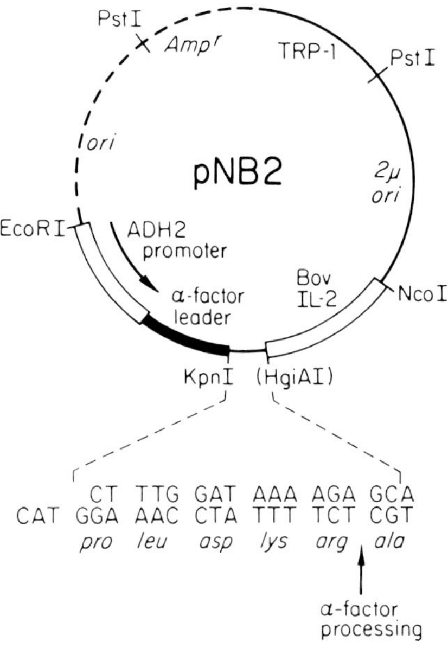

Figure 12 The yeast expression vector, pNB2. The yeast-*E. coli* shuttle vector, defined by the largest KpnI/NcoI portion of the vector, contains sequences from pBR322 that allow selection (Amp^r) and replication in *E. coli* (dashed lines), and the yeast *TRP*1 gene and 2 μ origin of replication for selection and autonomous replication in a TRP1 yeast strain (thin lines). The 1.2 kb EcoR1 to KpnI fragment (boxed) includes the yeast ADH2 promoter adjacent to the alpha-factor leader sequence. The alpha-factor leader was fused in-frame to the HgiA1 site near the NH_2-terminus of mature bovine IL-2 by means of a synthetic oligonucleotide (shown above). The bovine IL-2 gene was obtained on an HgiAI to SspI fragment, to which NcoI linkers were added. The DNA fragments plus the oligonucleotide were ligated together using standard methods (26), transformed into *E. coli* strain RR1, and the correct construction identified by restriction digest.

human IL-2 (27), we reasoned that application of this technique to the purification of recombinant bovine IL-2 (rBoIL-2) might be worthwhile. To this end, 6.9 L of yeast medium containing rBoIL-2 was filtered and pumped directly onto a Vydac C-4 15–20 μm PrepPAK column. Aqueous 0.1% TFA was then pumped through the column until the absorbance of the eluate was back to base-line levels, at which time a gradient of acetonitrile was initiated to elute proteins off the column. Fractions were collected and aliquots of each fraction were analyzed by SDS-PAGE and in the bovine microIL-2 assay for the presence of rBoIL-2. The bulk of the activity originally contained in 6.9 L of medium was found concentrated in two fractions (10 and 11) that eluted 28 and 29 min after the initiation of the acetonitrile gradient (Fig. 13). The yield of activity in these two fractions was 268% when compared with the starting material, which was likely due to the exclusion of inhibitory yeast products.

Purification of rBoIL-2 to homogeneity was achieved by chromatography of a portion of fractions 10 and 11 from this run, on the same column in 0.9 M acetic acid, 0.2 M pyridine. Proteins were eluted from the column with a gradient of propanol. A protein of 16,000 relative molecular weight, found preponderantly in fractions 30–32 (Fig. 14A), was the only protein detected in those fractions containing BoIL-2 activity (Fig. 14B). Recovery of activity in these fractions was 86% of that applied to this column.

Amino Acid Analysis

Samples were hydrolyzed in vacuo by constantly boiling HCl for 24 hr. After hydrolysis, samples were evaporated to dryness under vacuum and resuspended in 0.2 N sodium citrate, pH 2.2. Samples were injected onto an LKB model 4150-Alpha single-column amino acid analyzer, and residues were detected with ninhydrin. Peak areas were calculated using an LKB model 2220 recording integrator. Results (Table 2) were consistent with the amino acid composition predicted from the cDNA sequence.

Protein Sequencing

Protein sequencing was performed on an Applied Biosystems Model 470A Sequencer using the reagents and program supplied by the manufacturer. Phenylthiohydantoin amino acids were identified by reversed-phase HPLC as described previously (28). The protein sequence analysis confirmed that the protein was, indeed, bovine rIL-2 and that it was correctly

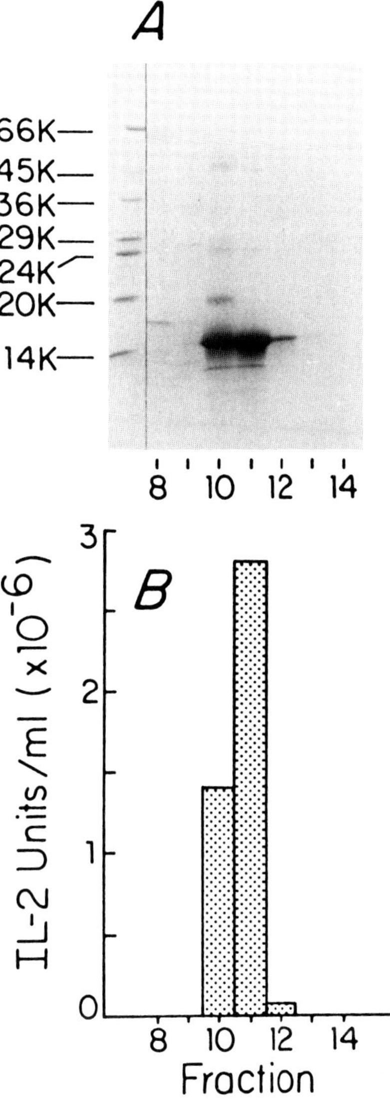

Figure 13 Concentration of recombinant bovine IL-2 by RP-HPLC. (A) Analysis by polyacrylamide gel electrophoresis of aliquots from fractions collected during the elution of the C-4 reversed-phase column with a gradient of acetonitrile. (B) Analysis of aliquots from the same fractions for the presence of biological activity in the bovine IL-2 assay.

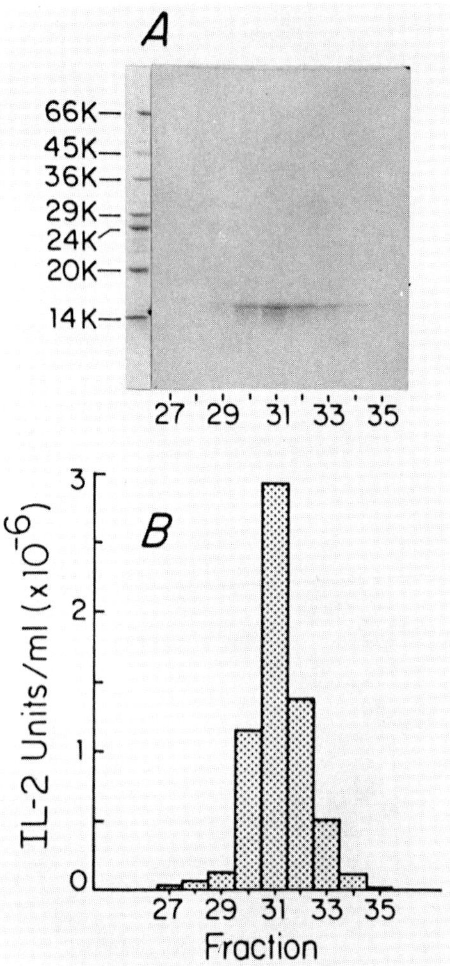

Figure 14 Purification of recombinant bovine IL-2 by RP-HPLC. (A) Fractions that contained bovine IL-2 from the first RP-HPLC run (fractions 10 and 11, Fig. 13A) were pooled, diluted 1:2 with 0.9 M acetic acid, 0.2 M pyridine, and applied to the same column that had been previously equilibrated in 0.9 M acetic acid, 0.2 M pyridine, and 20% n-propanol. Proteins were eluted with a gradient of n-propanol and aliquots of each fraction were analyzed by PAGE. (B) Aliquots from the same fractions were tested for biological activity in the bovine IL-2 assay.

Table 2 Comparison of the Predicted Amino Acid Composition of Recombinant Bovine IL-2 Versus the Experimentally Derived Composition

Amino acid	Experimental	Expected
Asn + Asp	15.6	16
Thr	10.6	11
Ser	9.6	10
Gln + Glu	16.7	16
Pro	5.5	5
Gly	2.8	2
Ala	5.8	5
Cys	3.2	3
Val	7.9	8
Met	3.2	4
Ile	3.9	5
Leu	22.4	22
Tyr	2.8	3
Phe	5.2	5
His	2.2	2
Lys	12.8	13
Arg	4.3	4

processed by the yeast to begin at alanine (Table 3). No other sequences were detected.

Bovine Interleukin-2 Receptors

The HPLC-purified bovine rIL-2 was lyophilized with sucrose (25 mg/1 mg IL-2) to remove pyridine-acetate-propanol buffer before radioiodination. Several vials were lyophilized and stored at 4°C for subsequent reconstitution with PBS. The bovine rIL-2 was radiolabeled using the Enzymobead radioiodination reagent (BioRad) essentially following the manufacturer's specifications. Fifty microliters of Enzymobead reagent, 20 μl of ^{125}I (2 mCi) and 10 μl of 2.5% beta-D-glucose were added to 5 μg of recombinant

Table 3 NH_2-Terminal Protein Sequencing of Recombinant Bovine IL-2

	CYCLE NUMBER (Values in pmol)																			
Amino Acid	1	2	3	4	5	6	7	8	9	10	11	12	13	14	15	16	17	18	19	20
Asn									38.9											
Ser				44.4	35.5	66.6									7.2					
Thr			96.7				47.0			27.5										
Gln																				
Gly								32.7												
His																				
Ala	245.1																			
Asp																			25.2	
Arg																				
Glu													11.6							
Tyr																				
Val																				
Pro		156.1																		
Met											16.7									
Ile																				
Leu																17.6	22.8	41.6		45.1
Phe																				
Trp																				
Lys												16.9		20.5						
Expected Sequences:																				
	Ala	Pro	Thr	Ser	Ser	Ser	Thr	Gly	Asn	Thr	Met	Lys	Glu	Lys	Ser	Leu	Leu	Leu	Asp	Leu

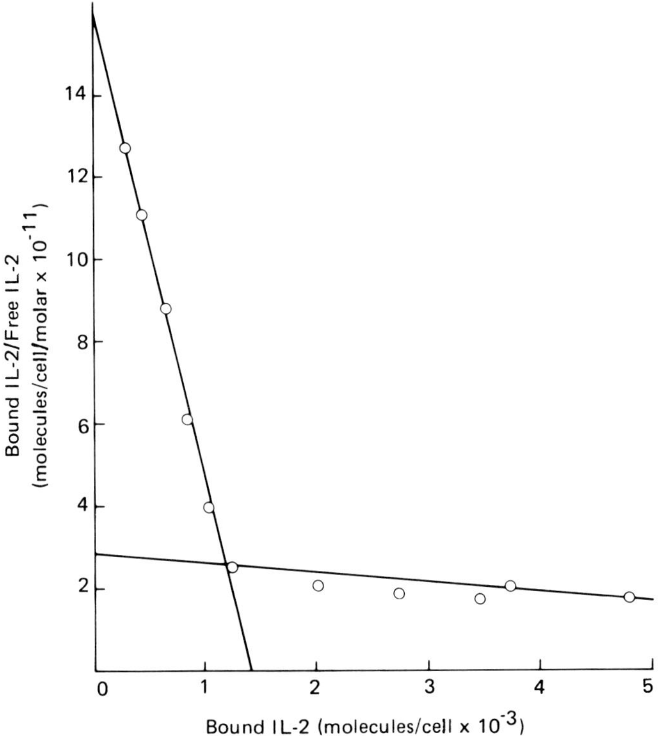

Figure 15 Scatchard representation of equilibrium binding of ^{125}I-labeled rIL-2 to the bovine IL-2-dependent T-cell line, BT2. BT2 cells were incubated with various concentrations of ^{125}I-labeled rIL-2 (specific radioactivity, 1.77×10^{15} cpm/mmol), and assayed for binding as described in the text. Data were corrected for nonspecific binding, measured in the presence of a 50-fold molar excess of unlabeled rBoIL-2, before computer analysis.

bovine IL-2 in 50 μl of 0.2 M $NaPO_4$ buffer, pH 7.2, and the mixture incubated at 25°C for 10 min. Sodium azide (20 μl of 25 mM) and sodium metabisulfite (10 μl of 5 mg/ml) were then added sequentially. After 5 min at 25°C, ^{125}I-labeled bovine IL-2 was separated from free ^{125}I by chromatography on a 2-ml Sephadex G-25 column, and equilibrated in 0.05 M sodium phosphate, pH 7.2, containing 0.01% bovine serum albumin. Fractions containing bovine IL-2 were pooled and stored at 4°C. Bioactivity of ^{125}I-labeled bovine rIL-2 was determined in the BT2 proliferation assay described earlier.

The BT2 cells (2×10^6) were incubated with this ^{125}I-labeled bovine rIL-2 in 150 μl RPMI 1640 containing 2.5% BSA, 20 mM HEPES buffer, and 0.2% sodium azide, pH 7.2 (binding medium). Incubations were carried out in 96-well microtiter plates maintained on a miniorbital shaker at 37°C for 30 min. Replicate 70-μl aliquots of incubation mixtures were then transferred to precooled 400-μl polyethylene centrifuge tubes containing 200 μl of a phthalate oil mixture, and cells plus bound ^{125}I-labeled bovine IL-2 were separated from unbound ^{125}I-labeled bovine IL-2 by centrifugation for 1.5 min in an Eppendorf Microfuge. Nonspecific binding of ^{125}I-labeled IL-2 was measured in the presence of a 50-fold or greater molar excess of unlabeled bovine rIL-2. Sodium azide (0.2%) was included in all binding assays to inhibit internalization and degradation of ^{125}I-labeled bovine IL-2 by cells at 37°C.

Binding of ^{125}I-labeled bovine IL-2 to cells was saturable and when equilibrium-binding data were plotted in the Scatchard coordinate system (Fig. 15) a biphasic curve was observed similar to that seen for human IL-2 (29). This suggested the presence of two classes of bovine IL-2 receptors; one with a K_a of 1.2×10^9 M^{-1} representing 1400 sites and one with a K_a of 1.7×10^7 M^{-1} representing 15,000 sites per cell.

SUMMARY

Human rIL-2 will induce proliferation of murine, as well as bovine, T-cell lines. This has led to speculation that human rIL-2 might find useful application in cattle. However in light of the large disparity between the human and bovine IL-2 amino acid sequences, it is likely that human IL-2 would be antigenic in cattle. Therefore we utilized a human IL-2 probe to isolate bovine IL-2 sequences from a cDNA library. We subsequently expressed bovine IL-2 in both bacteria and yeast. Using a rapid, two-step purification scheme, we have been able to isolate over 20 mg/L of homogeneous bovine rIL-2 secreted from the latter. The availability of sizable quantities of bovine rIL-2 should make it possible to ascertain potential therapeutic or prophylactic utility of this lymphokine in cattle. Additionally, the development of a means by which lymphokines might be released slowly over an extended period may make administration to cattle financially practical.

ACKNOWLEDGMENTS

For excellent technical help the authors thank Kathy Picha, June Little, Brian Davis, Ralph Klinke, Dirk Anderson, Steve Gimpel, Cathy Grubin, Janet Merriam, Noel Balantac, Toby Hemenway, and Kate McKereghan. For their part in contributing to this work by way of collaboration, the authors thank Drs. Linda Park, David Urdal, Carl March, Virginia Price, David Cosman, Alf Larsen, Michael Cantrell, Bruce Acres, Kenneth Grabstein, and Steve Gillis.

REFERENCES

1. Nickerson, S. and Heald, C. (1982). Cells in local reaction to experimental *Staphylococcus aureus* infection in the bovine mammary gland. *J. Dairy Sci. 65*:105–116.
2. Picha, K. and Baker P. (1986). Bovine T lymphocytes: 1. Generation and maintenance of an interleukin-2-dependent, cytotoxic T-lymphocyte cell line. *Immunology* (in press).
3. Bushman, H. and Pawlas, P. (1980). Characterization and separation of bovine lymphocytes. *Comp. Immunol. Microbiol. Infect. Dis. 3*:299–309.
4. Beldon, E., McCroskey-Rothwell, M., and Strelkauskas, A. (1981). Subpopulations of bovine lymphocytes separated by rosetting techniques. *Vet. Immunol. Immunopathol. 2*:467–474.
5. Beldon, E. and Strelkauskas, A. (1981). Mitogen and mixed lymphocyte culture responses of isolated bovine lymphocyte populations. *Am. J. Vet. Res. 42*:934–937.
6. Brownlie, J. and Scott, E. (1979). The response of bovine lymphocytes from lymph and blood to phytohemagglutinin. *Vet. Immunol. Immunopathol. 1*:5–13.
7. Davis, W., Perryman, L., and McGuire, T. (1984). In *Hybridoma Technology on Agricultural and Veterinary Research.* Edited by H. Gamble. Rowman Allanheld and Co., Totowa, N.J.

8. Wagner, H. and Feldman, M. (1972). Cell-mediated immune responses in vitro. I. A new in vitro system for the generation of cell-mediated cytotoxic activity. *Cell. Immunol. 3*:405–420.
9. Sondel, P. and Bach, F. (1975). Recognitive specificity of human cytotoxic T lymphocytes. I. Antigen-specific inhibition of human cell-mediated lympholysis. *J. Exp. Med. 142*:1339–1348.
10. Gillis, S., Ferm, M., Ou, W., and Smith, K. (1978). T cell growth factor: Parameters of production and a quantitative assay for activity. *J. Immunol. 120*:2027–2032.
11. Kashima, N., Nishi-Takaoka, C., Fujita, T., Taki, S., Yamada, G., Hamuro, J., and Taniguchi, T. (1985). Unique structure of murine interleukin-2 as deduced from cloned cDNAs. *Nature 313*:402–404.
12. Taniguchi, T., Mitsui, H., Fujita, T., Tukaoka, C., Kashima, N., Yoshimoto, R., and Hamuro, J. (1983). Structure and expression of a cloned cDNA for human interleukin-2. *Nature 302*:305–310.
13. March, C., Mosley, B., Larsen, A., Cerretti, D., Price, V., Braedt, G., Grabstein, K., Kronheim, S., Conlon, P., Henney, C., Gillis, S., Hopp, T., and Cosman, D. (1985). Cloning, sequence, and expression of two distinct human interleukin-1 (IL-1) cDNA's. *Nature 315*:641–647.
14. Wickens, M. and Stephenson, P. (1984). Role of conserved AAUAAA sequence: Four AAUAAA point mutants prevent messenger RNA 3′ end formation. *Science 226*:1045–1051.
15. Watson, M. (1984). Compilation of published signal sequences. *Nucl. Acid Res. 12*:5145–5164.
16. Marquis, D., Smolec, J., and Katz, D. (1985). Use of a portable ribosome binding site for studying the efficient expression of a eucaryotic gene under various procaryotic promoters. *J. Cell. Biochem.* (Suppl. 9B):221, Abstr. 990.
17. Jay, G., Khoury, G., Seth, A., and Jay, E. (1981). Construction of a general vector for efficient expression of mammalian proteins in bacteria: Use of a synthetic ribosome binding site. *Proc. Natl. Acad. Sci. USA 78*:5543–5548.
18. Cosman, D., Cerretti, D., Larsen, A., Park, L., March, C., Dower, S., Gillis, S., and Urdal, D. (1984). Cloning, sequence and expression of human interleukin-2 receptor. *Nature 312*:768–771.
19. Maeda, S., Nishino, N., Obaru, K., Mita, S., Nomiyama, H., Shimada, K., Fujimoto, K., Teranishi, T., Hirano, T., and Onoue, K. (1983). Cloning of interleukin 2 mRNAs from human tonsils. *Biochem. Biophys. Res. Commun. 115*:1040–1047.
20. Yokota, T., Arai, N., Lee, F., Rennick, D., Mosmann, T., and Arai, K.-I. (1985). Use of a cDNA expression vector for isolation of mouse interleukin 2 cDNA clones: Expression of T-cell growth-factor activity after transfection of monkey cells. *Proc. Natl. Acad. Sci. USA 82*:68–72.

21. Robb, R. (1984). Interleukin 2: The molecule and its function. *Immunol. Today 5*:203–209.
22. Clark, S., Arya, S., Wong-Staal, F., Matsumoto-Kobayashi, M., Kay, R., Kaufmann, R., Brown, E., Shoemaker, C., Copeland, T., Oroszlan, S., Smith, K., Sarngadharan, M., Linder, S., and Gallo, R. (1984). Human T-cell growth factor: Partial amino acid sequence, cDNA cloning, and organization and expression in normal and leukemic cells. *Proc. Natl. Acad. Sci. USA 81*:2543–2547.
23. Holbrook, N., Smith, K., Fornace, A., Comeau, C., Wiskocil, R., and Crabtree, G. (1984). T-cell growth factor: Complete nucleotide sequence and organization of the gene in normal and malignant cells. *Proc. Natl. Acad. Sci. USA 81*:1634–1638.
24. Brake, A., Merryweather, J., Coit, D., Heberlein, U., Masiarz, F., Mullenbach, G., Urdea, M., Valenzuela, P., and Barr, P. (1984). Alpha-factor-directed synthesis and secretion of mature foreign proteins in *Saccharomyces cerevisae. Proc. Natl. Acad. Sci. USA 81*:4642–4646.
25. Bitter, G., Chen, K., Banks, A., and Lai, P.-H. (1984). Secretion of foreign proteins from *Saccharomyces cerevisiae* directed by alpha-factor gene fusions. *Proc. Natl. Acad. Sci. USA 81*:5330–5334.
26. Maniatis, T., Fritsch, E., and Sambrook, J. (eds.) (1982). In *Molecular Cloning: A Laboratory Manual.* Cold Spring Harbor Publications, Cold Spring Harbor, N.Y.
27. Stern, A., Pan, Y.-C., Urdal, D., Mochizuki, D., DeChiara, S., Blacher, R., Wideman, J., and Gillis, S. (1984). Purification to homogeneity and partial characterization of interleukin-2 from a human T cell leukemia. *Proc. Natl. Acad. Sci. USA 81*:871–875.
28. Urdal, D., March, C., Gillis, S., Larsen, A., and Dower, S. (1984). Purification and chemical characterization of the receptor for interleukin 2 from activated human T lymphocytes and from a human T-cell lymphoma cell line. *Proc. Natl. Acad. Sci. USA 81*:6481–6485.
29. Robb, R., Greene, W., and Rusk, C. (1984). Low and high affinity cellular receptors for interleukin 2. *J. Exp. Med. 160*:1126–1146.

4
Cloning, Expression, and Characterization of the Human Interleukin-2 Receptor

DAVID L. URDAL, ROBERT W. OVERELL, BYRON M. GALLIS, ANDREW J. LEWIS, STEVEN K. DOWER, and DAVID J. COSMAN
Immunex Corporation, Seattle, Washington

INTRODUCTION

T cells require the presence of the lymphokine, interleukin-2 (IL-2) to proliferate in vitro (1,2). The cloning of a cDNA (3-5) that encodes the receptor for this molecule confirmed previous studies (6) suggesting that IL-2, like other polypeptide hormones, initiated its effects on cells by binding to a specific receptor glycoprotein in the plasma membrane. Neither IL-2 nor the receptor for this molecule are constitutively expressed by T cells. Rather, the genes encoding these proteins are transcribed in response to signals generated by antigen binding to the antigen receptor found on T cells, resulting in antigen-specific control of T-cell proliferation (6).

The possibility that IL-2 may play a much broader role in the immune system than has been previously anticipated, was suggested by the recent detection of the IL-2 receptor on B cells (7-9) and macrophages (10) and by the realization that IL-2 binding to the IL-2 receptor can result in events other than the stimulation of T-cell proliferation. These events include the induction of other lymphokines, such as gamma interferon (11-13), and the stimulation of new functional activities in cells involved in natural cell-mediated immunity (14,15).

Interleukin-2 has proved to be an effective treatment in a number of immunotherapy models (16), and the report of its efficacy in the treatment of human cancer (17) has reinforced the enthusiasm for the use of this molecule in the treatment of human disease. Similarly, reports that the treatment of animals with antibodies directed to the IL-2 receptor facilitates the acceptance by host animals of donor grafts has stimulated speculation that therapeutics directed at the IL-2 receptor will prove useful in the treatment of human organ transplantation (18). Finally, the presence of the IL-2 receptor only on activated T cells or on leukemias resulting from human T cell leukemia virus (HTLV) infection, has led to the suggestion that the detection of the IL-2 receptor may have diagnostic applications for the assessment of the immune status of patients and therapeutic applications in some cancer patients (19).

With these practical applications in mind and with the knowledge of the central role that this lymphokine receptor plays in the maintenance of a normal immune system, we will summarize the results of experiments we have conducted in our laboratory directed at achieving an understanding of the biochemistry of the IL-2 receptor.

CLONING OF THE INTERLEUKIN-2 RECEPTOR

Human T-cell leukemias caused by HTLV represent a pathological condition which, among other things, is characterized by the constitutive expression of high numbers of IL-2 receptors on the malignant cells (20). Cell lines, such as Hut-102 (21,22), can be established from leukemia cells isolated from such patients and provide a source from which both the IL-2 receptor protein and mRNA encoding the receptor can be isolated.

Purification of the IL-2 receptor was made possible by the generation of a monoclonal antibody, termed 2A3 (23), directed to this cell surface protein. An affinity column was prepared by coupling the antibody to activated Sepharose and used to purify receptor from detergent extracts of both Hut-102 cells and phytohemagglutinin (PHA)-activated peripheral blood lymphocytes (PBL) (24). The IL-2 receptors isolated from Hut-102 cells had a molecular mass of 55,000. Receptors isolated from activated PBL had a molecular mass of 60,000. Receptors from both sources had the same NH_2-terminal sequence of amino acids (24).

Oligonucleotide probes corresponding to amino acid residues 3 to 8 of the protein sequence of the IL-2 receptor (Cys-Asp-Asp-Asp-Pro-Pro) were synthesized and used to probe a cDNA library that had been constructed from polyadenylated mRNA isolated from Hut-102 cells (3). Two cDNA clones, designated pN1 and pN4, were selected for further study. A sequence of the two cDNAs, summarized in Fig. 1, revealed that pN1 and pN4 encoded closely related molecules. Both had a single large open-reading frame of 200 and 272 amino acids, respectively. However pN4 contained 216 nucleotides (Nos. 370-505) that were not found in pN1. Only pN4 encoded a functional IL-2 receptor when subcloned into an SV 40-based expression vector that was then transfected into COS monkey kidney cells (3).

The cDNA sequence of the IL-2 receptor predicted a small protein of molecular mass 28,428. There existed two potential N-linked glycosylation residues at Asn-49 and Asn-68, the glycosylation of which presumably contributes to the molecular weight (M_r) of 50,000-60,000 of the IL-2 receptor expressed on the cell surface. A conventional 21 amino acid transmembrane domain was present along with a short, 11 amino acid COOH-terminal cytoplasmic domain. This region appears to be too small to encode a protein domain that might have enzymatic function, such as the protein tyrosine kinase domain found on the cytoplasmic portion of the epidermal growth factor (EGF) receptor (25). The 216 base pair (bp) segment that was found to be missing from pN1, the inactive receptor, was homologous to the NH_2-terminal region of the cDNA clone and was flanked by 8 bp direct repeats suggesting the possibility that alternative RNA splicing could account for the two different cDNAs isolated. Analysis of genomic clones of the IL-2 receptor indeed confirmed this prediction and show the alignment of this region with a genomic exon (26). The IL-2 receptor can be phosphorylated in cells in response to the activation of protein kinase C with phorbol myristate acetate (27). The cDNA sequence shows a stretch of amino acids surrounding Ser-247 that conforms closely to a concensus protein kinase C phosphorylation site.

As previously mentioned, the IL-2 receptors found on malignant Hut-102 cells and on normal activated PBL displayed different relative molecular weights. To address the molecular basis of this heterogeneity in size, we wished to isolate an IL-2 receptor cDNA from a normal T-cell library to compare its sequence with the cDNAs isolated from HTLV-transformed cells. To this end, a cDNA library prepared from RNA extracted from mitogen-activated peripheral blood T cells was screened by hybridization with a probe from pN4 containing the mature coding region of the Hut-102-derived IL-2 receptor (28). One hybridizing cDNA clone, pTC, was isolated and characterized by nucleotide sequencing. Only four amino

PstI
5'--CTGCAGGCTTCACTGCCCCGGCTGGTCCCAAGGGTCAGGAAG

Met Asp Ser Tyr Leu Leu Met Trp Gly Leu Leu Thr Phe Ile Met Val Pro Gly Cys Gln -2
ATG GAT TCA TAC CTG CTG ATG TGG GGA CTG CTC ACG TTC ATC ATG GTG CCT GGC TGC CAG 60

SstI
Ala Glu Leu Cys Asp Asp Asp Pro Pro Glu Ile Pro His Ala Thr Phe Lys Ala Met Ala 19
GCA GAG CTC TGT GAC GAT GAC CCG CCA GAG ATC CCA CAC GCC ACA TTC AAA GCC ATG GCC 120

Tyr Lys Glu Gly Thr Met Leu Asn Cys Glu Cys Lys Arg Gly Phe Arg Arg Ile Lys Ser 39
TAC AAG GAA GGA ACC ATG TTG AAC TGT GAA TGC AAG AGA GGT TTC CGC AGA ATA AAA AGC 180
A
Lys

Gly Ser Leu Tyr Met Leu Cys Thr Gly Asn Ser Ser His Ser Ser Trp Asp Asn Gln Cys 59
GGA TCA CTC TAT ATG CTC TGT ACA GGA AAC TCT AGC CAC TCG TCC TGG GAC AAC CAA TGT 240
G

Gln Cys Thr Ser Ser Ala Thr Arg Asn Thr Thr Lys Gln Val Thr Pro Gln Pro Glu Glu 79
CAA TGC ACA AGC TCT GCC ACT CGG AAC ACA ACG AAA CAA GTG ACA CCT CAA CCT GAA GAA 300

Gln Lys Glu Arg Lys Thr Thr Lys Ile Gln Ser Pro Met Gln Pro Val Asp Gln Ala Ser 99
CAG AAA GAA AGG AAA ACC ACA AAA ATA CAA AGT CCA ATG CAG CCA GTG GAC CAA GCG AGC 360
G G
Glu Met

PstI
Leu Pro Gly His Cys Arg Glu Pro Pro Pro Trp Glu Asn Glu Ala Thr Glu Arg Ile Tyr 119
CTT CCA GGT CAC TGC AGG GAA CCT CCA CCA TGG GAA AAT GAA GCC ACA GAG AGA ATT TAT 420

His Phe Val Val Gly Gln Met Val Tyr Tyr Gln Cys Val Gln Gly Tyr Arg Ala Leu His 139
CAT TTC GTG GTG GGG CAG ATG GTT TAT TAT CAG TGC GTC CAG GGA TAC AGG GCT CTA CAC 480

Arg Gly Pro Ala Glu Ser Val Cys Lys Met Thr His Gly Lys Thr Arg Trp Thr Gln Pro 159
AGA GGT CCT GCT GAG AGC GTC TGC AAA ATG ACC CAC GGG AAG ACA AGG TGG ACC CAG CCC 540

Gln Leu Ile Cys Thr Gly Glu Met Glu Thr Ser Gln Phe Pro Gly Glu Glu Lys Pro Gln 179
CAG CTC ATA TGC ACA GGT GAA ATG GAG ACC AGT CAG TTT CCA GGT GAA GAG AAG CCT CAG 600

BglI
Ala Ser Pro Glu Gly Arg Pro Glu Ser Glu Thr Ser Cys Leu Val Thr Thr Thr Asp Phe 199
GCA AGC CCC GAA GGC CGT CCT GAG AGT GAG ACT TCC TGC CTC GTC ACA ACA ACA GAT TTT 660

Gln Ile Gln Thr Glu Met Ala Ala Thr Met Glu Thr Ser Ile Phe Thr Thr Glu Tyr Gln 219
CAA ATA CAG ACA GAA ATG GCT GCA ACC ATG GAG ACG TCC ATA TTT ACA ACA GAG TAC CAG 720

Val Ala Val Ala Gly Cys Val Phe Leu Leu Ile Ser Val Leu Leu Leu Ser Gly Leu Thr 239
GTA GCA GTG GCC GGC TGT GTT TTC CTG CTG ATC AGC GTC CTC CTC CTG AGT GGG CTC ACC 780

XbaI
Trp Gln Arg Arg Gln Arg Lys Ser Arg Arg Thr Ile End 251
TGG CAG CGG AGA CAG AGG AAG AGT AGA AGA ACA ATC TAG A--3' 862

Figure 1 The nucleotide sequence and predicted amino acid sequence of the IL-2 receptor. The nucleotide sequence shown is from pN4 except for sequences upstream from the arrow, which are derived from pN1 (3). The nucleotides are numbered from the position of the presumed initiator methionine codon, and the amino acids are numbered from the mature NH_2-terminus of the protein, the Glu residue marked with a star. The sequence of pN1 differs from pN4 at nucleotides 148, 183, 322, and 327. A 216-base-pair insert sequence is present in pN4 that is not present in pN1 (underlined in dots). The insert region and the NH_2-terminal region of the molecule are homologous as indicated by the boxed amino acid and nucleotide sequences. The 8-bp repeat flanking the insert is boxed. Underlined amino acid residues indicate those that were confirmed by protein sequence analysis, and triangles represent possible glycosylation sites.

Table 1 Summary of Predicted Amino Acid Residue Differences Between Human IL-2 Receptor cDNAs

DNA	Source of cDNA	Amino acid position				
		29	87	88	105	242
pN4	Hut-102 cells (3)	Glu	Lys	Ile	Arg	Arg
pTC	Activated PBL (28)	Glu	Glu	Met	Lys	Gln
pN1	Hut-102 cells (3)	Lys	Glu	Met	–	Arg
pIL2R-3	Hut-102 B2 cells (4)	Glu	Glu	Met	Arg	Arg
pTaC-2	MT-1 cells (5)	Glu	Glu	Met	Arg	Arg

Amino acid sequence differences among human IL-2 receptor cDNA clones. Amino acids are numbered according to Fig. 1.

acids were found to differ from those predicted from the cDNA sequence for the Hut-102 cDNA. A summary of sequence differences between cDNAs characterized by us and others is presented in Table 1. It is clear that only minor differences exist between the different clones suggesting that the differences seen between the receptor expressed in Hut cells and that in PBL probably are due to differences in posttranslational modifications of the protein.

EXPRESSION OF THE RECOMBINANT INTERLEUKIN-2 RECEPTOR

Having developed cDNAs that encoded the IL-2 receptor, we enjoyed the anticipation that we might now be able to approach an understanding of IL-2 receptor function by the expression of the IL-2 receptor in various cell lines and, through the technique of site-specific mutagenesis, to characterize more completely the molecular features of the molecule. Specifically, the putative protein kinase C phosphorylation site at Ser-247 was changed to an alanine residue (28) to test the notion that this residue might be involved in this posttranslational modification.

In order to express the recombinant IL-2 receptor in sufficient quantities so that we could examine its biochemical properties, the cDNAs encoding the IL-2 receptor from T cells, Hut-102 cells, and the Ala 247 mutant, were placed under the transcriptional control of the SV 40 early promoter and in front of SV 40-derived RNA processing signal sequences as has been described for the transient expression of pN4 in the COS cell system (3). The transcriptional unit was inserted into a bovine papilloma virus (BPV)-derived vector, p1-8 (29) (Fig. 2a). This vector includes the entire BPV genome, the ampicillin-resistance gene and origin of DNA replication from pML2d, and the neomycin-resistance gene from Tn5 under control of the mouse metallothionein promoter and Moloney sarcoma virus enhancer. The vector confers resistance to the neomycin-derivative G418 on mammalian cells. Accordingly, the three cDNAs engineered into this plasmid were transfected into C127 mouse mammary epithelial cells using a calcium phosphate procedure, and cells that were resistant to G418 were fractionated by fluorescence-activated cell sorting using the antireceptor monoclonal antibody 2A3 (28). Cells were selected for stable, high-level expression of receptors by this procedure and then were cloned to yield stable lines expressing from 2–6 $\times$ 10^6 receptors per cell. The results of one such sorting scheme are depicted in Table 2.

To express the recombinant IL-2 receptor in lymphoid cells, the IL-2 receptor cDNA was also inserted into two retrovirus vectors (Fig. 2b): SV(X) (30) and LSNL, a vector based on LSDL (31). The frequency of gene transfer in lymphoid and hematopoietic cells is, in general, much higher using retrovirus vectors than that obtained with protoplast fusion, clacium phosphate, or electroporation. The gene encoding neomycin resistance is incorporated into each of the retrovirus vectors to facilitate the selection of infected cells. The expression of the neomycin-resistance gene in the SV(X) vector relies on mRNA splicing to generate the appropriate transcript. An alternative strategy, which is used in the LSNL vector, is to drive transcription of the selectable marker (neo^r) from a second, internal promoter, in this case derived from SV 40 (Fig. 2b).

A PstI-XbaI fragment of the IL-2 receptor cDNA, containing the entire receptor-coding sequence, but lacking the polyadenylation signal, was ligated into the SV(X) and LSNL vectors using Bam-H1 linkers. The resulting plasmids were then transfected into the retrovirus packaging cell line, Ψ-2 (32). Neomycin-resistant clones isolated from such transfected cultures served as a stable source of recombinant retrovirus. The SV(X)-IL-2R vector was produced at consistently lower titer (1.2 $\times$ 10^3 neo^r colony forming units (CFU)/ml on Balb/c 3T3 cells) than was the LSNL-IL-2R construction (5 $\times$ 10^4 CFU/ml).

Table 2 Selection of Clones Expressing High Levels of IL-2 Receptor by Fluorescence-Activated Cell Sorting

Cells (C127/pN4/1-8)	Relative green fluorescence	Number of 2A3 binding sites/cell
Unsorted	.07	9×10^3
1st sort	1.87	4.6×10^4
2nd sort	3.20	7.8×10^4
3rd sort	5.40	1.6×10^5
4th sort	33.10	8.0×10^5
5th sort	155.70	7.4×10^5
6th sort	79.40	8.7×10^5
Clone B	166.50	2.7×10^6
Clone B2	509.50	4.5×10^6

The number of IL-2 receptors per cell was determined by ^{125}I-labeled 2A3 antibody binding to C127 cells that had been transfected with pN4/1-8 (23). Relative green fluorescence was determined on an EPICS-C flow cytometer following the staining of cells with biotinyl-2A3 and FITC-avidin as described (28).

The cloning experiment in Fig. 3 was performed to demonstrate that all clones of 3T3 cells that were transformed to drug resistance following such an infection also expressed IL-2 receptors, albeit to widely different degrees. Thus both vectors were capable of expressing the IL-2 receptor gene and the selectable marker concomitantly in the progeny of a single infected cell. A number of different cell lines were then infected with these retroviral vectors and the results are summarized in Table 3. Cells were infected with the vectors and then selected in G418 as bulk populations. Radiolabeled anti-receptor antibody was then used to quantitate the number of IL-2 receptors expressed on the G418-resistant infected cells.

The molecular basis of the variability in levels of receptor expression between the different cell lines (see Table 3) was examined by analysis of the levels of mRNA transcribed from the integrated provirus in the infected cells. Figure 4 summarizes the results of Northern blot analysis of RNA extracted from the cells listed in Table 3. The probe was antisense ^{32}P-labeled RNA specific for the *neo* gene and was generated by in vitro SP-6

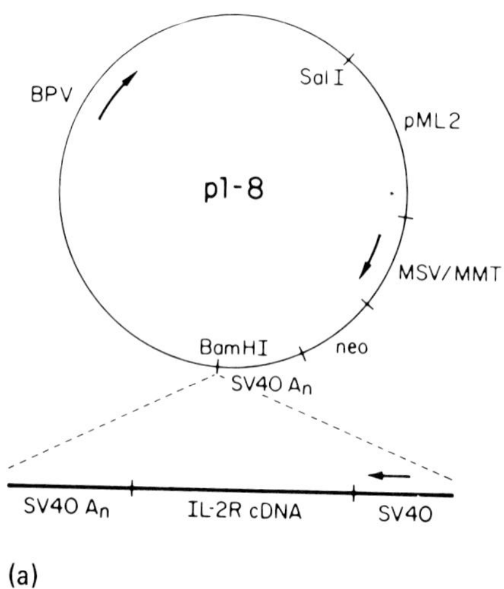

(a)

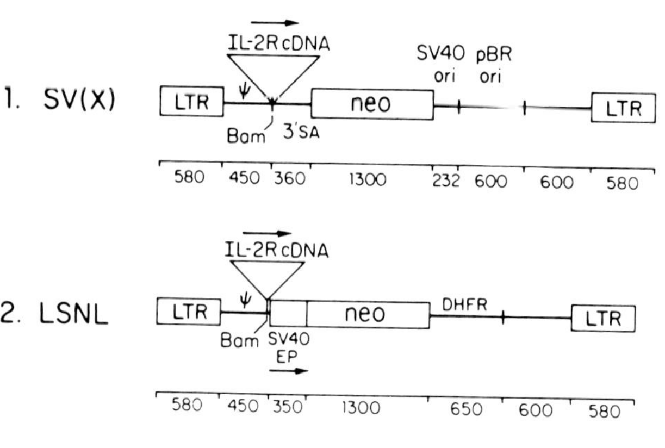

(b)

Figure 2 (a) Structure of the IL-2 receptor cDNA bovine papilloma virus (BPV) expression plasmid p1-8 (29). Arrows show the transcriptional orientation of BPV, the Moloney sarcoma virus enhancer linked to the metallothionein promoter (MSV/MMT), and the simian virus 40 early promoter (SV40). The region denoted pML2 contains sequences derived from the plasmid pBR322; *neo* refers to the neomycin-resistance gene from

RNA polymerase transcription. Two major species of mRNA were detected with this probe, in cells infected with either of the retroviral vectors used (see Fig. 4). For the LSNL-IL-2R vector, the upper band represents the full length mRNA transcribed from the promoter in the 5′ long terminal repeat (LTR) and encoding the IL-2 receptor, while the smaller mRNA is that driven from the internal SV 40 promoter (see Fig. 2B). Both messages hybridize with the *neo* probe because both mRNAs terminate in the 3′ LTR; however only the full-length RNA hybridizes with a probe specific for the IL-2 receptor cDNA (data not shown). Both species of message transcribed from the SV(X)-IL-2R vector (see Fig. 4) initiate in the 5′ LTR, the upper band representing the unspliced (receptor-encoding) and the lower band the spliced (*neo*-encoding) mRNAs (see Fig. 2B and also Ref. 30). These data show that differences in the steady-state levels of receptor-specific mRNA are sufficient to account for the observed variability in numbers of surface IL-2 receptors expressed on infected lymphoid cells (see Table 3 and Fig. 4).

Analysis of recombinant IL-2 receptor by surface labeling of drug-resistant cells is depicted in Fig. 5. Each of the three receptors encoded by Hut-102 cDNA, T-cell cDNA, and Ala-247 cDNA was expressed in the murine C127 epithelial cells as a band of approximately M_r 53,000. Similarly, receptor expressed in FDC-P2 cells infected with the LSNL-IL-2R was of M_r 53,000.

Tn5; SV40 A_h refers to SV 40-derived sequences containing RNA splice donor and acceptor sites and a polyadenylation site; and IL-2R cDNA designates the three IL-2 receptor cDNAs described in the text. (b) Structure of the IL-2 receptor cDNA retroviral vectors. (1) The SV(X) vector (30) relies on mRNA splicing to generate the transcript capable of expressing the *neo* gene. (2) The LSNL vector, which is derived from the vector LSDL (31), includes the SV40 early region promoter (SV40 EP) to drive the transcription of the selectable marker (*neo*). The *neo* gene (from Tn5) was the HindIII-SmaI fragment, and was inserted into the HindIII site of LSDL. In each case the IL-2 receptor cDNA is placed at the insert position at the Bam site. LTR, long terminal repeat; DHFR, dihydrofolate reductase. Figures represent approximate sizes of vector segments in base pairs.

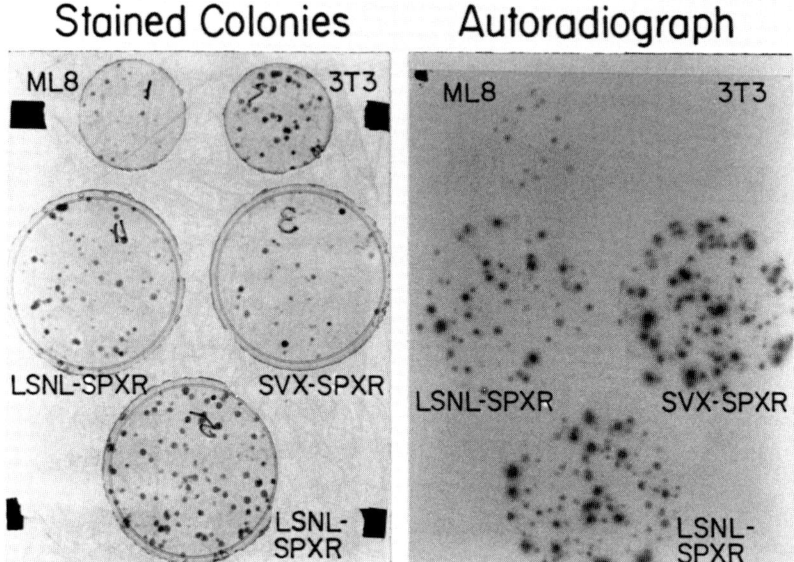

Figure 3 Coincidence of colonies of infected drug-resistant 3T3 cells with colonies of 3T3 cells that express the IL-2 receptor. Infected cells were plated at clonal density in 5- or 10-cm tissue culture dishes. After 11 days in culture, when colonies had grown to macroscopic size, plates were incubated with ^{125}I-labeled anti–IL-2 receptor monoclonal antibody (2A3) (10^{15} cpm/mmol, 5×10^{-10} M in RPMI containing 0.1% NaN_3, 2.5% BSP, 20 mM HEPES) for 2 hr at 8°C. The plates were then washed with phosphate-buffered saline (PBS), fixed with 2% glutaraldehyde, and stained with Geimsa. The plates were then applied to Kodak X-omat AR film and placed at −70°C with intensifying screens. The film was developed 4 hr later and radioactive colonies aligned with the stained colonies. Controls included 3T3 cells (receptor-negative) and ML8 cells, a clone of IL-2 receptor-positive 3T3 cells (approx. 10,000 receptors/cell) that had been obtained following calcium phosphate-mediated transfection of those cells with the IL-2 receptor cDNA in an SV 40-based expression vector (described in Ref. 3).

Table 3 Expression of IL-2 Receptor on Retroviral Vector-Infected Cells

Cells	Infected with (vector)	Neo^r population analyzed[a]	^{125}I-labeled 2A3 molecules bound/cell[b]
Balb/c 3T3	Control		NDR
	LSNL-IL2R	Bulk culture	65,520
	SV(X)-IL-2R	Bulk culture	192,070
CTLL-2[c]	Control		NDR
	LSNL-IL-2R	Clone R1	330
	LSNL-IL-2R	Clone R2.2	10,140
	LSNL-IL-2R	Clone R4.2	6,770
	LSNL-IL-2R	Clone R6.2	250
FDCP-2[d]	Control		NDR
	LSNL-IL-2R	Clone B9	12,560
	LSNL-IL-2R	Clone E4	17,160
HF[e]	Control		NDR
	LSNL-IL-2R	Bulk culture	16,370
	LSNL-IL-2R	Clone 2	17,570
	LSNL-IL-2R	Clone 5	22,160
BW5147[f]	Control		NDR
	SVX-IL-2R	Clone G1	160
	LSNL-IL-2R	12 independent clones	All <200

[a]Following infection by cocultivation with x-irradiated virus-producing $\Psi 2$ cells, target cells were grown for 24 hr, then selected in G418 (1 mg/ml active concentration). All binding figures are for infected cells, selected for drug resistance. Control cells were uninfected.

[b]Binding of ^{125}I-labeled 2A3 to intact cells was assayed as described (23) and expressed as molecules of antibody bound/cell. NDR, no detectable receptors.

[c]IL-2-dependent murine T cell line.

[d]IL-3-dependent murine hematopoeitic cell line.

[e]IL-2-dependent murine hematopoietic cell line derived from FDCP-2 according to Ref. 54.

[f]Growth factor-independent murine T-cell line.

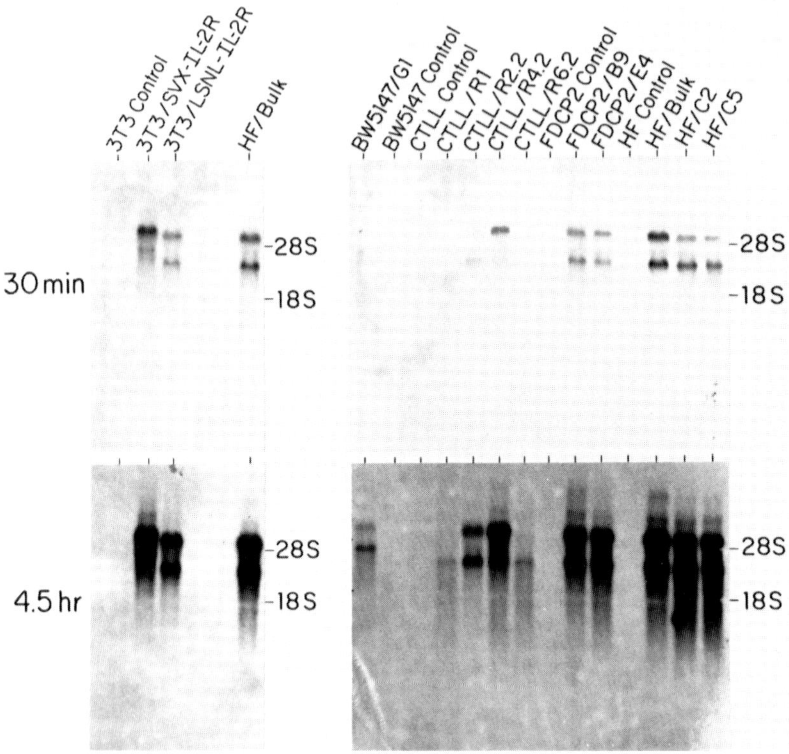

Figure 4 Total RNA was extracted from cells using the guanidinium isothiocyanate procedure (57). It was fractionated (5 μg/lane) on a 1.1% agarose-formaldehyde gel, transferred to Hybond (Amersham) and then probed with ^{32}P-labeled antisense RNA transcribed from the *neo* gene using SP-6 polymerase (Promega). Blots were hybridized at 63°C in Starks buffer (58) for 16 hr then washed in 0.1X SSC, 0.1% SDS for 30 min at 63°C and autoradiographed at −70°C using intensifying screens. The positions of the 28s and 18s ribosomal RNAs are indicated. The *neo* probe hybridizes to both messages from the two vectors. The approximate predicted transcript sizes (not including poly-A tails) are, for LSNL-IL-2R: 4900 nucleotides (full-length) and 3100 nucleotides (transcribed from the internal promoter), and for SV(X)-IL-2R: 5080 nucleotides (full-length) and 3730 nucleotides (spliced). Autoradiograms of two blots are presented; exposure times are indicated.

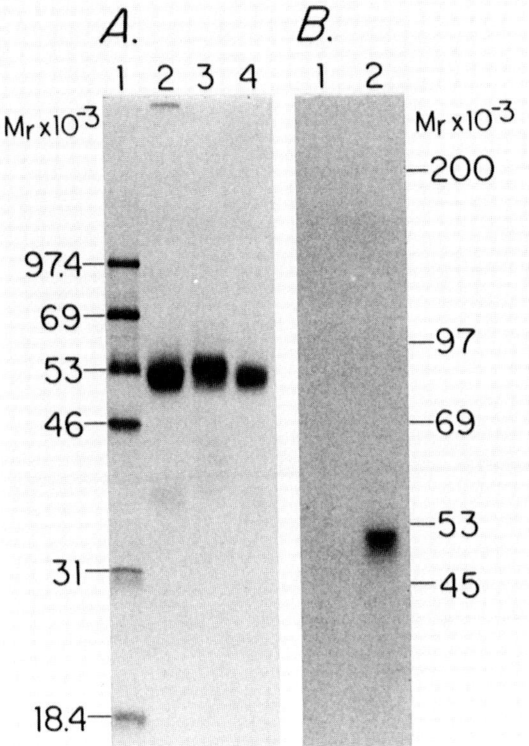

Figure 5 Analysis of recombinant human IL-2 receptor expression by ^{125}I surface-labeling followed by immunoprecipitation and SDS-PAGE. (A) C127 cells transfected with BPV vectors containing IL-2 receptor DNA. Lane 1, molecular weight standards; lane 2, C127 cells expressing the mutant Hut-102 Ala_{247} receptor; lane 3, C127 cells expressing the normal T-cell derived receptor (Ser-247), lane 4, C127 cells expressing the Hut-102 derived receptor (Ser-247). Cells were surface labeled with ^{125}I by the lactoperoxidase-glucose oxidase procedure. The cells were extracted with PBS containing 1% Triton X-100, 2 mM PMSF and ^{125}I-labeled receptor immunoprecipitated with 2A3 monoclonal antibody coupled to Affigel-10 beads (Biorad) as previously described (28). (B) FDCP-2 cells infected with the LSNL-IL-2R vector were surface-labeled as described in panel (A) and immunoprecipitated with: lane 1, control antibody coupled to Affigel-10; or lane 2, 2A3 antibody coupled to Affigel-10.

CHARACTERIZATION OF Ser-247 AS A PHOSPHORYLATION SITE

Protein phosphorylation is a means by which a cell may regulate enzyme activity, protein turnover, and signal transduction. Specifically, protein tyrosine kinases have been found to be integral domains of a number of growth factor and hormone receptors. This observation, coupled with the identity of several of the viral oncogenes as protein kinases has implicated these enzymes as important elements involved in the control of cell proliferation (34). Furthermore, other studies have shown that phosphorylation of membrane protein receptors can influence the surface expression and the ligand-binding properties of these molecules, thereby regulating the facility of signal transduction in these systems (35–39).

Treatment of T cells with phorbol myristate acetate (PMA), the primary target of which is protein kinase C (40), will cause the phosphorylation of the IL-2 receptor (27). Furthermore, it has been reported that protein kinase C is translocated from the cytosol to the plasma membrane within minutes following the stimulation of T cells with IL-2 (41) and that stimulation of T cells with IL-2 can induce the phosphorylation of the IL-2 receptor (42) and other proteins (42,43). These observations suggest that the transmission of the signal in response to IL-2 could well involve protein kinase C and that the phosphorylation of the IL-2 receptor could regulate aspects of this mechanism.

The ability to express IL-2 receptors at the level of several million molecules per cell in the BPV expression system described earlier, facilitated our study of the phosphorylation of the IL-2 receptor (44). Murine epithelial C127 cells, expressing IL-2 receptor were prelabeled with [^{32}P] PO_4 for 2 hr, incubated for an additional 10 min in the presence of PMA, and then extracted with detergent. The IL-2 receptor was immunoprecipitated from this solution with 2A3 antibody and analyzed by polyacrylamide gel electrophoresis. As shown in Fig. 6, an intense band of M_r 53,000 was detected by autoradiography (Fig. 6A, lane 5). If the cells were not incubated in the presence of PMA no ^{32}P-labeled band was detected (Fig. 6A, lane 4).

In contrast, when C127 cells expressing the mutant receptor (Ala-247) were labeled under similar conditions, no ^{32}P-labeled band could be detected in the presence or absence of PMA (Fig. 6A, lanes 1 and 2). Labeling of both the normal (Ser-247) and mutant (Ala-247) receptors by surface iodination could be readily detected (Fig. 6B, lanes 1 and 2) on cells in the same experiments indicating that the mutant receptor was

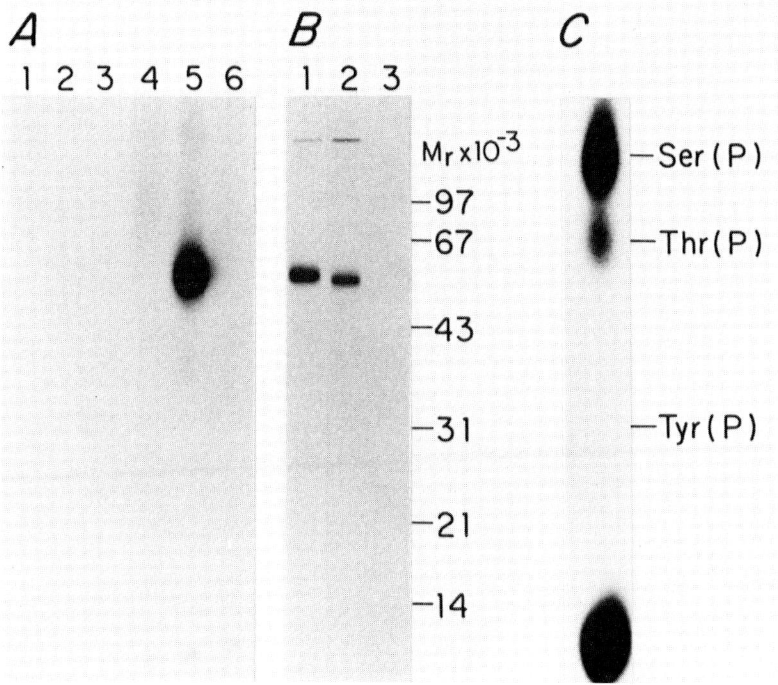

Figure 6 Phosphorylation of the human IL-2 receptor. (A) C127 cells expressing the mutant IL-2 receptor Ala-247, lanes 1, 2; and 3 or C127 cells expressing the natural IL-2 receptor Ser-247, lanes 4, 5, and 6 were incubated with $[^{32}P]PO_4$ in the presence (lanes, 2, 3, 5, and 6) or absence (lanes 1 and 4) of phorbol myristate acetate (PMA, 100 ng/ml). The cells were then extracted as previously described (44) and aliquots of the extract immunoprecipitated with control antibody coupled to beads (lanes 3 and 6) or with 2A3 antibody coupled to beads (lanes 1, 2, 4, and 5). (B) C127 cells from the same experiment depicted in panel (A) were surface labeled with ^{125}I as described in the legend to Fig. 5 and cell extracts immunoprecipitated with 2A3 coupled to Affigel-10 (lanes 1 and 2) or control antibody coupled to Affigel-10 (lane 3). Lane 1, C127 cells expressing the mutant receptor Ala-247; lane 2 and 3, C127 cells expressing the wild type receptor, Ser-247. (C) Phosphoamino acid content of IL-2 receptor phosphorylated in response to treatment with PMA of C127 cells expressing the wild type IL-2 receptor.

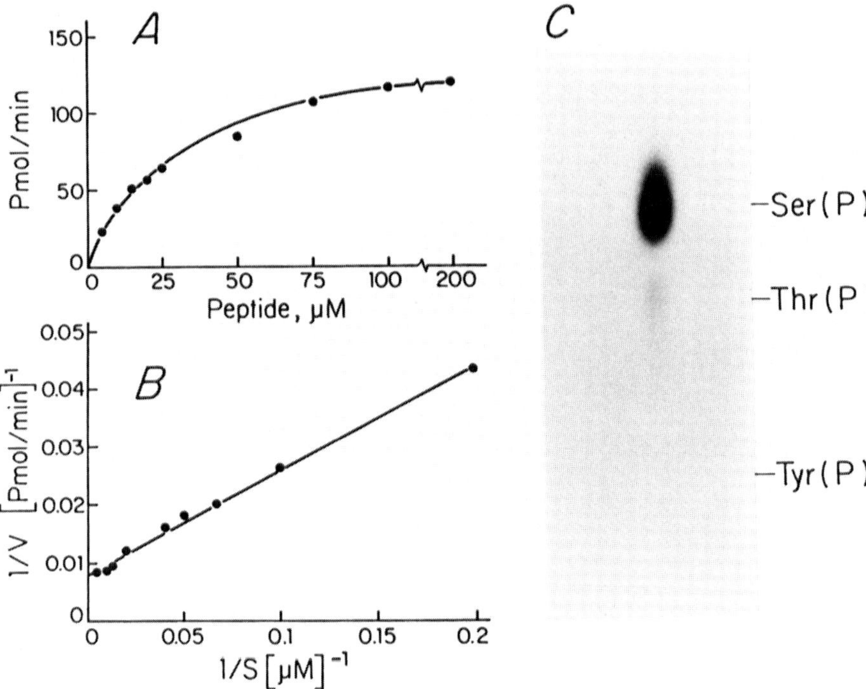

Figure 7 Phosphorylation of IL-2 receptor COOH-terminal synthetic peptide. (A) Rate of incorporation of ^{32}P onto IL-2 receptor COOH-terminal peptide as a function of peptide concentration. Reactions contained 20 μM HEPES (pH 7.8), 10 mM $MgCl_2$, 1.5 mM Ca^{2+}, 3 μg phosphatidyl serine, 0.3 μg of diolein, 2 mM DTT, and were for 10 min at 30°C during which time phosphorylation rates were linear. The ATP concentration was 200 μM (390 cpm/pmol). An aliquot (10 μl) was spotted in a 2-cm square of Whatman P-81 phosphocellulose paper and processed as previously described (44). (B) A plot of the data presented in (A) in the Lineweaver-Burke coordinate system. (C) Phosphoamino acid content of IL-2 receptor COOH-terminal peptide phosphorylated by protein kinase C. Reactions in which the peptide was phosphorylated to maximal stoichiometry (1 mole/mole) were subjected to phosphoamino acid analysis as previously described (44).

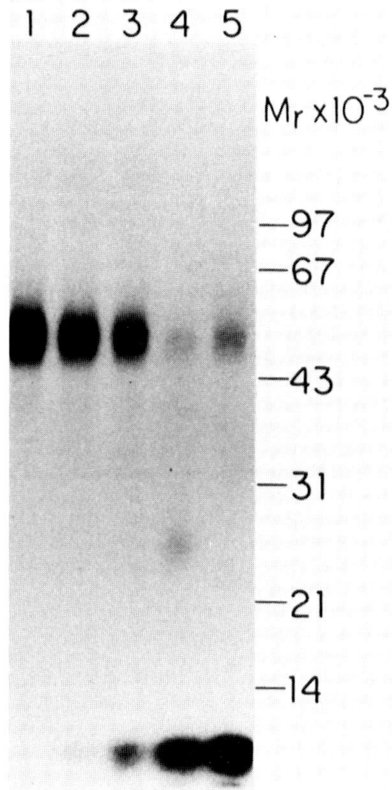

Figure 8 Inhibition of IL-2 receptor phosphorylation in membranes by synthetic IL-2 receptor COOH-terminal peptide. Cell membranes were prepared from C127 cells that expressed the wild type IL-2 receptor (44). Reactions contained 20 μg of membrane, 100 μM Na_3VO_4, 100 μM $CaCl_2$, and 40 μM [γ-^{32}P] ATP (10,000–20,000 cpm/mmol). The IL-2 receptor COOH-terminal peptide was included at a concentration of 0 μM (lane 1), 10 μM (lane 2), 20 μM (lane 3), 50 μM (lane 4) or 100 μM (lane 5). Reactions were terminated by addition of EGTA, EDTA, and RIPA buffer (50 mM Tris-HCl, pH 7.5, 1% NP40, 1% sodium deoxycholate, 0.1% SDS), and IL-2 receptor was immunoprecipitated with 2A3 antibody coupled to Affigel-10.

expressed in the plasma membrane. These results suggested that the alteration of Ser-247 to an alanine residue obviated the capacity of the receptor to be phosphorylated in response to PMA treatment of cells. Phosphoamino acid analysis of the ^{32}P-labeled normal receptor showed that the label was incorporated predominantly into serine (Fig. 6C). Serine and alanine differ only at the β carbon atom where the hydroxyl group in serine is replaced by a hydrogen in alanine. Although it is possible that this subtle change in a single amino acid resulted in a change in the conformation of the receptor that prevented its phosphorylation elsewhere, we concluded that the more likely explanation was that Ser-247 is the residue in the IL-2 receptor that is phosphorylated in response to PMA treatment of the cells.

Because protein kinase C is considered the primary receptor for PMA in cells and serine was the residue derivatized with ^{32}P in cells treated with PMA, we looked more closely at the role of protein kinase C in this reaction. A polypeptide was synthesized that corresponded to the COOH-terminal 11 amino acids of the IL-2 receptor. The peptide was found to serve as an excellent substrate for protein kinase C purified from rat brain. As shown in Fig. 7, protein kinase C catalyzed the phosphorylation of this peptide with a K_m of 23 μM and serine was the predominant site of phosphorylation (Fig. 7C). Finally, when the COOH-terminal peptide was included in phosphorylation experiments on membranes isolated from murine epithelial cells expressing the IL-2 receptor, phosphorylation of the IL-2 receptor was inhibited (Fig. 8). A concentration of 20 μM inhibited the incorporation of ^{32}P into the IL-2 receptor by 50%. These results confirmed the conclusions drawn from the experiments using the mutant receptor and suggested that the COOH-terminal domain of the IL-2 receptor contained the substrate for the C127 kinase and that the activity of this kinase correlated with that of protein kinase C.

IN SEARCH OF A FUNCTIONAL RECOMBINANT INTERLEUKIN-2 RECEPTOR

The significance of phosphorylation at Ser-247 may be revealed once we understand more fully the mechanism through which IL-2 binding to its receptor delivers a signal to the cell. A fundamental paradox surrounding the IL-2 receptor was revealed by the early observations demonstrating that the number of IL-2 receptors detected by radiolabeled IL-2 binding were always lower (at the level of 10%) than the number of receptor molecules detected by radiolabeled antibodies directed at the IL-2 receptor (45), and yet both IL-2 and antibody recognized the same protein on cells (46). The paradox was resolved when it was demonstrated that radiolabeled IL-2 binding to IL–2-dependent cells was characterized by the presence of two distinct classes of IL-2 receptors, each distinguished by having a different affinity for radiolabeled IL-2 (47). In contrast, monoclonal antibodies to the IL-2 receptor see a single class of molecules, the total number of members of which corresponds to the sum of the high- and low-affinity sites detected by radiolabeled IL-2. Figure 9 illustrates the biphasic nature of radiolabeled IL-2 binding to CTLL cells, a murine IL–2-dependent T-cell lines. Early experiments were performed at IL-2 concentrations at which only the high-affinity sites could be detected. The low-affinity sites were detected only when higher concentrations of radiolabeled IL-2 were used.

It has since been suggested that the high-affinity class of interleukin-2 receptor is the class of sites that most closely correlates with the minimum concentration of IL-2 sufficient to allow the proliferation of T cells, and the ability of T cells to respond to IL-2 corresponds better to the concentration of high-affinity sites present on responding cells than to the number of total IL-2 receptors found on responding cell populations (46). More recently it has been reported that it is only the high-affinity class of IL-2 receptors that is internalized by the cell upon binding IL-2 (49,50).

It soon became evident that when the IL-2 receptor cDNA was expressed in fibroblast (3T3) or epithelial cells (C127), only low-affinity IL-2 binding was detected (28,51). Figure 9b summarizes the results of ^{125}I-labeled IL–2-binding experiments performed on C127 cells. It is clear from analysis of these data that although the IL-2 receptor is expressed at high levels in these cells, there is no evidence of high-affinity IL-2 binding. Furthermore the binding of IL-2 to the native IL-2 receptor (Ser-247), the IL-2 receptor cloned from normal T cells (also Ser-247), and the mutant receptor (Ala-247), was identical suggesting that phosphorylation at serine-247 did not by itself influence the affinity with which IL-2 bound to the receptor.

One possible resolution to this enigma as outlined is that the IL–2-binding protein as cloned and described is only part of a receptor complex. The COOH-terminal domain of the receptor is small and may need to associate with other components in the cell to form a receptor complex that can transduce a signal upon binding IL-2. Furthermore, this complex may be found only in lymphoid or hematopoietic cells, because expression

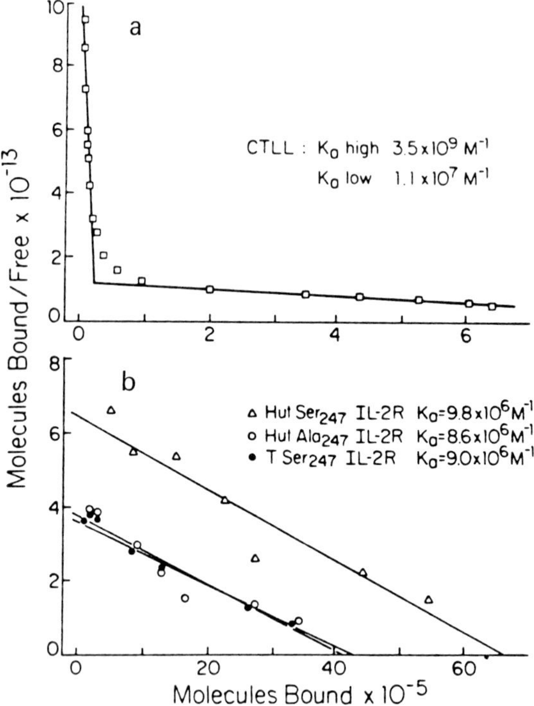

Figure 9 Equilibrium binding of ^{125}I-labeled IL-2 to murine CTLL cells (a) and to recombinant receptor expressed in C127 cells (b). (a) Binding was performed as previously described (28). The curves defined by the data obtained from the equilibrium binding experiment was fitted using RS/1, a commercially available scientific processing package operating on a VAX 11/750 computer under the VMS operating system. This curve was then replotted in the Scatchard coordinate system depicted in the figure. (b) Scatchard analysis of ^{125}I-labeled IL-2 binding to C127 cells expressing the wild type Hut-102 derived IL-2 receptor (triangle), the mutant Ala_{247} IL-2 receptor (circle), and to C127 cells expressing the wild type normal T cell-derived receptor (closed circle).

of the IL-2 receptor in other cell types does not result in the presence of high-affinity IL-2 binding.

As described previously, the use of recombinant retroviruses expressing the IL-2 receptor cDNA has allowed us to infect a variety of hematopoietic and lymphoid cell lines. Interleukin–2-dependent murine cells, such as CTLL and HF, can be infected in this way and will express the human IL-2 receptor as detected by antibodies directed to the IL-2 receptor (see Table 3). The detection of high-affinity human IL-2 receptors is complicated however by the constitutive presence of high numbers of endogenous murine IL-2 receptors on these cells. Binding experiments in the presence of murine IL-2 to block only murine IL-2 receptors have been ambiguous and difficult to interpret. Other workers (52) have done similar experiments and report that these cells will respond specifically to human IL-2 under conditions in which the murine receptors are blocked by specific antibodies. The authors conclude that the human IL-2 receptor is expressed in a functional manner in these cells.

We also infected an IL–3-dependent cell line, FDC-P2, with the IL-2 receptor containing retroviral vector. This cell line has been reported to respond to IL-3 in a fashion similar to the way that IL–2-dependent cells respond to IL-2. Protein kinase C is reported to localize in the plasma membrane following the binding of IL-3 to the cell surface (53). The FDCP-2 cell line has also been reported to "switch" to IL-2 dependence following the appropriate culture conditions (54). Both observations, coupled with the similarity in molecular weight between the IL-2 and IL-3 receptors (55), have led to the suggestion that the two receptors may share similar signal mechanisms. The IL-2 receptors were expressed on these cells, as detected by monoclonal antibody 2A3 (see Table 3), but no evidence for high-affinity IL-2 binding was detected, nor was any biological response to IL-2 measurable, suggesting that the two receptor systems act independently of each other.

In contrast, when EL-4 cells, a murine T-cell lymphoma, were transfected with the human IL-2 receptor, high-affinity receptors were detected on the cells (56). These cells did not express endogenous murine IL-2 receptors, and thus this experiment constitutes the most convincing evidence that an IL-2 receptor complex might be responsible for high-affinity IL-2 binding. Interestingly, the IL-2 receptor-positive EL-4 cells responded to IL-2 by demonstrating an IL–2-dependent inhibition of cell proliferation.

These results have reinforced the idea that the IL-2 receptor must be present or synthesized in the appropriate cellular environment before it can function as a receptor capable of binding IL-2 with high affinity and of transmitting a signal across the plasma membrane. They have also stimulated the search for possible candidates that might fill the role as members of the IL-2 receptor complex. We believe that the identification and characterization of these other proteins will resolve the nature of the high-affinity IL-2 receptor and should go a long way toward increasing our understanding of the elements involved in the control of T-cell proliferation, the response to IL-2 and, possibly the factors that can contribute to malignancy in these cells.

ACKNOWLEDGMENTS

We thank Judy Reaveley and Linda Troup for their help in the preparation of the manuscript. We also thank Janis Wignall, Alan Alpert, and Karen Weisser for their excellent technical assistance, and Linda Park, Tom Hopp, Carl March, Alf Larsen, and Doug Cerretti for helpful discussions and contributions to the project.

REFERENCES

1. Morgan, D. A., Ruscetti, F. W., and Gallo, R. C. (1976). Selective in vitro growth of T lymphocytes from normal human bone marrows. *Science 193*:1007.
2. Gillis, S. and Smith, K. A. (1977). Long-term culture of tumor-specific cytotoxic T cells. *Nature 268*:154.
3. Cosman, D., Cerretti, D. P., Larsen, A., Park, L., March, C., Dower, S., Gillis, S., and Urdal, D. (1984). Cloning, sequence and expression of human interleukin-2 receptor. *Nature 312*:768.
4. Leonard, W. J., Depper, J. M., Crabtree, G. R., Rudikoff, S., Pumphrey, J., Robb, R. J., Kronke, M., Svetlik, P. B., Peffer, N. J., Waldmann, T. A., and Greene, W. C. (1984). Molecular cloning and expression of cDNAs for the human interleukin-2 receptor. *Nature 311*:626.
5. Nikaido, T., Shimizu, A., Ishida, N., Sabe, H., Teshigawara, K., Maeda, M., Uchiyama, T., Yodoi, J., and Honjo, T. (1984). Molecular cloning of cDNA encoding human interleukin-2 receptor. *Nature 311*:631.
6. Robb, R. J., Munck, A., and Smith, K. A. (1981). T cell growth factor receptors. Quantitation, specificity and biological relevance. *J. Exp. Med. 154*:1455.
7. Waldmann, T., Goldman, C. K., Robb, R. J., Depper, J. M., Leonard, W. J., Sharrow, S. O., Bongiovanni, K. F., Korsmeyer, S. J., and Greene, W. C. (1984). Expression of interleukin 2 receptors on activated human B cells. *J. Exp. Med. 160*:1450.

8. Boyd, A. W., Fisher, D. C., Fox, D. A., Schlossman, S. F., and Nadler, L. M. (1985). Structural and functional characterization of IL-2 receptors on activated human B cells. *J. Immunol. 134*:2387.
9. Mittler, R., Rao, P., Olini, G., Westbrook, E., Newman, W., Hoffman, M., and Goldstein, G. (1985). Activated human B cells display a functional IL-2 receptor. *J. Immunol. 134*:2393.
10. Hermann, F., Cannistra, S. A., Levine, H., and Griffin, J. D. (1985). Expression of interleukin 2 receptors and binding of interleukin 2 by gamma interferon-induced human leukemic and normal monocytic cells. *J. Exp. Med. 162*:1111.
11. Grabstein, K., Dower, S., Gillis, S., Urdal, D., and Larsen, A. (1986). Expression of interleukin-2, interferon γ, and the IL-2 receptor by human peripheral blood lymphocytes. *J. Immunol. 136*:4503.
12. Reem, G. H. and Yeh, N.-H. (1984). Interleukin 2 regulates expression of its receptor and synthesis of gamma interferon by human T lymphocytes. *Science 225*:429.
13. Farrar, W. L., Johnson, H. M., and Farrar, J. J. (1981). Regulation of the production of murine interferon and cytotoxic T lymphocytes by interleukin 2. *J. Immunol. 126*:1120.
14. Grimm, E. A., Robb, R. J., Roth, J. A., Neckers, L. M., Lachman, L. B., Wilson, D. J., and Rosenberg, S. A. (1983). Lymphokine-activated killer cell phenomenon. III. Evidence that IL-2 is sufficient for direct activation of peripheral blood lymphocytes into lymphokine-activated killer cells. *J. Exp. Med. 158*:1356.
15. Brooks, C. G., Holscher, M., and Urdal, D. (1984). Natural killer cell activity in cloned cytotoxic T lymphocytes: Regulation by interleukin 2, interferon and specific antigen. *J. Immunol. 135*:1145.
16. Gillis, S., Conlon, P. J., Cosman, D., Hopp, T., Dower, S. K., Price, V., Mochizuki, D., and Urdal, D. (1986). Lymphokines: From conjecture to the clinic. *Semin. Oncol. 13*:218–227.
17. Rosenberg, S. A., Lotze, M., Muul, L., Leitman, S., Chang, A., Ettinghausen, S., Matory, Y., Skibber, J., Shiloni, E., Vetto, J., Seipp, C., Simpson, C., and Reichert, C. (1985). Observation on the systemic administration of autologous lymphokine-activated killer cells and recombinant interleukin-2 to patients with metastatic cancer. *N. Engl. J. Med. 313*:1485.
18. Kirkman, R. L., Barrett, L. V., Gaulton, G., Kelley, V., Ythier, A., and Strom, T. (1985). Administration of an anti-interleukin 2 receptor monoclonal antibody prolongs cardiac allograft survival in mice. *J. Exp. Med. 162*:358.
19. Waldmann, T. A. (1986). The structure, function and expression of interleukin-2 receptors on normal and malignant lymphocytes. *Science 232*:727.

20. Depper, J. M., Leonard, W. J., Kronke, M., Waldmann, T. A., and Greene, W. C. (1984). Augmented T cell growth factor expression in HTLV-1 infected human leukemic T cells. *J. Immunol. 133*:1691.
21. Gazdar, A. F., Karney, D. N., Bunn, P. A., Russell, E. K., Jaffe, E. S., Schecter, G. P., and Guccion, C. G. (1980). Mitogen requirements for in vitro propagation of cutaneous T cell lymphomas. *Blood 55*:409.
22. Gootenberg, J. E., Ruscetti, F. W., Mier, J. W., Gazdar, A., and Gallo, F. C. (1981). Human cutaneous T cell lymphoma and leukemia cell lines produce and respond to T cell growth factor. *J. Exp. Med. 154*: 1403.
23. Dower, S. K., Hefeneider, S. H., Alpert, A. R., and Urdal, D. L. (1985). Quantitative measurement of human interleukin-2 receptor levels with intact and detergent-solubilized human T cells. *Mol. Immunol. 22*:937.
24. Urdal, D. L., March, C. J., Gillis, S., Larsen, A., and Dower, S. K. (1984). Purification and chemical characterization of the receptor for interleukin 2 from activated human T lymphocytes and from a human T-cell lymphoma cell line. *Proc. Natl. Acad. Sci. USA 81*:6481.
25. Downward, J., Yarden, Y., Mayes, E., Scrace, G., Totty, N., Stockwell, P., Ullrich, A., Schlessinger, J., and Waterfield, M. (1984). Close similarity of epidermal growth factor receptor and v-*erb*-B oncogene protein sequences. *Nature 307*:521.
26. Leonard, W. J., Depper, J. M., Kanehisa, M., Kronke, M., Peffer, N. J., Svetlik, P. B., Sullivan, M., and Greene, W. C. (1985). Structure of the human interleukin-2 receptor gene. *Science 230*:633.
27. Shackelford, D. A. and Trowbridge, I. S. (1984). Induction of expression and phosphorylation of the human interleukin 2 receptor by a phorbol diester. *J. Biol. Chem. 259*:11706.
28. Cosman, D., Wignall, J., Lewis, A., Alpert, A., Cerretti, D. P., Park, L., Dower, S. K., Gillis, S., and Urdal, D. (1986). High level stable expression of human interleukin 2 receptors in mouse cells generates only low affinity interleukin-2 binding sites. *Mol. Immunol. 23*:935.
29. Sarver, N., Ricca, G. A., Hood, M., Link, J., Tarr, J. C., and Drohan, W. N. (1985). Sustained high level expression of recombinant human gamma interferon using a bovine papilloma virus vector. In *Papilloma Viruses: Molecular and Clinical Aspects.* Edited by P. M. Howley and T. R. Broker. A. R. Liss, New York.
30. Cepko, C., Roberts, B., and Mulligan, R. (1984). Construction and applications of a highly transmissible murine retrovirus shuttle vector. *Cell 37*:1053.
31. Miller, A. D., Law, M.-F., and Verma, I. (1985). Generation of helper-free amphotrophic retrovirus that transduce a dominant-acting methotrexate-resistant dihydrofolate reductase gene. *Mol. Cell. Biol. 5*:431.

32. Mann, R., Mulligan, R. C., and Baltimore, D. (1983). Construction of a retrovirus packaging mutant and its use to produce helper-free defective retrovirus. *Cell 33*:453.
33. Emerman, M. and Temin, H. (1984). Genes with promoters in retrovirus vectors can be independently suppressed by an epigenetic mechanism. *Cell 39*:459.
34. Hunter, T. and Cooper, J. A. (1985). Protein-tyrosine kinases. *Ann. Rev. Biochem. 54*:897.
35. Takayama, S., White, M. F., Lauris, V., and Kahn, C. R. (1984). Phorbol esters modulate insulin receptor phosphorylation and insulin action in cultured hepatoma cells. *Proc. Natl. Acad. Sci. USA 81*:7757.
36. Davis, R. J. and Czech, M. P. (1985). Tumor-promoting phorbol diesters cause the phosphorylation of epidermal growth factor receptors in normal human fibroblasts at threonine-654. *Proc. Natl. Acad. Sci. USA 82*:1974.
37. Cochet, C., Gill, G. N., Meisenhelder, J., Cooper, J. A., and Hunter, T. (1984). C-kinase phosphorylates the epidermal growth factor receptor and reduces its epidermal growth factor stimulated tyrosine protein kinase activity. *J. Biol. Chem. 259*:2553.
38. Thomopoulos, P., Testa, N., Gourdin, M.-F., Hervy, C., Titeux, M., and Vainchenker, N. (1982). Inhibition of insulin receptor binding by phorbol esters. *Eur. J. Biochem. 129*:389.
39. King, A. C. and Cuatrecasas, P. (1982). Resolution of high and low affinity epidermal growth factor receptors. Inhibition of high affinity component by low temperature, cyclohexamide and phorbol esters. *J. Biol. Chem. 257*:3053.
40. Nishizuka, Y. (1984). Turnover of inositol phospholipids and signal transduction. *Science 225*:1365.
41. Farrar, W. L. and Anderson, W. B. (1985). Interleukin-2 stimulation of protein kinase C plasma membrane association. *Nature 315*:233.
42. Gaulton, G. N. and Eardley, D. (1986). Interleukin-2 dependent phosphorylation of interleukin-2 receptors and other T cell membrane proteins. *J. Immunol. 136*:2470.
43. Ishii, T., Sugamura, K., Nakamura, M., and Hinuma, Y. (1986). IL-2 rapidly induces phosphorylation of a cellular protein, PP67, in an IL-2 dependent murine cell line. *Biochem. Biophys. Res. Commun. 135*:487.
44. Gallis, B., Lewis, A., Wignall, J., Alpert, A., Mochizuki, D., Cosman, D., Hopp, T., and Urdal, D. (1986). Phosphorylation of the human interleukin-2 receptor and a synthetic peptide identical to its C-terminal, cytoplasmic domain. *J. Biol. Chem. 261*:5075.
45. Greene, W. C. and Robb, R. (1984). Receptors for T-cell growth factor: Structure, function and expression on normal and neoplastic cells. *Contemp. Top. Mol. Immunol. 10*:1.

46. Robb, R. J. and Greene, W. C. (1983). Direct demonstration of the identity of T cell growth factor binding protein and the Tac antigen. *J. Exp. Med. 158*:1332.
47. Robb, R. J., Greene, W. C., and Rusk, C. M. (1984). Low and high affinity cellular receptors for interleukin 2. *J. Exp. Med. 160*:1126.
48. Smith, K. and Cantrell, D. A. (1985). Interleukin-2 regulates its own receptors. *Proc. Natl. Acad. Sci. USA 82*:864.
49. Fuji, M., Sugamura, K., Sano, K., Nakai, M., Sugita, K., and Hinuma, Y. (1986). High affinity receptor-mediated internalization and degradation of interleukin 2 in human T cells. *J. Exp. Med. 163*:550.
50. Weissman, A., Harford, J., Svetlik, P., Leonard, W., Depper, J., Waldmann, T., Greene, W., and Klausner, R. (1986). Only high affinity receptors for interleukin 2 mediate internalization of ligand. *Proc. Natl. Acad. Sci. USA 83*:1463.
51. Greene, W. C., Robb, R., Svetlik, P., Rusk, C., Depper, J., and Leonard, W. (1985). Stable expression of cDNA encoding the human interleukin 2 receptor in eukaryotic cells. *J. Exp. Med. 162*:363.
52. Kondo, S., Shimizu, A., Maeda, M., Tagaya, Y., Yodoi, J., and Honjo, T. (1986). Expression of functional human interleukin 2 receptor in mouse T cells by cDNA transfection. *Nature 320*:75.
53. Farrar, W. L., Anderson, T. P., and Anderson, W. B. (1985). Altered cytosol/membrane enzyme redistribution on interleukin 3 activation of protein kinase C. *Nature 315*:235.
54. LeGros, G. S., Gillis, S., and Watson, J. (1985). Induction of IL-2 responsiveness in a murine IL-3 dependent cell line. *J. Immunol. 135*: 4009.
55. Park, L. S., Friend, D., Gillis, S., and Urdal, D. (1986). Characterization of the cell surface receptor for a multi-lineage colony-stimulating factor (CSF-2α). *J. Biol. Chem. 261*:205.
56. Hatakeyama, M., Minamoto, S., Uchiyama, T., Hardy, R., Yamada, G., and Taniguchi, T. (1986). Reconstitution of functional receptor for human interleukin-2 in mouse cells. *Nature 318*:467.
57. Maniatis, T., Fritsch, E. F., and Sambrook, J. (1982). In *Molecular Cloning, A Laboratory Manual.* Cold Spring Harbor Laboratory, New York.
58. Wahl, G., Stern, M., and Stark, G. (1979). Efficient transfer of large DNA fragment from agarose gels to diazobenzyloxymethyl paper and rapid hybridization by using dextran sulfate. *Proc. Natl. Acad. Sci. USA 76*:3683.

5

Molecular Analysis of the Murine Interleukin-2 Receptor

KATHLEEN N. MC KEREGHAN, ALAN R. ALPERT, KENNETH GRABSTEIN, DAVID J. COSMAN, and DOUGLAS PAT CERRETTI
Immunex Corporation, Seattle, Washington

INTRODUCTION

T lymphocytes, essential for the generation of a normal immune response, require the presence of the lymphokine interleukin-2 (IL-2) to proliferate (1,2). The proliferation of T cells is initiated by the binding of IL-2 to its cell surface receptor (3,4). With the aid of affinity columns made with a monoclonal antibody specific for the human IL-2 receptor (5,6), sufficient quantities of the protein were purified so that an amino acid sequence from the amino end could be determined (7). Based on this sequence, synthetic oligonucleotide probes were synthesized and used to screen cDNA libraries resulting in the isolation of clones encoding the human IL-2 receptor (8-10). More recently, genomic clones of the human IL-2 receptor have been isolated (11,12).

The gene for the human IL-2 receptor encodes a protein of 272 amino acids including an amino-terminal signal sequence of 21 amino acids, a 219 amino acid extracellular domain, a membrane-spanning domain composed of 22 hydrophobic amino acids, followed by a cytoplasmic domain of 10 amino acids. The cytoplasmic portion of the IL-2 receptor would presumably be responsible for transmission of a proliferative signal in response to IL-2. Because this region is relatively short, it has been speculated that other proteins may be required in association with the IL-2 receptor to transmit this signal.

To understand more fully the mechanism of action of the IL-2 receptor, we have isolated a cDNA clone encoding the murine IL-2 receptor. By comparing the amino acid sequences of the human and murine receptor we hope to identify highly conserved regions that may function in the binding of IL-2 and in signal transduction.

MATERIALS AND METHODS

Construction and Analysis of a Complementary DNA Library

Polyadenylated mRNA was isolated from the IL–2-dependent murine T-cell line CTLL-2, which is known to express high levels of IL-2 receptor (4). Procedures for RNA purification and cDNA library construction have been described (14,15). Small-scale plasmid DNA preparations from 15 pools representing approximately 10^5 total transformants were digested with PstI, electrophoresed on 0.8% agarose gels, blotted onto nitrocellulose filters, and hybridized with a ^{32}P-labeled human IL-2 receptor cDNA probe. The probe was obtained by nick-translating a 1340 base pair (bp) fragment representing the IL-2 receptor insert from pN1/N4-S (8). Hybridizations were for 16 hr at 55°C in 6X NaCl/Cit (1X NaCl/Cit = 0.15 M NaCl/ 0.015 M sodium citrate, pH 7) containing 0.1% Sarcosyl; 5X Denhardt's solution (1X = 0.02% polyvinylpyrrolidone/0.01% Ficoll/0.02% bovine serum albumin); 0.5% Nonidet P-40; 100 μg/ml denatured salmon sperm DNA; and probe at 10^6 cpm/ml. Filters were washed extensively in 6X NaCl/Cit at room temperature, and then washed for 1 hr at 42°C and for 1.5 hr at 55°C before autoradiography. Positive pools containing the largest hybridizing cDNAs were subdivided, and the process was repeated on pools of 2000 transformants. Positive pools were then used in colony filter hybridization experiments to identify transformants that hybridized strongly with the probe. The inserts from the cDNA clones were subcloned into M13mp18 and mp19 (16) and sequenced by the chain-termination method (17,18). Computer analysis of DNA and protein sequences was performed by software designed by the University of Wisconsin Genetics Computer Group (19).

Construction of a Recombinant Murine Interleukin-2 Receptor Expression Plasmid

An expression vector was constructed by inserting a 923 bp Sau3A fragment from pMrec-1, containing the entire coding region of the murine

IL-2 receptor (Fig. 1), into the Bg1II site of pMLSV (8) in the correct orientation for expression from the SV40 promoter. The resulting plasmid, pMLSV-Mrec-1, was digested with BamH1 and the fragment containing the SV40 promoter, the murine IL-2 receptor coding region, and SV40 splicing and polyadenylation signals was purified and ligated to BamH1 digested p1-8, resulting in plasmid pMrec-1/1-8. p1-8 is a bovine papilloma virus-derived vector (a gift of N. Sarver) and has been described previously (20). The transcriptional orientation of the IL-2 receptor cDNA was the same as that of the BPV early region (21).

Transfection of C127 Cells

One million murine mammary epithelial cells (C127 cells) were transfected with 5 μg of plasmid DNA and 20 μg of carrier salmon sperm DNA as described (22,23). After 4 hr the cells were given a 15% glycerol shock. The following day the cultures were trypsinized and replated at a 1:4 dilution in medium containing 2 mg/ml G418 (Gibco). The G418-resistant cell lines were maintained in medium containing 500 μg/ml G418.

Analysis and Fluorescence-Activated Sorting of Cells

Analysis and sorting of C127 cells expressing the murine IL-2 receptor were accomplished using monoclonal antibody 7D4 (24). Antibody 7D4 binds to murine IL-2 receptors located on the cell surface. A total of $1–2 \times 10^7$ cells were incubated with a saturating amount of 7D4 culture supernatant for 30 min at 4°C. After two washes with phosphate buffered saline (PBS)/1% bovine serum albumin (BSA), the cells were stained by further incubation with fluoroscein isothiocyanate (FITC)-rabbit-antirat IgG plus IgM (H + L) (Zymed Labs, Burlingame, California) as a second-step antibody for 30 min at 4°C. The samples were washed and centrifuged twice, resuspended in PBS/BSA, and propidium iodide was added at a final concentration of 5 μg/ml to aid in gating out nonviable cells.

Samples were run on an EPICS-C flow cytometer (Coulter Corp.), utilizing an argon laser at 488-nm excitation and a constant power of 300 mw. The top 1.0% of the viable 7D4-stained cells were collected and cultured in G418-containing medium until the next sort. After the seventh cycle of sorting, 7D4-positive cells were cloned at one and three cells per well (96-well Costar culture dishes) using a Coulter Autoclone.

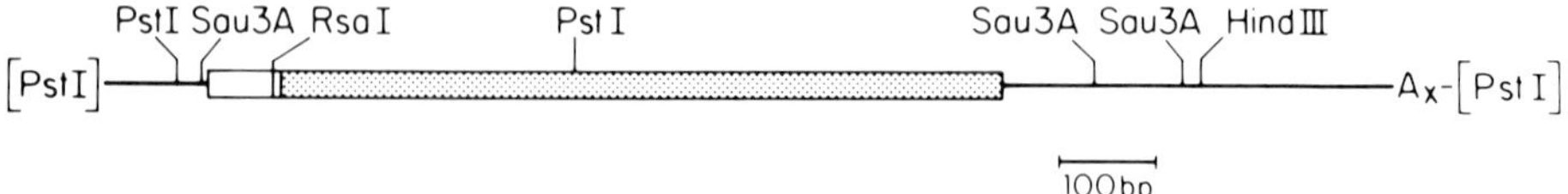

Figure 1 Partial restriction map of the cDNA insert encoding murine IL-2 receptor. Coding sequences are boxed. The open box represents the proposed signal sequence, and the shaded box represents the coding region for mature protein. PstI sites in brackets were generated by the cloning procedure.

RNA Analysis

Total RNA was isolated from murine CTLL-2 cells, mixed lymphocyte cultures (MLC), concanavalin A (Con A)-stimulated spleen cells and human HL-60 cells as described (8). Each RNA (5 μg) was glyoxalated and electrophoresed in 1.1% agarose gels containing 10 mM $NaPO_4$, pH 7, transferred to a nitrocellulose filter (Schleicher and Schuel), and hybridized with a ^{32}P-labeled RNA probe transcribed with Sp6 polymerase. The [^{32}P] RNA probe was synthesized from a plasmid containing a 875 bp RsaI/HindIII fragment (isolated from pMrec-1) inserted into pSP64 (Promega Biotec). Hybridization and washing of blots was as described (8).

Genomic DNA Analysis

Genomic DNA was isolated from 2×10^8 spleen cells by standard techniques (25). The DNA (10 μg) was digested with various restriction endonucleases and electrophoresed in 0.7% agarose gels, blotted, and hybridized at high stringency to a murine IL-2 receptor probe (25). The ^{32}P-labeled IL-2 receptor probe was obtained by nick-translating the internal PstI/HindIII fragment isolated from pMrec-1.

RESULTS

Cloning and Sequence of Murine Interleukin-2 Receptor

A cDNA library was made with mRNA isolated from the IL–2-dependent murine T-cell line, CTLL-2, which synthesizes high levels of IL-2 receptor. Screening of this library with a human IL-2 receptor probe resulted in several hybridizing clones, one of which, pMrec-1, was further characterized.

A partial restriction endonuclease map and the sequence of the cDNA insert is shown in Figs. 1 and 2, respectively. The cDNA insert of pMrec-1 contains 1350 bp including a stretch of adenylate residues at the 3′ end (data not shown) corresponding to the poly-A tail of mRNA. The cDNA clone also contains an open-reading frame of 272 amino acids starting with a Met codon at nucleotide 1 and a termination codon at nucleotide 945. Comparison of the amino acid sequence with that of the human IL-2 receptor (7) indicates the amino-terminal end of murine IL-2 receptor may be Glu-1. Thus the mature protein would be composed of 248 amino acids and have a nonglycosylated relative molecular weight of 28,375. The 5′ end of the open-reading frame would encode 25 amino acids with many characteristics expected of a signal peptide for secreted or membrane proteins (26).

Expression of Recombinant Murine Interleukin-2 Receptor

To determine if the cDNA insert in pMrec-1 codes for the murine IL-2 receptor, a recombinant expression system was used to direct synthesis of the IL-2 receptor. The bovine papilloma virus (BPV)-derived vector p1-8 (20) was used to generate cell lines that would stably express the murine IL-2 receptor. A DNA fragment (isolated from pMrec-1) containing the entire open-reading frame was inserted into the BglII site of pMLSV (8). This construction places the murine IL-2 receptor under the transcriptional control of the SV40 early promoter followed by SV40 RNA-processing signals. The entire cassette was then inserted into the BamHI site of p1-8 to give pMrec-1/1-8 (Fig. 3). Transfection into C127 cells, selection of G418-resistant cells, and multiple rounds of fluorescence-activated cell sorting using a monoclonal antibody (7D4) against the mouse IL-2 receptor (24), allowed the generation of cell lines expressing high levels of the mouse IL-2 receptor, as can be seen in Fig. 4. After seven cycles of sorting, clonally derived cell lines were isolated that stably express high levels of IL-2 receptor as detected by a monoclonal antibody specific for the murine IL-2 receptor. Preliminary experiments indicate that these cells express approximately 10^6 receptors per cell and, as has been reported for the human receptor (13,27), the recombinant murine IL-2 receptors were all of low affinity for IL-2.

Messenger RNA and Genomic DNA Analysis

The expression of IL-2 receptor mRNA was studied by Northern blot analysis of mRNA isolated from CTLL-2 cells, concanavalin A

```
Human                                                                     ATG
                                                                          Met   -21
Murine
                                                          Met Cys Gln Glu Asp   -21
                                                          ATG TGC CAG GAA GAT
-60  GAT TCA TAC CTG CTG ATG TGG GGA CTG CTC ACG TTC ATC ATG GTG CCT GGC TGC CAG GCA
     Asp Ser Tyr Leu Leu Met Trp Gly Leu Leu Thr Phe Ile Met Val Pro Gly Cys Gln Ala   -1

     Gly Ala Thr Leu Leu Met Leu Gly Phe Leu Ser Leu Thr Ile Val Pro Ser Cys Arg Ala   -1
-60  GGA GCC ACG TTG CTG ATG TTG GGG TTT CTC TCA TTA ACC ATA GTA CCC AGT TGT CGG GCA

1    GAG CTC TGT GAC GAT GAC CCG CCA GAG ATC CCA CAC GCC ACA TTC AAA GCC ATG GCC TAC
     Glu Leu Cys Asp Asp Asp Pro Pro Glu Ile Pro His Ala Thr Phe Lys Ala Met Ala Tyr   20

     Glu Leu Cys Leu Tyr Asp Pro Pro Glu Val Pro Asn Ala Thr Phe Lys Ala Leu Ser Tyr   20
1    GAA CTG TGT CTG TAT GAC CCA CCC GAG GTC CCC AAT GCC ACA TTC AAA GCC CTC TCC TAC

61   AAG GAA GGA ACC ATG TTG AAC TGT GAA TGC AAG AGA GGT TTC CGC AGA ATA AAA AGC GGG
     Lys Glu Gly Thr Met Leu Asn Cys Glu Cys Lys Arg Gly Phe Arg Arg Ile Lys Ser Gly   40

     Lys Asn Gly Thr Ile Leu Asn Cys Glu Cys Lys Arg Gly Phe Arg Arg Leu Lys ... Glu   39
61   AAG AAC GGC ACC ATC CTA AAC TGT GAA TGC AAG AGA GGT TTC CGA AGA CTA AAG ... GAA

121  TCA CTC TAT ATG CTC TGT ACA GGA AAC TCT AGC CAC TCG TCC TGG GAC AAC CAA TGT CAA
     Ser Leu Tyr Met Leu Cys Thr Gly Asn Ser Ser His Ser Ser Trp Asp Asn Gln Cys Gln   60

     Leu Val Tyr Met Arg Cys Leu Gly Asn ... ... ... ... Ser Trp Ser Ser Asn Cys Gln   55
118  TTG GTC TAT ATG CGT TGC TTA GGA AAC ... ... ... ... TCC TGG AGC AGC AAC TGC CAG

181  TGC ACA AGC TCT GCC ACT CGG AAC ACA ACG AAA CAA GTG ACA CCT CAA CCT GAA GAA CAG
     Cys Thr Ser Ser Ala Thr Arg Asn Thr Thr Lys Gln Val Thr Pro Gln Pro Glu Glu Gln   80

     Cys Thr Ser Asn Ser His Asp Lys Ser Arg Lys Gln Val Thr Ala Gln Leu Glu His Gln   75
166  TGC ACC AGC AAC TCC CAT GAC AAA TCG AGA AAG CAA GTT ACA GCT CAA CTT GAA CAC CAG

241  AAA GAA AGG AAA ACC ACA ... AAA ATA CAA AGT CCA ATG CAG CCA GTG GAC CAA GCG AGC
     Lys Glu Arg Lys Thr Thr ... Lys Ile Gln Ser Pro Met Gln Pro Val Asp Gln Ala Ser   99

     Lys Glu Gln Gln Thr Thr Thr Asp Met Gln Lys Pro Thr Gln Ser Met His Gln Glu Asn   95
226  AAA GAG CAA CAA ACC ACA ACA GAC ATG CAG AAG CCA ACA CAG TCT ATG CAC CAA GAG AAC

298  CTT CCA GGT CAC TGC AGG GAA CCT CCA CCA TGG GAA AAT GAA GCC ACA GAG AGA ATT TAT
     Leu Pro Gly His Cys Arg Glu Pro Pro Pro Trp Glu Asn Glu Ala Thr Glu Arg Ile Tyr   119

     Leu Thr Gly His Cys Arg Glu Pro Pro Pro Trp Lys His Glu Asp Ser Lys Arg Ile Tyr   115
286  CTT ACA GGT CAC TGC AGG GAG CCA CCT CCT TGG AAA CAT GAA GAT TCC AAG AGA ATC TAT

358  CAT TTC GTG GTG GGG CAG ATG GTT TAT TAT CAG TGC GTC CAG GGA TAC AGG GCT CTA CAC
     His Phe Val Val Gly Gln Met Val Tyr Tyr Gln Cys Val Gln Gly Tyr Arg Ala Leu His   139

     His Phe Val Glu Gly Gln Ser Val His Tyr Glu Cys Ile Pro Gly Tyr Lys Ala Leu Gln   135
346  CAT TTC GTG GAA GGA CAG AGT GTT CAC TAC GAG TGT ATT CCG GGA TAC AAG GCT CTA CAG

418  AGA GGT CCT GCT GAG AGC GTC TGC AAA ATG ACC CAC GGG AAG ACA AGG TGG ACC CAG CCC
     Arg Gly Pro Ala Glu Ser Val Cys Lys Met Thr His Gly Lys Thr Arg Trp Thr Gln Pro   159

     Arg Gly Pro Ala Ile Ser Ile Cys Lys Met Lys Cys Gly Lys Thr Gly Trp Thr Gln Pro   155
406  AGA GGT CCT GCT ATT AGC ATC TGC AAG ATG AAG TGT GGG AAA ACG GGG TGG ACT CAG CCC

478  CAG CTC ATA TGC ACA GGT GAA ATG GAG ACC AGT CAG TTT CCA GGT GAA GAG AAG CCT CAG
     Gln Leu Ile Cys Thr Gly Glu Met Glu Thr Ser Gln Phe Pro Gly Glu Glu Lys Pro Gln   179

     Gln Leu Thr Cys Val Asp Glu Arg Glu His His Arg Phe Leu Ala Ser Glu Glu Ser Gln   175
466  CAG CTC ACA TGT GTA GAT GAA AGA GAA CAC CAC CGA TTT CTG GCT AGT GAG GAA TCT CAA

538  GCA AGC CCC GAA GGC CGT CCT GAG AGT GAG ACT TCC TGC CTC GTC ACA ACA ACA GAT TTT
     Ala Ser Pro Glu Gly Arg Pro Glu Ser Glu Thr Ser Cys Leu Val Thr Thr Thr Asp Phe   199

     Gly Ser Arg Asn Ser Ser Pro Glu Ser Glu Thr Ser Cys Pro Ile Thr Thr Thr Asp Phe   195
526  GGA AGC AGA AAT TCT TCT CCC GAG AGT GAG ACT TCC TGC CCC ATA ACC ACC ACA GAC TTC

598  CAA ATA CAG ACA GAA ATG GCT GCA ACC ATG GAG ACG TCC ATA TTT ACA ACA GAG TAC CAG
     Gln Ile Gln Thr Glu Met Ala Ala Thr Met Glu Thr Ser Ile Phe Thr Thr Glu Tyr Gln   219

     Pro Gln Pro Thr Glu Thr Thr Ala Met Thr Glu Thr Phe Val Leu Thr Met Glu Tyr Lys   215
586  CCA CAA CCC ACA GAA ACA ACT GCA ATG ACG GAG ACA TTT GTG CTC ACA ATG GAG TAT AAG

658  GTA GCA GTG GCC GGC TGT GTT TTC CTG CTG ATC AGC GTC CTC CTC CTG AGT GGG CTC ACC
     Val Ala Val Ala Gly Cys Val Phe Leu Leu Ile Ser Val Leu Leu Leu Ser Gly Leu Thr   239

     Val Ala Val Ala Ser Cys Leu Phe Leu Leu Ile Ser Ile Leu Leu leu Ser Gly Leu Thr   235
646  GTA GCA GTG GCC AGC TGC CTC TTC CTG CTC ATC AGC ATC CTC CTC CTG AGC GGG CTC ACC

718  TGG CAG CGG AGA CAG AGG AAG AGT AGA AGA ACA ATC TAG
     Trp Gln Arg Arg Gln Arg Lys Ser Arg Arg Thr Ile End                               251

     Trp Gln His Arg Trp Arg Lys Ser Arg Arg Thr Ile End                               247
706  TGG CAA CAC AGA TGG AGG AAG AGC AGA AGA ACC ATC TAG
```

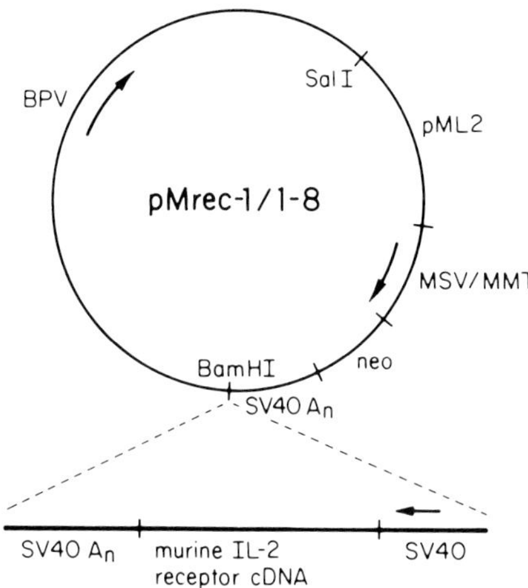

Figure 3 Structure of murine IL-2 receptor cDNA expression plasmid, pMrec-1/1-8. Arrows show the transcriptional orientation of: BPV (bovine papilloma virus), MSV/MMT (the Moloney sarcoma virus enhancer linked to the mouse metallothionein promoter), and SV40 (the simian virus 40 early promoter). pML2 contains sequences derived from the plasmid pBR322, *neo* refers to the neomycin-resistance gene from Tn5, SV40 A_n refers to SV40-derived sequences containing RNA splice donor and acceptor sites and a polyadenylation site, and murine IL-2 receptor cDNA designates the region encoding the murine IL-2 receptor.

Figure 2 Nucleotide sequences and predicted amino acid sequences of human (8) and murine IL-2 receptors. Nucleotides are numbered from the initiator Met codon and amino acids are numbered from the amino-terminus of the mature proteins. Homologous amino acid residues are boxed, closed circles indicate homologous cysteinyl residues and heavily boxed cysteinyl residues are those conserved in the intramolecular homology. Dashed lines indicate sequences deleted in the truncated human IL-2 receptor cDNA clone and the bar represents the presumed transmembrane region.

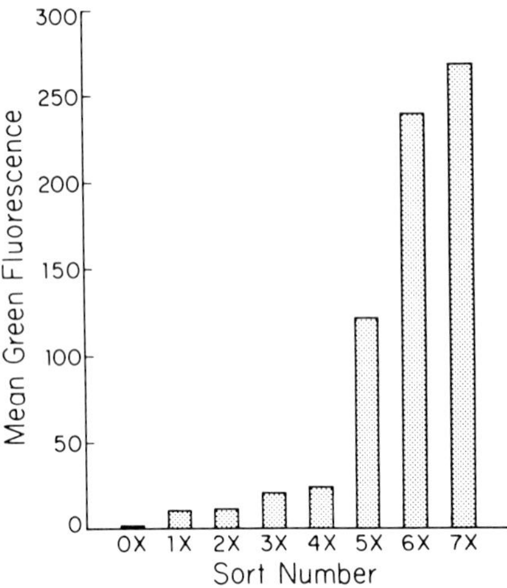

Figure 4 Analysis of C127 cells transfected with the murine IL-2 receptor cDNA expression vector (pMrec-1/1-8), during repetitive cycles of fluorescence-activated cell sorting. The relative green fluorescence is shown for the starting population of cells and at each of seven sorts. Background fluorescence has been subtracted from the fluorescence values obtained with 7D4, a monoclonal antibody specific for the murine IL-2 receptor.

(Con A)-stimulated murine spleen cells and MLC cells using a murine IL-2 receptor probe. Ribonucleic acid, isolated from human HL-60 cells, was also analyzed as a negative control (Fig. 5A). At least four mRNA species of 4.3, 3.7, 2.7, and 1.5 kb were found in the murine cell lines with the 3.7-kb species being the most abundant. No hybridizing mRNA was detectable in the human cells. The nature of the four transcripts are not known. However two of the transcripts (3.7 and 1.5 kp) may correspond to the transcripts (3.4 and 1.4 kb) found for the human IL-2 receptor (8–10). The different-sized classes of mRNA found in humans have been attributed to different polyadenylation sites (9). This may also be the case for the four mRNA-sized classes found in murine cells.

The four mRNA species found in the mouse could also be explained by additional gene copies of the IL-2 receptor. To address this question, a murine IL-2 receptor probe was hybridized to Southern blots of genomic DNA digested with various restriction endonucleases (Fig. 5B). Digestions

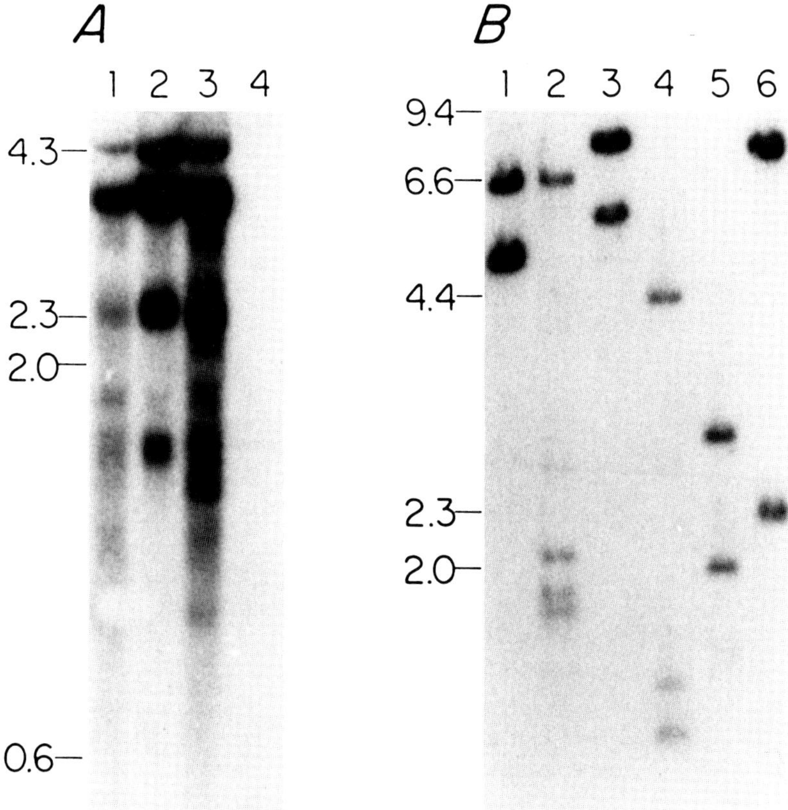

Figure 5 (A) Autoradiographs of Northern blots of murine IL-2 receptor mRNA. Hybridization of IL-2 receptor probe to blots of RNA isolated from: Con A-stimulated murine spleen cells (lane 1), CTLL-2 cells (lane 2), murine mixed lymphocyte cultures (lane 3) and human HL-60 cells (lane 4). The size markers (in kilobase pairs) are from HindIII digested bacteriophage lambda DNA. (B) Autoradiograph of hybridizations with murine IL-2 receptor probe to Southern blots of murine genomic DNA digested with BamHI (lane 1), EcoR1 (lane 2), Hind III (lane 3), PstI (lane 4), PvuII (lane 5), and XbaI (lane 6). The size markers (in kilobase pairs) are as above.

with EcoR1 and PstI resulted in four and three bands, respectively, while digestions with BamHI, HindIII, PvuII, and XbaI resulted in two bands each. While not definitive, these results indicate that the gene for the murine IL-2 receptor probably exists as a single copy.

DISCUSSION

The gene encoding the murine IL-2 receptor has been isolated by screening a murine cDNA library with a human IL-2 receptor probe. The cDNA library was made from mRNA isolated from the IL–2-dependent cell line CTLL-2. In addition the cDNA clone was shown to encode the IL-2 receptor by its ability to synthesize, in a recombinant expression system, a cell surface antigen recognized by the monoclonal antibody, 7D4, that is specific for the murine IL-2 receptor.

Two other laboratories have isolated cDNA clones encoding the murine IL-2 receptor using a similar procedure (28,29). The amino acid sequence as predicted from the DNA sequence of the mature IL-2 receptor agrees with the sequence of Miller et al. (28), but differs at six positions with the sequence determined by Shimuzu et al. (29). These are at positions 78 (Glu), 79 (Glu), 97 (Ala), 119 (Val), 195 (Leu), and 206 (Val). A unique feature of pMrec-1 is that the signal sequence is four amino acids longer (positions –24 to –21) than that described by other groups. Alignment of the murine and human IL-2 receptor sequences (see Fig. 2) shows a high degree of homology at the DNA (68%) and amino acid (60%) levels. The homology of the mature receptor is dispersed throughout the molecule but there are regions that are especially well conserved. These regions are: at the NH_2-terminal end (amino acids 1 to 38), where there are 29 identities out of 38; in the middle of the protein (amino acids 96 to 106), where there are 10 identities out of 11; the predicted transmembrane domain (amino acids 216 to 327, Fig. 2, bar), where there are 19 identities out of 22; and the COOH-terminal or cytoplasmic domain (amino acids 238 to 247), where there are nine identities out of 10. It is these highly conserved regions that may play an important role in the function of the IL-2 receptor. Interestingly, the alignment of 12 out of 13 cysteinyl residues (Fig. 2, closed circles) in the murine protein is conserved when compared with the human, indicating that disulfide bridges play an important role in the structure of the IL-2 receptor. Note also that one of the conserved cysteinyl residues occurs within the transmembrane region. This residue might form disulfide bonds with other membrane proteins involved in the transfer of the signal initiated by IL-2 binding to the receptor. A nonconserved feature of the two proteins is that the murine receptor has twice the number of possible *N*-linked glycosylation sites (positions 12, 22, 95, and 179) than does the human homologue, and their positions are not conserved.

It was first noted by Cosman et al. (8) that a substantial degree of homology exists intramolecularly between two regions of the human IL-2 receptor. Region 1 corresponds to amino acids 1 to 102, and region 2 to amino acids 103 to 174. This intramolecular homology also exists in the murine receptor. These internal repeats in the murine protein correspond to amino acids 1 to 97 and 98 to 170. When these two regions are aligned an interesting feature is that the positions of four cysteinyl residues are conserved (see Fig. 2, heavy boxed Cys residues). Because of the substantial degree of homology found between these two regions, it is possible that they are a result of a duplication of an ancestral gene. A similar observation has been made in other receptors including the insulin receptor (30,31), the low-density lipoprotein (LDL) receptor (32), the epidermal growth factor (EGF) receptor (33) and the EGF receptor-related oncogene *neu* or v-*erb*-B-2 (34,35). In these receptor proteins it was suggested that two cysteinyl-rich domains form intramolecular or intermolecular disulfide bridges resulting in the structural scaffolding required for ligand binding and possibly for signal transmission. It is tempting to speculate that the two homologous domains in the human and murine IL-2 receptor play a similar role.

When the human IL-2 receptor cDNA clone was isolated a second clone was found (8,9) that is essentially identical with the IL-2 receptor except for a deletion of 216 bp coding for 72 amino acids (see Fig. 2, dashed line). When this "truncated" human IL-2 receptor was inserted into a SV40-based expression vector and transfected into COS monkey kidney cells, expression of IL-2 receptors was not detected as judged by binding of the monoclonal antibody 2A3 and binding of radiolabeled IL-2 (8). Thus the function of this truncated form of the IL-2 receptor, if any, is not known. Recently, the sequence for the gene of the human IL-2 receptor was determined, and it was found that these 216 bp correspond exactly to exon 4 (11,12). Thus the cDNA clone of the truncated receptor may simply be an artifact caused by alternate splicing of the mRNA primary transcript (joining of exon 3 to exon 5) and has no function in the binding of IL-2. This is supported by the fact that a cDNA, coding for the truncated receptor, has not been isolated from murine cells (this work, 28,29).

In addition S1 nuclease analysis has indicated that a mRNA for a truncated receptor does not exist at detectable levels in murine cells (data not shown).

With the isolation of a gene encoding the murine IL-2 receptor, a detailed analysis can be made of regions of high homology that may be directly involved in the function of the IL-2 receptor, binding of IL-2, and signal transmission. Particularly, the transmembrane region and cytoplasmic end of the IL-2 receptor will be the focus of extensive work in the future.

ACKNOWLEDGMENTS

We thank Steve Gimpel for excellent technical assistance, Janis Wignall for murine genomic DNA preparations, and Judy Byce for preparation of the manuscript.

REFERENCES

1. Morgan, D. A., Ruscetti, F. W., and Gallo, R. C. (1976). Selective in vitro growth of T-lymphocytes from normal human bone marrow. *Science 193*:1007–1008.
2. Gillis, S. and Smith, K. S. (1977). Long term culture of tumor-specific cytotoxic T-cells. *Nature 268*:154–156.
3. Bonnard, G. D. D., Yosaka, D., and Jacobson, D. (1979). Ligand activated T cell growth factor-induced proliferation: Absorption of T cell growth factor by activated T cells. *J. Immunol. 123*:2704–2708.
4. Robb, R. J., Munck, A., and Smith, K. A. (1981). T cell growth factor receptors. Quantitation, specificity and biological relevance. *J. Exp. Med. 154*:1455–1474.
5. Dower, S. K., Hefeneider, S. H., Alpert, A. R., and Urdal, D. L. (1985). Quantitative measurement of human interleukin 2 receptor levels with intact and detergent-solubilized human T-cells. *Mol. Immunol. 22*: 937–947.
6. Uchiyama, T., Broker, S., and Waldmann, T. A. (1981). A monoclonal antibody (anti-Tac) reactive with activated and functionally mature T cells. I. Production of anti-Tac monoclonal antibody and distribution of Tac (+) cells. *J. Immunol. 126*:1393–1397.
7. Urdal, D. L., March, C. J., Gillis, S., Larsen, A., and Dower, S. K. (1984). Purification and chemical characterization of the receptor for interleukin 2 from activated human T lymphocytes and from a human T-cell lymphoma cell line. *Proc. Natl. Acad. Sci. USA 81*:6481–6485.

8. Cosman, D., Cerretti, D. P., Larsen, A., Park, L., March, C., Dower, S., Gillis, S., and Urdal, D. (1984). Cloning, sequence and expression of human interleukin-2 receptor. *Nature 312*:768–772.
9. Leonard, W. J., Depper, J. M., Crabtree, G. R., Rudikoff, S., Pumphrey, J., Robb, R. J., Kronke, M., Svetlik, P. B., Peffer, N. J., Waldmann, T. A., and Greene, W. C. (1984). Molecular cloning and expression of cDNAs for the human interleukin-2 receptor. *Nature 311*:626–631.
10. Nikaido, T., Shimizu, A., Ishida, N., Sabe, H., Teshigawara, K., Maeda, M., Uchiyama, T., Todoi, J., and Honjo, T. (1984). Molecular cloning of cDNA encoding human interleukin-2 receptor. *Nature 311*:631–635.
11. Leonard, W. J., Depper, J. M., Kanehisa, M., Kronke, M., Peffer, N. J., Svetlik, P. B., Sullivan, M., and Greene, W. C. (1985). Structure of the human interleukin-2 receptor gene. *Science 230*:633–639.
12. Ishida, N., Kanamori, H., Noma, T., Nikaido, T., Sabe, H., Suzuki, N., Shimizu, A., and Honjo, T. (1985). Molecular cloning and structure of the human interleukin-2 receptor gene. *Nucl. Acid. Res. 13*:7579–7589.
13. Cosman, D., Wignall, J., Lewis, A., Albert, A., Cerretti, D. P., Park, L., Dower, S. K., Gillis, S., and Urdal, D. L. (1986). High level stable expression of human interleukin-2 receptors in mouse cells generates only low affinity interleukin-2 binding sites. *Mol. Immunol. 23*:935–941.
14. March, C., Mosley, B., Larsen, A., Cerretti, D., Price, V., Braedt, G., Grabstein, K., Kronheim, S., Conlon, P., Henney, C., Gillis, S., Hopp, T., and Cosman, D. (1985). Cloning, sequence, and expression of two distinct human interleukin-1 (IL-1) cDNAs. *Nature 315*:641–647.
15. Cantrell, M. A., Anderson, D., Cerretti, D. P., Price, V., McKereghan, K., Tushinski, R. J., Mochizuki, D. Y., Larsen, A., Grabstein, K., Gillis, S., and Cosman, D. (1985). Cloning, sequence, and expression of a human granulocyte/macrophage colony-stimulating factor. *Proc. Natl. Acad. Sci. USA 82*:6250–6254.
16. Norrander, J., Kempe, T., and Messing, J. (1983). Construction of improved M13 vectors using oligodeoxynucleotide-directed mutagenesis. *Gene 26*:101–106.
17. Sanger, F., Nicklen, B., and Coulson, A. R. (1977). DNA sequencing with chain-terminating inhibitors. *Proc. Natl. Acad. Sci. USA 74*:5463–5467.
18. Biggin, M. D., Gibson, T. J., and Hong, G. F. (1983). Buffer gradient gels and ^{35}S label as an aid to rapid DNA sequencing. *Proc. Natl. Acad. Sci. USA 80*:3963–3965.
19. Devereux, J., Haeberli, P., and Smithies, O. (1984). A comprehensive set of sequence analysis programs for the Vax. *Nucl. Acid. Res. 12*:387–395.
20. Sarver, N., Ricca, C. A., Hood, M., Link, J., Tarr, J. C., and Drohan, W. N. (1985). Sustained high level expression of recombinant human gamma interferon using a bovine papilloma virus vector. In *Papilloma*

Viruses: Molecular and Clinical Aspects. Edited by P. M. Howley and T. R. Broker. A. R. Liss, New York.

21. Heilman, C. H., Engel, L., Lowy, D. R., and Howley, P. M. (1982). Virus specific transcription in bovine papilloma virus transformed mouse cells. *Virology 119*:22–34.
22. Sarver, N., Gruss, P., Law, M.-F., Khoury, G., and Howley, P. M. (1981). Bovine papilloma virus deoxyribonucleic acid: A novel eucaryotic cloning vector. *Mol. Cell. Biol. 1*:486–496.
23. Sarver, N., Byrne, J. C., and Howley, P. M. (1982). Transformation and replication in mouse cells of a bovine papilloma virus pML2 plasmid vector that can be rescued in bacteria. *Proc. Natl. Acad. Sci. USA 79*: 7147–7151.
24. Malek, T. R., Robb, R. J., and Shevach, E. M. (1983). Identification and initial characterization of a rat monoclonal antibody reactive with the murine interleukin 2 receptor-ligand complex. *Proc. Natl. Acad. Sci. USA 80*:5694–5698.
25. Maniatis, T., Fritsch, E. F., and Sambrook, J. (1982). In *Molecular Cloning, A Laboratory Manual.* Cold Spring Harbor Laboratory, New York.
26. Watson, M. E. E. (1984). Compilation of published signal sequences. *Nucl. Acid. Res. 12*:5145–5164.
27. Greene, W. C., Robb, R. J., Svetlik, P. B., Rusk, C. M., Depper, J. M., and Leonard, W. J. (1985). Stable expression of cDNA encoding the human interleukin 2 receptor in eukaryotic cells. *J. Exp. Med. 162*:363–368.
28. Miller, J., Malek, T. R., Leonard, W. J., Greene, W. C., Shevach, E. M., and Germain, R. N. (1985). Nucleotide sequence and expression of a mouse interleukin 2 receptor cDNA. *J. Immunol. 134*:4212–4217.
29. Shimuzu, A., Kondo, S., Takeda, S.-I., Yodoi, J., Ishida, N., Sabe, H., Osawa, H., Diamantstein, T., Nikaido, T., and Honjo, T. (1985). Nucleotide sequence of mouse IL-2 receptor cDNA and its comparison with the human IL-2 receptor sequence. *Nucl. Acid. Res. 13*:1505–1516.
30. Ullrich, A., Bell, J. R., Chen, E. Y., Herrera, R., Petruzzelli, L. M., Dull, T. J., Gray, A., Coussens, L., Kiao, Y.-C., Tsubokawa, M., Mason, A., Seeburg, P. H., Grunfeld, C., Rosen, O. M., and Ramachandran, J. (1985). Human insulin receptor and its relationship to the tyrosine kinase family of oncogenes. *Nature 313*:756–761.
31. Ebina, Y., Ellis, L., Jarnagin, K., Edery, M., Craf, L., Clauser, E., Ou, J.-H., Masiarz, F., Kan, Y. W., Goldfine, I. D., Roth, R. A., and Rutter, W. J. (1985). The human insulin receptor cDNA: The structural basis for hormone-activated transmembrane signalling. *Cell 40*:747–758.
32. Yamamoto, T., Davis, C. G., Brown, M. S., Schneider, W. J., Casey, M. L., Goldstein, J. L., and Russell, D. W. (1984). The human LDL receptor: A cysteine-rich protein with multiple Alu sequences in its mRNA. *Cell 39*:27–38.

33. Ullrich, A., Coussens, L., Hayflick, J. S., Dull, T. J., Gray, A., Tam, A. W., Lee, J., Yarden, Y., Libermann, T. A., Schlessinger, J., Downward, J., Mayes, E. L. V., Whittle, N., Waterfield, M. D., and Seeburg, P. H. (1984). Human epidermal growth factor receptor cDNA sequence and aberrant expression of the amplified gene in A431 epidermoid carcinoma cells. *Nature 309*:418–425.
34. Bargmann, C. I., Hung, M.-C., and Weinberg, R. A. (1986). The *neu* oncogene encodes an epidermal growth factor receptor-related protein. *Nature 319*:226–230.
35. Yamamoto, T., Ikawa, S., Akiyama, T., Semba, K., Nomura, N., Miyajima, N., Saito, T., and Toyoshima, K. (1986). Similarity of protein encoded by the human c-*erb*-B-2 gene to epidermal growth factor receptor. *Nature 319*:230–234.

6

Interleukin-1α: Cloning, Expression, and Biological Activities

DAVID J. COSMAN, MICHAEL C. DEELEY, SHIRLEY R. KRONHEIM, THOMAS P. HOPP, PAUL J. CONLON, STEVEN GILLIS, and BRUCE MOSLEY
Immunex Corporation, Seattle, Washington

The biological entity known as interleukin-1 is an important mediator of inflammatory responses. It is released by activated macrophages, Epstein-Barr virus (EBV)-infected B cells, Langerhans cells, astrocytes, endothelial cells, keratinocytes, and mesangeal cells and has been reported to have a wide range of activities (1,2). These include induction of interleukin-2 release by T cells, stimulation of B-lymphocyte proliferation and secretion of antibody, fibroblast and endothelial cell growth factor activity, induction of acute-phase protein synthesis by hepatocytes, stimulation of collagenase release from synovial cells, bone resorption via osteoclast activation, and increase of collagen synthesis by epithelial cells (1,2).

For such an array of biological activities to be possessed by one molecule would be highly unusual. The IL-1 activities have been reported to be associated with proteins of molecular weights ranging from very small to very large, although the majority of investigators have assigned relative molecular weights of around 15,000 or 30,000 (1,2). Thus until recently, it was not clear if IL-1 was a single protein or more than one molecule.

We wished to understand the molecular biology and biological properties of interleukin-1 and have therefore isolated two distinct human cDNAs that encode proteins with IL-1 activity, termed IL-1α and IL-1β (3). These two proteins are only 26% homologous in their amino acid sequences, but they share many biological properties. In this chapter we focus mainly on IL-1α.

RESULTS

Interleukin-1α cDNAs were isolated from a cDNA library prepared from RNA extracted from human macrophages that had been activated with lipopolysaccharide (LPS) (3). The RNA had been sized on the basis of its ability to direct IL-1 synthesis by frog (*Xenopus*) oocytes. From a library of 20,000 transformants, 5000 were selected for further analysis. Elimination of the plasmids lacking inserts and of those hybridizing to cDNA made from unstimulated macrophage RNA, left 2000 transformants. Of these, 768 were screened in pools of 48 for their ability to select biologically active IL-1 RNA. We assayed biologically active IL-1 from RNA translated in vitro by a rabbit reticulocyte lysate, because we had found that the levels of IL-1 activity produced in this system were higher and more reproducible than those produced after oocyte injection. Using this hybrid selection assay, we were able to isolate two cDNA clones containing partial copies of IL-1α mRNA, and then to use these as probes to identify IL-1α cDNAs encompassing almost the entire message. The sequence of IL-1α is shown in Fig. 1. It contains a single, large, open-reading frame of 271 amino acids, encoding a protein of predicted relative molecular weight of 30,606. Although IL-1 is thought to be a secreted protein, the predicted sequence does not contain a classic NH_2-terminal signal sequence or internal hydrophobic amino acid sequences. Human IL-1α has 62% amino acid homology to murine IL-1 (4) and 64% amino acid homology to rabbit IL-1 (5), suggesting that these genes are homologues. Protein sequence data on mouse IL-1 suggested that the secreted, 17 kilodalton (kDa) form of the molecule is the COOH-terminal portion of the 30 kDa primary translation product, beginning at Ser-115 (4). This aligns with Ser-113 of the human IL-1α molecule. Accordingly, we have constructed a number of expression vectors designed to produce the primary translation product ("full-length" IL-1α) or the COOH-terminal 159 amino acids starting at Ser-113 ("mature" IL-1α). These will be described in more detail later.

Expression in *Escherichia coli*

An IL-1α expression vector was constructed using the P_L promoter from phage λ, synthetic oligonucleotides specifying a ribosome-binding site, a methionine initiation codon, and a few amino acids of IL-1α as shown in Fig. 2. The remainder of mature IL-1α was provided by an AluI-HincII restriction endonuclease fragment isolated from p10A (3). The plasmid pLT IL-1α was transformed into *E. coli* containing pRK248cIts, a plasmid that bears a thermolabile repressor of P_L transcription. Cultures harboring the two plasmids were grown at 30°C to a cell density of 2 × 10^7 cells/ml and then shifted to 42°C for 20 hr. Total proteins were extracted in sodium dodecyl sulfate (SDS) and analyzed on an SDS-polyacrylamide gel (SDS-PAGE) (Fig. 3). Compared with extracts from cells bearing a control plasmid, a protein band corresponding to mature IL-1α can be seen. For comparison, an extract from *E. coli* expressing mature IL-1β is shown (6). Equivalent samples were tested for biological activity in the LBRM-1A5 conversion assay as described (13). A high level of IL-1 activity was detected after heat induction of transcription from the P_L promoter in cells bearing pLTIL-1α. The identity of the mature IL-1α band was verified by Western blot analysis using monoclonal antibodies directed against IL-1α (data not shown).

Purification

Recombinant IL-1α could be extracted from *E. coli* by lysozyme/EDTA treatment at pH 8 followed by lowering the pH to 2.8. Following a high-speed centrifugation, IL-1α was prepared from the supernatant by sequential chromatography on Sulphapropyl Sephadex C-25, DEAE Sephacel and phenyl-Sepharose CL4-B which yielded homogeneous IL-1α as described elsewhere (6). Mature IL-1β was also expressed in *E. coli* and purified to homogeneity (6). The purified proteins are shown in Fig. 3.

Comparison of Biological Activities of Interleukin-1α and Interleukin-1β

The availability of homogeneous recombinant IL-1α and IL-1β (6) enabled us to make a comparison of the biological activities of these proteins. The concentrations of the two molecules were quantitated by amino acid analysis, and they were titrated in three assay systems: mouse thymocyte comitogenesis, direct thymocyte proliferation, and the LBRM-33-1A5 conversion assay. All three assays measure the IL-1-induced release of IL-2 by T cells. The results (Table 1) show that, within the limits of these assays, the specific activities of IL-1α and IL-1β were identical and that the recombinant IL-1s were at least as active as natural IL-1β. However the activities of the recombinant IL-1s in a bone resorption assay were different.

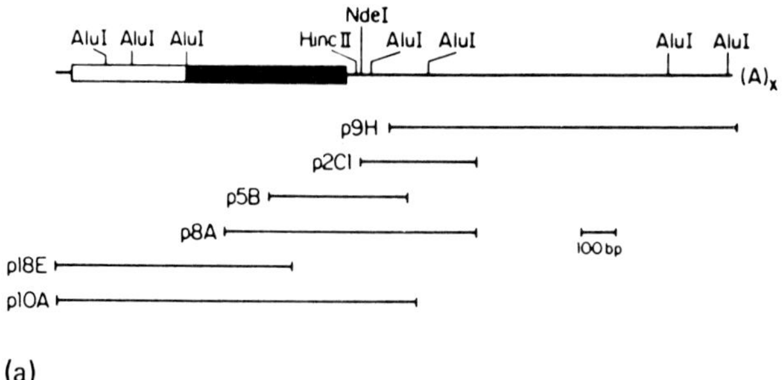

(a)

```
                                5'--TGAGGGAGTCATTTCATTGGCGTTTGAGTCAGCAAAGAAGTCAAG      -1

ATG GCC AAA GTT CCA GAC ATG TTT GAA GAC CTG AAG AAC TGT TAC AGT GAA AAT GAA GAA    60
Met Ala Lys Val Pro Asp Met Phe Glu Asp Leu Lys Asn Cys Tyr Ser Glu Asn Glu Glu    20

GAC AGT TCC TCC ATT GAT CAT CTG TCT CTG AAT CAG AAA TCC TTC TAT CAT GTA AGC TAT   120
Asp Ser Ser Ser Ile Asp His Leu Ser Leu Asn Gln Lys Ser Phe Tyr His Val Ser Tyr    40

GGC CCA CTC CAT GAA GGC TGC ATG GAT CAA TCT GTG TCT CTG AGT ATC TCT GAA ACC TCT   180
Gly Pro Leu His Glu Gly Cys Met Asp Gln Ser Val Ser Leu Ser Ile Ser Glu Thr Ser    60

AAA ACA TCC AAG CTT ACC TTC AAG GAG AGC ATG GTG GTA GTA GCA ACC AAC GGG AAG GTT   240
Lys Thr Ser Lys Leu Thr Phe Lys Glu Ser Met Val Val Val Ala Thr Asn Gly Lys Val    80

CTG AAG AAG AGA CGG TTG AGT TTA AGC CAA TCC ATC ACT GAT GAT GAC CTG GAG GCC ATC   300
Leu Lys Lys Arg Arg Leu Ser Leu Ser Gln Ser Ile Thr Asp Asp Asp Leu Glu Ala Ile   100

                                                            AluI
GCC AAT GAC TCA GAG GAA GAA ATC ATC AAG CCT AGG TCA GCA CCT TTT AGC TTC CTG AGC   360
Ala Asn Asp Ser Glu Glu Glu Ile Ile Lys Pro Arg Ser Ala Pro Phe Ser Phe Leu Ser   120
                                     C            *
                                    Asn

AAT GTG AAA TAC AAC TTT ATG AGG ATC ATC AAA TAC GAA TTC ATC CTG AAT GAC GCC CTC   420
Asn Val Lys Tyr Asn Phe Met Arg Ile Ile Lys Tyr Glu Phe Ile Leu Asn Asp Ala Leu   140

AAT CAA AGT ATA ATT CGA GCC AAT GAT CAG TAC CTC ACG GCT GCT GCA TTA CAT AAT CTG   480
Asn Gln Ser Ile Ile Arg Ala Asn Asp Gln Tyr Leu Thr Ala Ala Ala Leu His Asn Leu   160

GAT GAA GCA GTG AAA TTT GAC ATG GGT GCT TAT AAG TCA TCA AAG GAT GAT GCT AAA ATT   540
Asp Glu Ala Val Lys Phe Asp Met Gly Ala Tyr Lys Ser Ser Lys Asp Asp Ala Lys Ile   180

ACC GTG ATT CTA AGA ATC TCA AAA ACT CAA TTG TAT GTG ACT GCC CAA GAT GAA GAC CAA   600
Thr Val Ile Leu Arg Ile Ser Lys Thr Gln Leu Tyr Val Thr Ala Gln Asp Glu Asp Gln   200

CCA GTG CTG CTG AAG GAG ATG CCT GAG ATA CCC AAA ACC ATC ACA GGT AGT GAG ACC AAC   660
Pro Val Leu Leu Lys Glu Met Pro Glu Ile Pro Lys Thr Ile Thr Gly Ser Glu Thr Asn   220

CTC CTC TTC TTC TGG GAA ACT CAC GGC ACT AAG AAC TAT TTC ACA TCA GTT GCC CAT CCA   720
Leu Leu Phe Phe Trp Glu Thr His Gly Thr Lys Asn Tyr Phe Thr Ser Val Ala His Pro   240

AAC TTG TTT ATT GCC ACA AAG CAA GAC TAC TGG GTG TGC TTG GCA GGG GGG CCA CCC TCT   780
Asn Leu Phe Ile Ala Thr Lys Gln Asp Tyr Trp Val Cys Leu Ala Gly Gly Pro Pro Ser   260

ATC ACT GAC TTT CAG ATA CTG GAA AAC CAG GCG TAG GTCTGGAGTCTCACTTGTCTCACTTGTGCAG   847
Ile Thr Asp Phe Gln Ile Leu Glu Asn Gln Ala End                                   271

 Hinc2     NdeI
TGTTGACAGTTCATATGTACCATGTACATGAAGAAGCTAAATCCTTTACTGTTAGTCATTTGCTGAGCATGTACTGAGC   926

CTTGTAATTCTAAATGAATGTTTACACTCTTTGTAAGAGTGGAACCAACACTAACATATAATGTTGTTATTTAAAGAAC  1005

ACCCTATATTTTGCATAGTACCAATCATTTTAATTATTATTCTTCATAACAATTTTAGGAGGACCAGAGCTACTGACTA  1084

TGGCTACCAAAAAGACTCTACCCATATTACAGATGGGCAAATTAAGGCATAAGAAAACTAAGAAATATGCACAATAGCA  1163

GTTGAAACAAGAAGCCACAGACCTAGGATTTCATGATTTCATTTCAACTGTTTGCCTTCTGCTTTTAAGTTGCTGATGA  1242

ACTCTTAATCAAATAGCATAAGTTTCTGGGACCTCAGTTTTATCATTTTCAAAATGGAGGGAATAATACCTAAGCCTTC  1321

CTGCCGCAACAGTTTTTTATGCTAATCAGGGAGGTCATTTTGGTAAAATACTTCTCGAAGCCGAGCCTCAAGATGAAGG  1400

CAAAGCACGAAATGTTATTTTTTAATTATTATTTATATATGTATTTATAAATATATTTAAGATAATTATAATATACTAT  1479

ATTTATGGGAACCCCTTCATCCTCTGAGTGTGACCAGGCATCCTCCACAATAGCAGACAGTGTTTTCTGGGATAAGTAA  1558

GTTTGATTTCATTAATACAGGGCATTTTGGTCCAAGTTGTGCTTATCCCATAGCCAGGAAACTCTGCATTCTAGTACTT  1637

GGGAGACCTGTAATCATATAATAAATGTACATTAATTACCTTGAGCCAGTAATTGGTCCGATCTTTGACTCTTTTGCCA  1716

TTAAACTTACCTGGGCATTCTTGTTTCATTCAATTCCACCTGCAATCAAGTCCTACAAGCTAAAATTAGATGAACTCAA  1795

CTTTGACAACCATAGACCACTGTTATCAAAACTTTCTTTTCTGGAATGTAATCAATGTTTCTTCTAGGTTCTAAAAATT  1874

GTGATCAGACCATAATGTTACATTATTATCAACAATAGTGATTGATAGAGTGTTATCAGTCATAACTAAATAAAGCTTG  1953

CAAGAAAAAAAAAAAAAAAAAAAAAA--3'                                                   1979
```

(b)

In this assay (7), rat fetal long bones were labeled with ^{45}Ca in vivo, extracted, and then incubated in vitro with or without IL-1. The amount of ^{45}Ca released into the medium is quantitated, and the results are expressed as the ratio of cpm released with IL-1 to that released without IL-1. The results (Fig. 4), over a wide range of IL-1 concentrations, show that IL-1β is much more active in this assay than IL-1α. Not only is the concentration needed for half maximal activity 100-fold less for IL-1β than IL-1α, but the maximum amount of ^{45}Ca released is greater for IL-1β than for IL-1α. Thus IL-1β is a more potent bone-resorbing agent than IL-1α. This difference in biological activity is the first to be demonstrated between IL-1α and IL-1β. Other assay systems are currently being investigated.

Activities of Full-Length and Mature Interleukin-1α and Interleukin-1β

Both IL-1α and IL-1β are initially synthesized as 30 kDa precursors and yet are found in macrophage supernatants as 17 kDa, COOH-terminal, biologically active fragments. This raises several questions, one of which is that of the biological activities of the precursors. We previously demonstrated that full-length IL-1β, when translated in a rabbit reticulocyte lysate, was biologically inactive. Full-length IL-1α, in contrast, appeared to be fully active (3). However the possibility that IL-1α was efficiently converted to the mature form in the reticulocyte lysate or during the bioassay could not be eliminated. To address this issue in a more definitive way, we constructed a series of vectors designed to express IL-1 molecules at high levels in an in vitro translation system. Full-length and

---

Figure 1 (a) Restriction endonuclease map of human IL-1α. Coding sequences are boxed. Shaded boxed region represents the presumptive form of IL-1α. Below are shown the cDNA clones used for sequencing. One clone, p10A, contains the entire coding region. Each cDNA clone begins and ends with PstI sites, generated by the cloning procedures. (b) Nucleotide sequence and predicted amino acid sequence of IL-1α. Nucleotides and amino acids are numbered from the presumed initiator codon. The star under Ser-113 indicates the position of the presumed mature NH_2-terminal. The nucleotide sequence differs between p18E and p10A at base 330 (G→C) which would cause an amino acid change, Lys-110→Asn. The 3′ maturation signal is underlined. Coordinates of cDNA clones shown in A are: p18E, nucleotides -45–652; p10A, -35–1075; p8A, 447–1195; p5B, 591–995; p2C1, 860–1194; p9H, 928–1979.

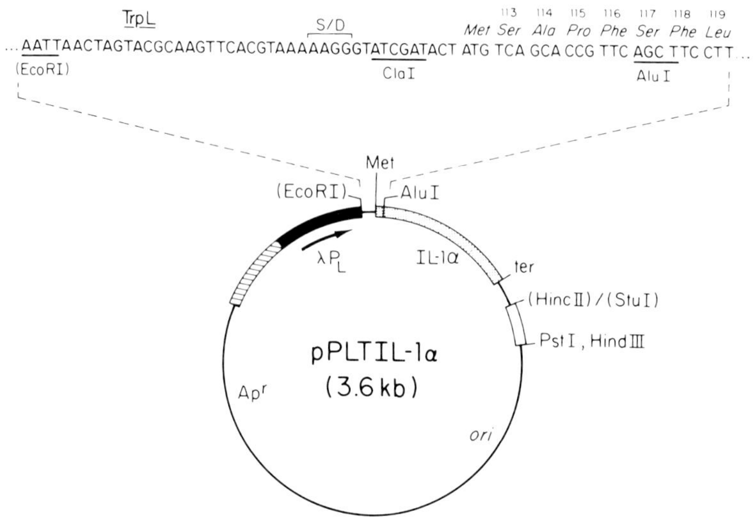

Figure 2 The structure of the mature IL-1α expression vector, pPLT IL-1α. λ P_L represents the leftward promoter of phage λ. The synthetic oligonucleotides are shown that specify the leader sequence from the *trp* operon (*Trp L*), the Shine/Dalgarno concensus ribosome initiation sequence (S/D), and the first five amino acids of mature IL-1α. The remainder of IL-1α is encoded in the AluI-HincII fragment that is shown as a stippled bar. Ap^R is the ampicillin resistance gene of pBR322. Ori is the origin of replication from pBR322. The striped and open boxes contain irrelevant sequences from bacteriophage λ and the 3′ noncoding region of human IL-2, respectively.

mature IL-1α and IL-1β were each inserted downstream of the promoter sequence for the SP6 RNA polymerase to construct the series of plasmids shown in Fig. 5. In vitro transcription of each of these plasmids, following linearization of the DNA downstream of the IL-1-coding sequences, gave rise to large amounts of IL-1-specific RNA that could then be used as a template for protein synthesis in a rabbit reticulocyte lysate in vitro translation system, supplemented with [^{35}S] methionine. The preponderant labeled protein product in each case was full-length or mature IL-1α or IL-1β (Fig. 6). The activity of these proteins was measured in three assay systems. The first was a biological assay for IL-1; the second tested their

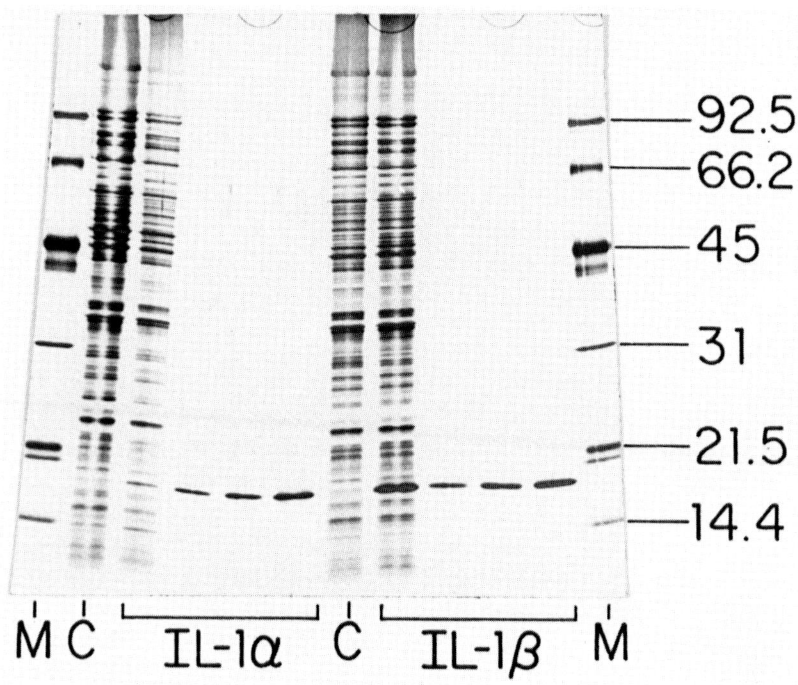

Figure 3 Expression of IL-1α and IL-1β in *E. coli.* The *E. coli*, strain RR1, was grown and induced as described in the text. The bacteria were pelleted, and proteins analyzed on SDS-PAGE. M represents molecular weight standards, and C represents extracts from bacteria bearing a control plasmid. The lanes marked IL-1α and IL-1β show extracts from bacteria containing pPLTIL-1α and pLNIL-1β, followed by increasing amounts of purified IL-1α and IL-1β, respectively (*Source*: from Ref. 6).

Table 1 Recombinant Human IL-1s: Specific Activities (U/mg Protein)[a]

	Thymocyte mitogenesis	Thymocyte Co mitogenesis	1A5 conversion assay
Recombinant HuIL-1α	1.5×10^8	2.1×10^8	8.1×10^{10}
Recombinant HuIL-1β	1.0×10^8	1.6×10^8	7.6×10^{10}
Natural HuIL-1β	1.5×10^7	4.4×10^7	5.7×10^{10}

[a]Assays were as described in Refs. 12 and 13.

ability to compete the binding of ^{125}I-labeled natural IL-1α to its receptor. Note that both IL-1α and IL-1β compete for binding to the same receptor (8). In the third assay, the ^{35}S-labeled IL-1 molecules were incubated with cells bearing IL-1 receptors, the cells were washed free of unbound IL-1, lysed, and run on SDS-PAGE. This analysis served to detect IL-1 molecules that bound specifically to the IL-1 receptor, and determined if the full-length IL-1 molecules were capable of binding to the IL-1 receptor and mediating biological activity. The results (Table 2) show unequivocally that both the mature IL-1s and full-length IL-1α are biologically active,

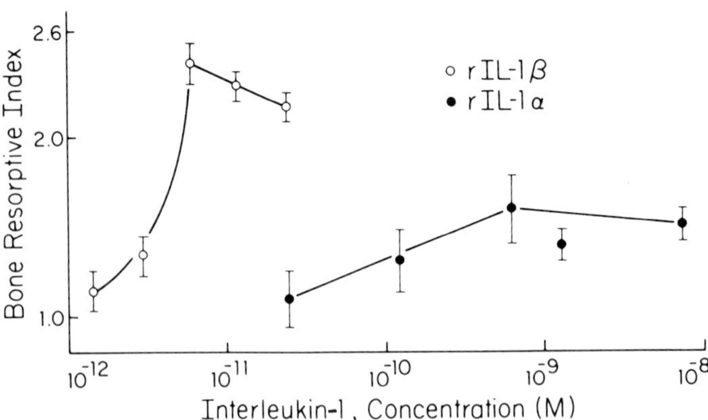

Figure 4 Bone resorption effects of recombinant interleukin-1α and interleukin-1β. Bone resorption assays were performed as described (7).

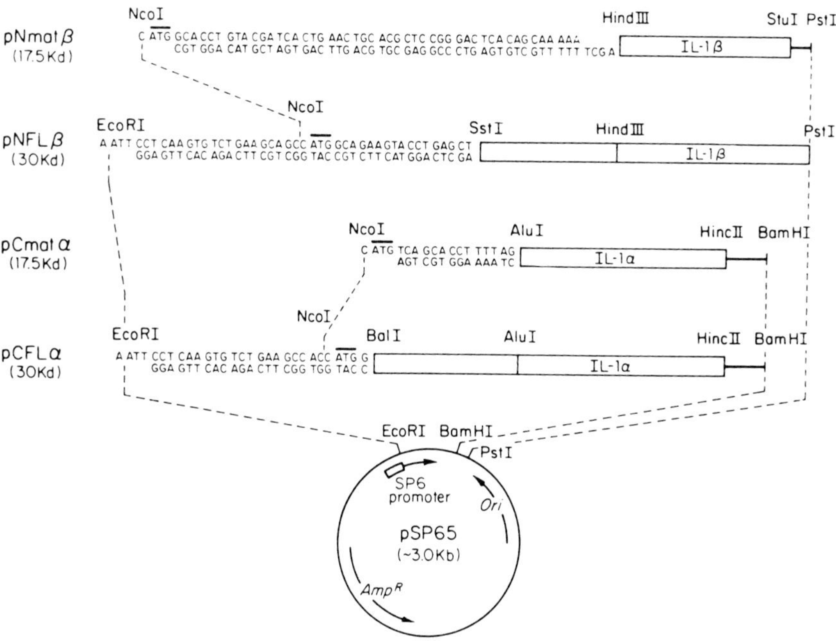

Figure 5 Structure of plasmids designed to express IL-1 in vitro. The plasmid backbone in each case is pSP65 (Promega Biotec) containing the SP6 promoter. The indicated oligonucleotides and restriction fragments of IL-1α and IL-1β were inserted into the polylinker downstream of the promoter. pNmatβ, pNFLβ, pCmatα, and pCFLα are designed to express, respectively, mature IL-1β, full-length IL-1β, mature IL-1α, and full-length IL-1α.

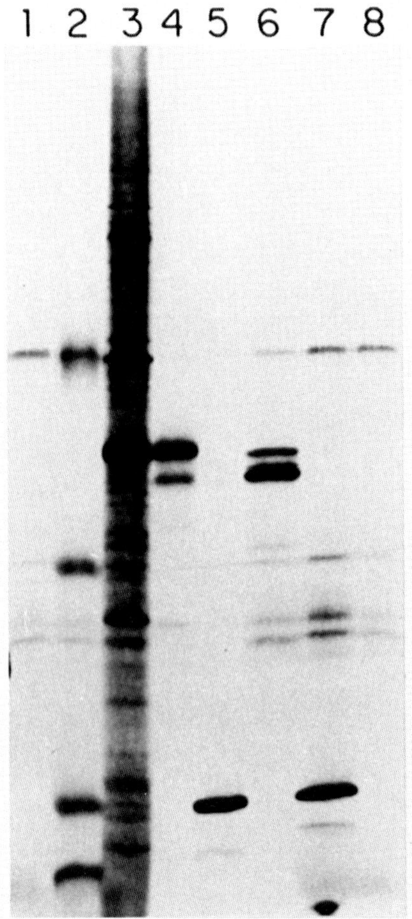

Figure 6 Interleukin-1 proteins produced in vitro. The plasmids described in Fig. 5 were transcribed with SP6 RNA polymerase and the RNA was translated in a rabbit-reticulocyte lysate supplemented with [^{35}S] methionine as described (14). The labeled proteins were analyzed on SDS-PAGE. Lanes 1 and 8 are from lysates with no added RNA, lane 2 contains molecular weight standards of 46, 31, 18.3, and 12.3 kDa, lane 3 shows the translation productions of RNA extracted from human peripheral blood monocytes stimulated with LPS, and lanes 4–7 show the translation products of RNA transcribed from the plasmids pNFLβ, pNmatβ, pCFLα, and pCmatα, respectively.

Table 2 Properties of IL-1 In Vitro Translation Products

RNA	Number of methionine residues	^{35}S incorporated into protein[a] [(cpm/μl) × 10^{-3}]	Biological activity (U/ml)[b]
17.5 kDa IL-1α	4	7.5	1.8×10^6
30 kDa IL-1α	7	11.5	4.8×10^6
17.5 kDa IL-1β	7	16.5	1.1×10^7
30 kDa IL-1β	12	41.5	<1000
EL-4 pA$^+$	–	21	<1000
pBM pA$^+$	–	20	8.0×10^3
None	–	4.3	<1000

[a]Incorporation of [^{35}S] methionine into protein was assayed by TCA purification.
[b]Biological activity was assayed in the LBRM-1A5 conversion assay (13).

whereas full-length IL-1β, in contrast, is biologically inactive. Results, presented elsewhere in this volume (Chap. 8) using the same IL-1 preparations as are shown here, demonstrate that full-length IL-1α can both bind to cells in an intact form and block the binding of mature IL-1 to its receptor. Full-length IL-1β is unable to do either.

DISCUSSION

The role of IL-1 as a central mediator in the inflammatory response has emerged from many years of research. The cloning of two distinct but distantly related IL-1 genes has opened up several research possibilities. First, homogeneous recombinant IL-1 proteins can be used to determine which of the many biological activities ascribed to impure preparations of IL-1 are, in fact, due to IL-1. Second, it will now be possible to examine if IL-1α and IL-1β are equally potent in these assays. Third, IL-1 probes can be used to determine exactly which cell types produce IL-1, whether they produce IL-1α or IL-1β or both, and at what level the expression of IL-1 activity is regulated. Fourth, the definition of the amino acid sequences of IL-1α and IL-1β has produced the surprising result that, although both proteins are apparently secreted by activated macrophages and other cell types, there are no apparent signal peptide sequences characteristic of other secreted proteins. This observation has led us to investigate how the 30-kDa full-length IL-1 precursors are processed by the cell and the mechanisms by which 17-kDa mature IL-1s are produced in cell supernatants. We are pursuing all of these approaches, and the work reported here represents progress along these lines.

The generation of appropriate reagents has been the first priority. The cloning of IL-1α and IL-1β cDNAs has given us the first tool; sensitive probes for the expression of IL-1 mRNAs (3). This has enabled us to detect IL-1α and IL-1β transcripts in both human T and B cells (9,10). Here and elsewhere (6) we report the high-level expression of the mature forms of IL-1 in *E. coli* and their purification to homogeneity. These pure proteins have been used in some of the many biological systems that respond to IL-1. Results presented here show that recombinant IL-1α and IL-1β have similar specific activities when measured in three assays that involve the induction of IL-2 release by murine T cells. The specific activities are comparable with those previously determined for purified, natural IL-1β, suggesting that the recombinant products are fully active.

In contrast, there is a clear difference between the activities of the two recombinant IL-1s in a bone resorption assay: IL-1β is the more potent as judged not only by the concentration needed to achieve half maximal activity but also by the higher maximum ^{45}Ca release mediated by IL-1β. This result demonstrates the first known difference between the two IL-1 molecules, and may indicate that IL-1β is more involved in the pathogenicity of arthritis previously attributed to IL-1. However it remains a formal possibility that, as we are using human IL-1 in a rat fetal long-bone assay, the differences we measure are solely due to a lesser ability of IL-1α to bind to the rat IL-1 receptor than that of IL-1β.

The other difference between IL-1α and IL-1β that we have addressed concerns the biological activities of their respective 30 kDa precursors. Many reports have characterized molecules of approximately 30 kDa having IL-1 biological activity (1,2). However we had previously found that full-length IL-1β, translated in a reticulocyte lysate following hybrid selection of mRNA, was inactive (3). Here we extend those results by expression of considerable quantities of full-length IL-1β in a coupled in vitro SP6 transcription/reticulocyte lysate translation system and show that it is indeed biologically inactive and incapable of blocking the binding of mature IL-1 to its receptor (see Chap. 8). In contrast, full-length IL-1α, when expressed in the same system, appears to be as active as mature IL-1α. The full-length IL-1α molecule is, in addition, capable of binding to cells and blocking the binding of mature IL-1 (see Chap. 8). We would therefore suggest that previous reports of 30 kDa IL-1 activity were probably measuring IL-1α precursor and not IL-1β precursor. It also follows from these results that any other IL-1α molecules initiating between amino acid 1 and 113 will also probably be biologically active. We have confirmed this for an IL-1α molecule starting at amino acid 71. However an IL-1β molecule starting at amino acid 71 is still biologically inactive (Mosley et al., manuscript in preparation). These results are in conflict with the claim of Matsushima et al. to have detected a 23-kDa biologically active form of IL-1β (11). We would suggest that the IL-1 activity migrating at 23 kDa on their gel filtration column was, in fact, IL-1α related. Further studies will be needed to elucidate the mechanism by which the precursors of IL-1α and IL-1β are processed to the final 17.5 kDa forms.

ACKNOWLEDGMENTS

We thank Dr. Anthony Allison and the Institute for Biological Science at Syntex, Palo Alto, for performing the bone resorption assays; Dirk Anderson, Toby Hemenway, Paula Glackin, Terri Washkewicz, and Sue Tyler for technical assistance; and Linda Troup for preparation of the manuscript.

REFERENCES

1. Durum, S. K., Schmidt, J. A., and Oppenheim, J. J. (1985). Interleukin 1: An immunological perspective. *Ann. Rev. Immunol. 3*:263.
2. Dinarello, C. A. (1984). Interleukin 1. *Rev. Infect. Dis. 6*:51.
3. March, C. J., Mosley, B., Larsen, A., Cerretti, D. P., Braedt, G., Price, V., Gillis, S., Henney, C. S., Kronheim, S. R., Grabstein, K., Conlon, P. J., Hopp, T. P., and Cosman, D. (1985). Cloning, sequence and expression of two distinct human interleukin-1 cDNAs. *Nature 315*: 641.
4. Lomedico, P. T., Gubler, V., Hellman, C. P., Dukovich, M., Giri, J. G., Pan, Y.-C. E., Collins, K., Semionow, R., Chua, A. O., and Mizel, S. B. (1984). Cloning and expression of murine interleukin-1 cDNA in *Escherichia coli. Nature 312*:458.
5. Furutani, Y., Notake, M., Yamayoshi, M., Yamagishi, J., Nomura, H., Ohue, M., Furata, R., Fukui, T., Yamada, M., and Nakamura, S. (1985). Cloning and characterization of the cDNAs for human and rabbit interleukin-1 precursor. *Nucleic Acids Res. 13*:5869.

6. Kronheim, S. R., Cantrell, M. A., Deeley, M. C., March, C. J., Glackin, P. J., Anderson, D. M., Hemenway, T., Merriam, J. E., Cosman, D., and Hopp, T. P. (1986). Purification and characterization of human interleukin-1 expressed in *Escherichia coli. Biotechnology 4*:1078.
7. Horton, J. E., Raisz, L. G., Simmons, H. A., Oppenheim, J. J., and Mergenhagen, S. E. (1972). Bone resorbing activity in supernatant fluid from cultured human peripheral blood leukocytes. *Science 177*: 793.
8. Dower, S. K., Kronheim, S. R., Cantrell, M. A., Gillis, S., Henney, C. S., and Urdal, D. L. (1986). Human interleukin-1α and interleukin-1β interact with the same cell surface receptor. *Nature 324*:266.
9. Acres, R. B., Larsen, A., Gillis, S., and Conlon, P. J. (1987). Production of IL-1α and IL-1β by clones of EBV transformed human B cells: Effects on antigen presentation. *Mol. Immunol.* (in press).
10. Acres, R. B., Larsen, A., and Conlon, P. J. (1987). Interleukin-1 expression in a clone of human T cells. *J. Immunol.* (in press).
11. Matsushima, K., Taguchi, M., Kovacs, E. J., Young, H. A., and Oppenheim, J. J. (1986). Intracellular location of human monocyte associated interleukin-1 activity and release of biologically active IL-1 from monocytes by trypsin and plasmin. *J. Immunol. 136*:2883.
12. Kronheim, S. R., March, C. J., Erb, S. K., Conlon, P. J., Mochizuki, D. Y., and Hopp, T. P. (1985). Human interleukin-1, purification to homogeneity. *J. Exp. Med. 161*:490.
13. Conlon, P. J. (1983). A rapid biologic assay for the detection of interleukin-1. *J. Immunol. 131*:1280.
14. Mosley, B., Urdal, D. L., Larsen, A., Cosman, D., Conlon, P. J., Gillis, S., and Dower, S. K. (1987). The IL-1 receptor binds the human IL-1α precursor but not the IL-1β precursor. *J. Biol. Chem.* (in press).

7
Molecular Organization and Expression of the Prointerleukin-1β Gene

ANDREW C. WEBB
Wellesley College, Wellesley, Massachusetts

LANNY J. ROSENWASSER
The New England Medical Center and Tufts University School of Medicine, Boston, Massachusetts

PHILIP E. AURON
Harvard-M.I.T. Division of Health Sciences and Technology, Cambridge, Massachusetts; The New England Medical Center and Tufts University School of Medicine, Boston, Massachusetts

Multiplicity of function, diversity of cellular origin, and molecular variability have been the hallmarks of well over a decade of study into the hormonelike cytokine known as interleukin-1 (IL-1) (1). As with other lymphokines, the advent of recombinant DNA techniques has facilitated major advances in our understanding of the molecular biology of IL-1. Post-cloning progress in IL-1 biology has been swift and the subject of a number of recent reviews (2–4). Consequently, this chapter will not attempt to duplicate these efforts, but merely serve to provide a brief synopsis of the latest observations that have been made by our group into the structure and function of the human IL-1β gene.

Ever since the revelation that essentially all IL-1 is probably the product of only two genes (now designated as IL-1α and IL-1β, Ref. 5), each being translated into a high-molecular-weight precursor polypeptide (proIL-1) carrying an inefficient secretory signal sequence (5–7), we have viewed the control of IL-1 expression as a potentially multilevel process. From a physiological standpoint, one might expect the expression of a protein as potent as IL-1 to be under rigid control at several levels from gene transcription through cellular release of protein. Experimental evidence is accumulating to suggest that this is indeed the case for IL-1 in human monocytes. Large quantities of proIL-1 are synthesized by monocytes in rapid response to a wide variety of stimulants (3,8), but over 80% of this protein remains within the cytosol (9), approximately 3% becomes membrane bound (10), and the remainder contributes to the rather modest levels of extracellular, biologically active IL-1β protein. Therefore the classic hormonal functions of IL-1, with their attendant metabolic impact (1), are satisfied at most by 20% of the proIL-1 synthesized by the monocyte.

GENOMIC STRUCTURE AND ORGANIZATION

The paradox of the existence and functioning of two IL-1 genes (alpha and beta) clearly defined on the basis of distinct isoelectric points (pI) for the mature 17 kilodalton (kDa) polypeptide products (namely pI 5 and pI 7, respectively), but with seemingly indistinguishable biological profiles (4), has raised the issue of what selective forces led to the maintenance of these two loci in the genome. This enigma is further compounded by the finding that there appears to be differential expression of these IL-1 gene counterparts, because human monocytes transcribe the IL-1β gene 10–50 times more efficiently than the IL-1α sequence (5), and consequently produce about 10 times more pI 7 than pI 5 IL-1 (3). A similar situation appears to exist with regard to the murine cell line PU5-1.8, in which a five- to tenfold greater amount of beta than alpha mRNA is transcribed (47). However the murine macrophage cell line $P388D_1$ has been reported to produce predominantly pI 5 IL-1 extracellularly following lipopolysaccharide (LPS) stimulation (11), even though both IL-1α and IL-1β mRNA can be detected in these cells (3).

Our initial approach to clarifying the molecular basis for control of IL-1β gene expression has been to examine the primary structure of the transcriptional unit. Our group has recently cloned and determined the nucleotide sequence for the human IL-1β gene (12). A similar analysis for the IL-1α gene was recently reported by Furutani et al. (13). Comparison of these two gene sequences revealed a striking similarity of genomic organization for these two members of the IL-1 gene family. With the complete nucleotide sequences for both the human IL-1α and IL-1β genes now available, it was natural to ask whether any obvious differences in primary structural elements might be invoked to account for the marked difference observed in the expression levels for human monocytes.

In our study, the isolation of bacteriophage lambda genomic clones from two different human tissue libraries (i.e., fetal liver and leukocyte), and comparison to Southern analysis of total human DNA derived from various sources, confirmed the presence of a single IL-1β locus, which we had previously localized to the long arm of human chromosome 2 (2q13-2q21) (14). Both the IL-1α and IL-1β genes are split into seven exons, but consistent with the relative mRNA sizes (1.6 kb for beta and 2.2 kb for alpha), the primary transcription product of the beta gene was found to be 7.0 kb in length compared with the 10.2 kb alpha transcript). Despite relatively poor overall amino acid homology (25%), close comparison of the two human IL-1 genes for both exon size and the positions within the peptides of splice junctions, revealed a remarkable conservation of organization (Table 1). Particularly striking was the precise registration within both alpha and beta genomic sequences of protein domains that we had previously hypothesized as being representative of functional delineation within the polypeptides (15). The implication from this observation is that the evolutionary constraints on this genomic pattern of organization have been maintained in the face of considerable sequence divergence (45% exon nucleotide homology).

This remarkable degree of structural conservation between alpha and beta genes suggested that the origin of a second IL-1 gene might be the consequence of a gene duplication event. Consequently, it was with some considerable interest that we discovered the molecular signatures of retrotransposition flanking the IL-1β genomic sequence. Specifically, the gene was delineated by both upstream and downstream direct repeats and possessed a 3′ poly-A tail. We have hypothesized, therefore, that the IL-1α gene represents the ancestral sequence that was duplicated to create an active retroposon in the form of the IL-1β gene (12). Because both IL-1 genes have now been identified in mice, reverse transcriptase-mediated retrotransposition obviously took place before divergence of the rodent and primate lineages some 75–100 million years ago. There are a number of precedents in the literature for retroposons, but the rodent preproinsulin I gene represents the only clear example of an active retroposon reported to date (16). In order for such a gene duplication to yield a functional sequence, there

Table 1 Comparison of ProIL-1 Exon Boundaries

	ProIL-1α[a]		ProIL-1β[b]	
Exon number	Inclusive amino acids	Protein homology regions	Inclusive amino acids	Protein homology regions
2	1–16	A	1–16	A
3	17–32	–	17–33	–
4	33–106	B	34–100	B
5	107–163	N	101–155	N
6	164–205	C–D_1	156–199	C–D_1
7	206–271	E	200–269	E

Source: Data from Ref. 13 (a) and Ref. 12 (b).

presumably must have been genomic reinsertion of either a normal length primary transcript downstream of a novel promoter, or a 5′ elongated transcript carrying its own promoter sequences. Comparison of the IL-1α and IL-1β gene upstream sequences reveals sufficient homology to suggest that the beta gene may have been derived from an alpha transcript that initiated at a cryptic, probably inefficient, upstream promoter. Such an abnormally long transcript would contain a cDNA copy of the normal promoter, which would be carried along during retrotransposition. Although transcription initiation from a cryptic upstream promoter is likely to have been a rare event, the retrotransposition of the IL-1 gene via this mechanism is a reasonable scenario and is analagous to the proposed origin of the rodent preproinsulin I gene from preproinsulin II (16,17). Figure 1 schematically illustrates the relationship between the two human IL-1 genes. The IL-1β upstream regulatory elements (e.g., TATA and CAT boxes), unlike those found in the IL-1α gene, bear strong homology to the consensus sequences for conventional, high-efficiency eukaryotic promoters (18). Superficially, this structural difference alone might contribute to the transcriptional superiority of the beta gene observed in monocytes. Clearly experimental confirmation of this supposition will require both an analysis of the transcriptional effects of site-specific mutagenesis in the IL-1β upstream sequences and a better understanding of the mechanisms transducing the monocyte stimulatory signal from the cell membrane, through the cytoplasm, to the nucleus.

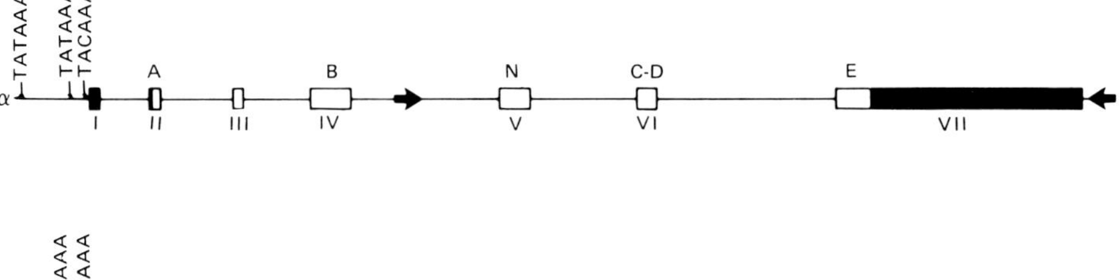

Figure 1 Schematic representation of human proIL-1 genes. The upper and lower lines represent the organization of IL-1α and IL-1β, respectively. The horizontal lines each represent the extent of the nucleotide sequence; open and closed boxes represent translated and untranslated exon sequences, respectively, large arrows locate *Alu*-like sequences; in IL-1β small arrows and the A near the downstream end of the gene represent, respectively, direct repeats and the location of an oligo(A) tract associated with retrotransposition. Letter nomenclature above exon boxes designate protein homology regions contained within (A–E as in Fig. 2). N designates the exon coding for the mature amino terminus of 17-kDa IL-1. Also indicated are the locations of potential promoter sequences (i.e., TATAAA or TACAAA).

MINIMAL SEQUENCE THAT CONTAINS INTERLEUKIN-1 ACTIVITY

Our original hypothesis that homology analysis of the IL-1α and IL-1β polypeptides revealed highly conserved functional domains within the sequence (15) has to a large extent been borne out by experimentation (23) and the recent confirmation from additional cDNA sequences in the mouse and rabbit (5–7,19,47). Figure 2 shows the alignment of all five IL-1 sequences using the National Biomedical Research Foundation (NBRF) program ALIGN (20). Indicated in the figure are intra- and interclass regions of homology. The two different classes have been designated as IL-1α and IL-1β (5). Intraclass comparison between human and murine forms reveals about 65% perfect amino acid homology, whereas the interclass homology between the alpha and beta molecules has demonstrated a more distant relationship of less than 30% (15), suggesting that IL-1α and IL-1β are members of a gene family.

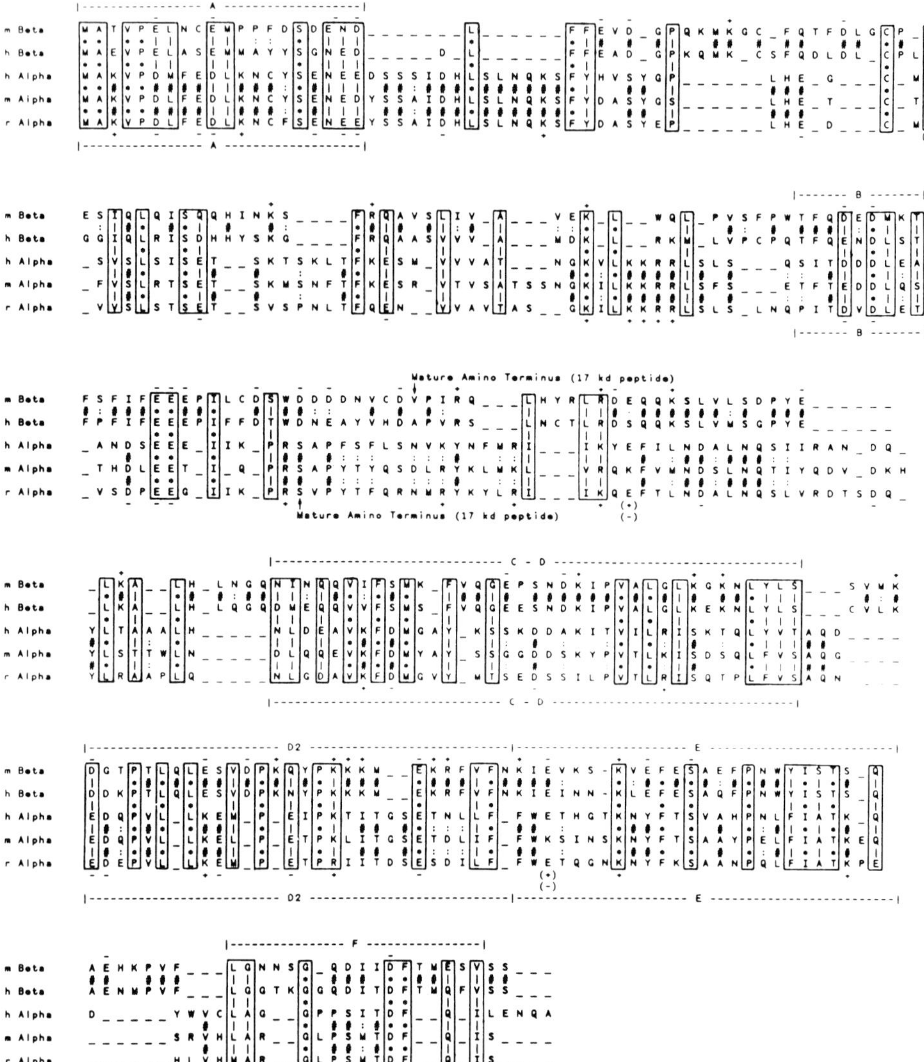

Figure 2 Homology alignment of proIL-1 amino acid sequences. Alignment using the NBRF program ALIGN generated gapped alignments in which homology among the five known proIL-1 sequences could be judged (h = human, m = murine, and r = rabbit). Following alignment, residues judged to be highly homologous were marked according to the degree of homology and with regard to intra- or interclass relationship (i.e., alpha or beta). Key: *, perfect interclass; |, conservative interclass; #, perfect intraclass; :, conservative intraclass. All interclass homologies are enclosed within boxes, and regions of clustered interclass homology designated as A through F. Conserved intraclass charged residues are indicated by + or –.

Because the alpha and beta forms share all IL-1 biological activities (4), common structural elements essential to function may be found within the two classes. In Fig. 3 the alignment data of Fig. 2 is displayed in a concise form by plotting the values of PAM_{250} (parameter for accepted mutations over 250 million years of evolution) (20,21). These values are used by the NBRF ALIGN program to derive the relationship as a function of alignment position shown in Fig. 2. In panel (a), the only PAM values shown are those associated with amino acids absolutely conserved among all five sequences. The different amplitudes reflect the differential degree of conservation recognized for amino acids in related proteins (20). Panel (b) contains all the data shown in panel (a), but in addition reveals the scores of imperfect, conservative, homology of the type described by Toh et al. (22), which classifies amino acids according to structural similarities. The plotted values shown in (b) are labeled as PAM_{250min} because they represent the summation of interclass values for the minimum PAM_{250} derived by comparison of the human form with the other members within each class. In panel (c) all $PAM_{250 min}$ values for the alignments are plotted using a penalty (–20 PAM) for gaps that relate to insertions or deletions in the aligned sequence. Such a plot reveals the common location of intraclass conservation, suggesting the existence of conserved "spacer" structures. When the data in Fig. 3, panels (a) and (b) are examined, it is obvious that the greatest degree of conservative structure is located within the carboxyl half of the proIL-1 molecule, corresponding to the portion contained within the mature, 17 kDa peptide. In addition to the PAM_{250} values for conserved residues, Fig. 3, panel (b) also indicates the locations of important conserved amino acid types, such as charged residues (+ or –), obligatory bends (proline residues, P), and the only conserved internal methionine residue (M). It has been demonstrated that conserved, charged residues in related proteins are often found at the protein surface in association with ligand-binding sites. Therefore, it is possible that the conserved, charged amino acids found within highly homologous portions of the mature peptide, in the proximity of absolutely conserved peptide backbone bends, may represent sites important for biological activity.

Using the homology data as a guide, our first experiments utilized deletion subclones of human IL-1β cDNA for transfection into simian COS cells (23). This revealed that lymphocyte-activating factor (LAF) activity was resident within a 7-kDa subpeptide located between residues 136 and 197 of the 269 amino acid proIL-1β sequence corresponding to the C and D_1 homology regions. The importance of the C-D homology region for

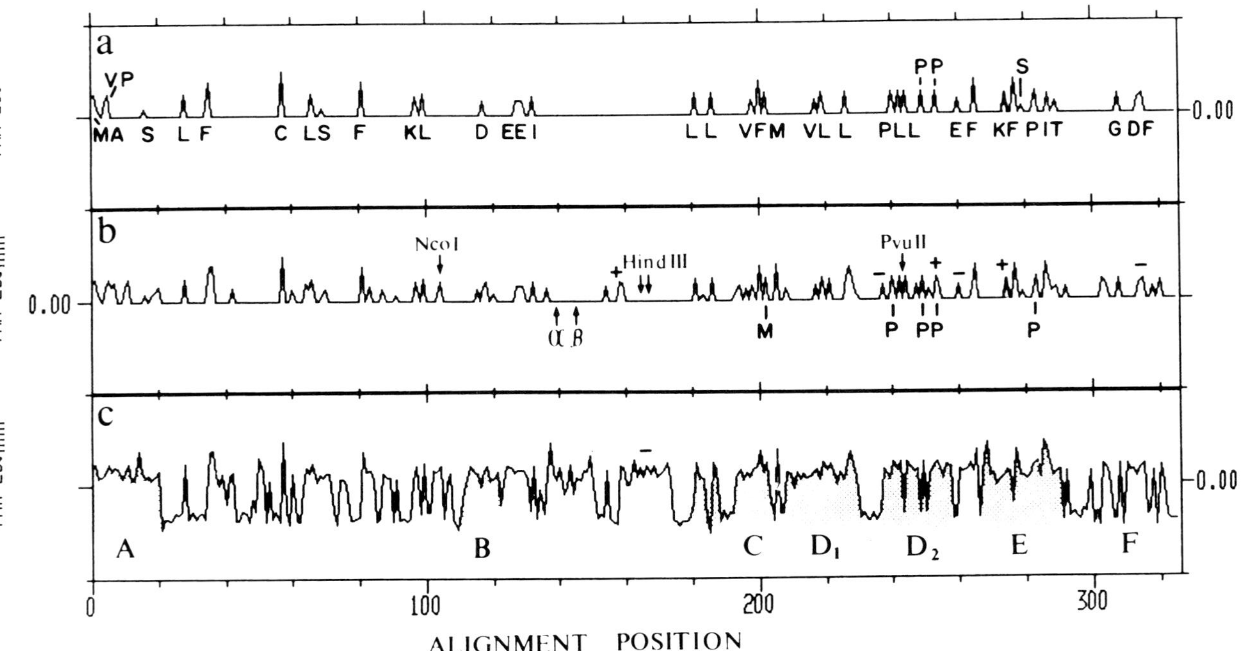

Figure 3 Protein kinship among the proIL-1 sequences. Relationships among the proteins are plotted as PAM_{250} values (see text). The alignment position is directly related to amino acid position but contains placeholders for gaps as shown in Fig. 2. (a) selectively shows PAM_{250} values for perfectly conserved residues among all five proIL-1 sequences. (b) shows the minimum relative PAM_{250} for perfect as well as conserved residues. (c) shows the minimum relative PAM_{250} for all residues, including a −20 penalty for gaps. Shaded regions locate interesting homology regions. Absolutely conserved residues of interest are designated by single-letter amino acid codes. Absolutely conserved charge residues are designated by + or −.

maintenance of thymocyte proliferative activity has been subsequently confirmed by the finding that a nanopeptide from residues 163–171 (within homology region D_1, see Figs. 2 and 3) of the proIL-1β sequence, when used at concentrations as high as 200 μg/ml, can elicit LAF activity (24).

However some recent experiments utilizing an SP6 vector system to generate synthetic mRNA for subsequent translation into IL-1β subpeptides in rabbit reticulocyte lysates, have cast some doubt on our original assignment of the "active site" to within the C-D domain (25). Although the precise constructs in these later experiments differ slightly from those used in the COS cell transfection assay system, little LAF activity has now been consistently recovered in peptides located carboxyl to residue 133. The reason for this discrepancy is presently unclear, but differences between the two experimental systems used in terms of product stability, translational efficiencies, as well as the possibility that COS cells are activated by the subpeptides to produce either IL-1 or IL-1-like factors are all being considered.

REGULATION OF PROINTERLEUKIN-1β GENE EXPRESSION

Transcriptional Regulation

We have recently undertaken an extensive study of the kinetics of IL-1β gene transcription in the human monocytic leukemia cell line THP-1 (26) stimulated with LPS. A somewhat unexpected finding of this study was that IL-1β cytoplasmic mRNA induction was extremely rapid, being detectable within 1 hr, and reaching a maximum at least two orders of magnitude above that detected in unstimulated cells within 4 hr after LPS stimulation (27). This was also reflected in a similar, but even more rapid, response within the nucleus as analyzed by both equilibrium nuclear mRNA levels and run-off transcriptional studies. The turnover of IL-1β mRNA synthesized during this induction was similarly rapid, but not complete, reaching a plateau 20- to 30-fold over background within 6 hr after stimulation. These kinetics correlate well with the synthesis of IL-1 activity by human monocytes and THP-1 cells following exposure to LPS, in which intracellular IL-1 activity has been detected within 1 hr and high levels of both intra- and extracellular IL-1 are reached 3 hr after stimulation (3). The LPS-induced increase in IL-1 synthesis by monocytes was both actinomycin D and cycloheximide (CH) sensitive, ruling out a major contribution to IL-1 production by either preformed mRNA or protein. Our studies further indicated that CH inhibition of de novo protein synthesis results in an elevated or "superinduced" level of IL-1β mRNA (400- to 600-fold over background) with rates of accumulation and decay kinetics both being identical (Fig. 4). Interestingly, these features of proIL-1β mRNA synthesis are shared by several protooncogenes (e.g., *c-myc, c-fos*) (28,29) and "competence factors" (30) that have been implicated in cellular differentiation. The inclusion of IL-1β in this category of transiently expressed, tightly regulated genes may imply a novel role for proIL-1β in monocyte differentiation, particularly when one considers that most of the IL-1β synthesized remains inside the cell (9).

Given these data, we have hypothesized that IL-1β gene expression is dependent upon specific protein factors that exert their control at two discrete levels. The proIL-1β promoter appears to be under the positive control of a transcriptional activator (TA) protein preexisting in THP-1 cells. The rapid induction of the IL-1β gene by LPS stimulation is mediated by a conversion of this TA from its prestimulatory, inactive state to an active form. The model further predicts the existence of a separate repressor protein ("transcriptional clamp"; TC), the synthesis of which is also responsive to LPS stimulation. However treatment of the THP-1 cells with inhibitors of protein synthesis (e.g., CH) distinguishes between these two regulatory factors and seems to explain the superinducibility of the IL-1β gene. Specifically, TA function is refractory to CH, whereas the repressor function is dependent upon its synthesis following LPS stimulation. Both an inherently short half-life for IL-1β mRNA (about 2 hr) and the existence of a rigid transcriptional control system of the type proposed by our two-stage model are consistent with cellular regulation of a potent biological molecule.

More recent work in our laboratory indicates that the kinetics of IL-1β expression by THP-1 cells is stimulant specific. For example, phorbol myristic acetate (PMA) stimulation leads to a much slower appearance and decay of IL-1β mRNA, somewhat reminiscent to the response of the histiocytic lymphoma line U937 which is refractory to LPS stimulation, but responsive to PMA. These observations suggest that the membrane receptor/transduction system for LPS and PMA stimulants are likely to be quite separate. Since PMA induction is thought to be mediated by protein kinase C (31), it is possible that LPS induction is manifested by an alternate mechanism. Consistent with the data is a model in which LPS directly induces both the IL-1β and the TC genes, whereas PMA induces the IL-1β gene much less effectively than LPS, and down-regulates or has no effect on TC activation. Additional work will be required to prove this model and to relate it to the various aspects of IL-1 induction.

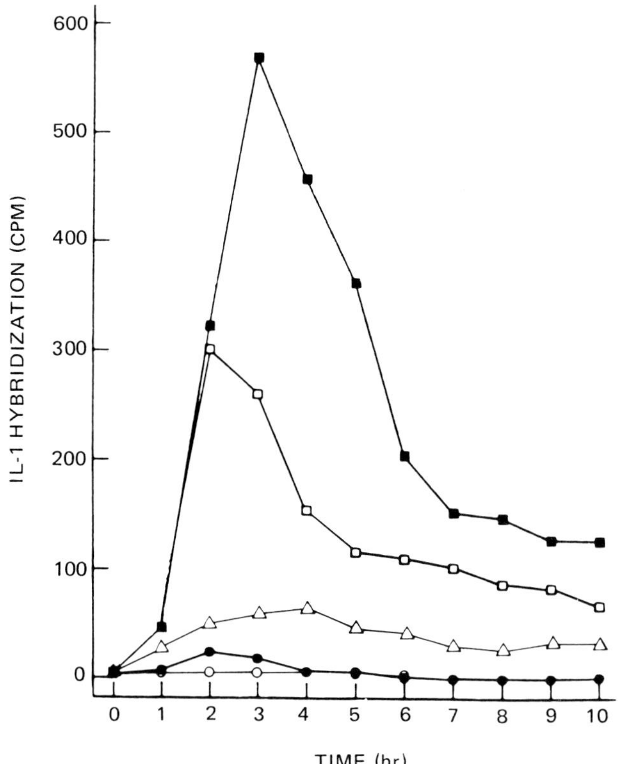

Figure 4 ProIL-1β mRNA production in the THP-1 monocyte cell line. Cytoplasmic mRNA was isolated by the method of White and Bancroft (46) and analyzed by dot blot hybridization using a radiolabeled IL-1β cDNA probe. Cells were analyzed either in the absence (open symbols) or presence (closed symbols) of cycloheximide (CH). Key: control (open circles); 0.5 μg/ml LPS (open triangles); 10 μg/ml LPS (open squares); 1.0 μg/ml CH alone (closed circles); 2 μg/ml LPS + 0.1 μg/ml CH.

Posttranscriptional Regulation

Control of gene expression via alternate splicing pathways for precursor nuclear (hn) RNA is now a well-established phenomenon (32). With IL-1β, the genomic sequence indicated a number of potential alternate splice donor/acceptor sites (12). However we have not yet observed extensive heterogeneity of mRNA species on Northern blot analyses that might indicate the common utilization of such alternate splicing in IL-1β gene expression, with two exceptions. The first example relates to the observation on Northern blot analysis that the mRNA species in guanidinium isothiocyanate preparations of keratinocytes are markedly different in both molecular weight and number from that seen in various monocyte/macrophage extracts (e.g., blood monocytes, THP-1, and U937 cell lines) (2). The second variation in IL-1β mRNA that we have identified is synthesized both constitutively and upon LPS stimulation of endothelial cells from the human umbilical cord (33). Although the release of IL-1 activity by stimulated endothelial cells has been reported on several occasions (34-36), the identification of IL-1β gene expression by these cells is relatively recent. Interestingly however, unlike the studies reported using saphenous vein endothelial cells (37), we have determined that the mRNA synthesized by umbilical cord endothelial cells that hybridizes to the IL-1β cDNA probe is consistently 50-100 nucleotides shorter than the IL-1β mRNA from monocytes. We are now pursuing studies to distinguish between explanations for this result based upon either an alternate splicing of legitimate IL-1β mRNA in these particular endothelial cells or a transcription of yet another closely related IL-1 sequence.

Two other recent observations are important. First, the finding that human amniotic fluid is rich in IL-1 is consistent both with umbilical cord endothelial cells expressing high levels of IL-1β mRNA and also a variation in the posttranscriptional processing of the mRNA specific to tissue of fetal origin. Second, human fibroblasts stimulated with TNF have been shown by S1 nuclease mapping to synthesize a shorter IL-1α mRNA than the normal 2.2 kb species (38).

Prointerleukin-1 Activity and Posttranslational Processing

It now seems to be generally accepted that the high degree of molecular variability exhibited by IL-1 activities, be they of differing molecular size or variations in protein isoelectric points, are mostly a manifestation of posttranslational proteolysis of the proIL-1 peptides (2,3). For a molecule that has evolved to function in the decidely unfavorable environment posed by the site of inflammation, maintenance of biological activity even under extreme proteolysis would be clearly advantageous. However controversy appears to be rampant over the issues of whether or not the full-length precursor to IL-1β has IL-1 activity, and whether the intact protein is a purely intracellular form of IL-1 that is reduced to the major processed intermediate of 23-kDa on the way to the "mature" 17-kDa polypeptide during or after transport through the monocyte membrane. We have recently obtained experimental evidence relevant to both these questions.

First, the issue of 31-kDa proIL-1 biological activity appears to have been resolved by experiments in collaboration with Dr. Lee Gehrke at the Massachusetts Institute of Technology in which IL-1β synthesized and radiolabeled by reticulocyte translation of SP6-generated full-length cDNA transcripts has been monitored in the LAF assay. An SDS-PAGE analysis of the [^{35}S] methionine-labeled IL-1β indicates that the proIL-1β polypeptide remains undegraded throughout the time course of the murine D10.G4.1 comitogenic assay while retaining biological activity, albeit at a level approximately one-quarter that of the mature 17-kDa polypeptide synthesized and assayed under the same conditions in vitro.

One of the most surprising findings that resulted from molecular cloning of the cDNAs for IL-1 was the absence of conventional hydrophobic signal sequences (39) that would have allowed for the efficient transport of the cytokine to the extracellular environment, where most of its hormonelike actions were anticipated to occur. The demonstration of IL-1 activity in association with the undegraded 31-kDa proIL-1 molecule correlates well with the presence of LAF activity in the cell lysates of both stimulated human monocytes and mammalian cells transfected with the IL-1β cDNA clone. In other words, proteolysis of the precursor to the more potent 17-kDa form must take place either during or after transport out of the cell by some as yet ill-defined mechanism. Experiments using the in vitro-labeled proIL-1 favor a model of processing during export from the cell rather than extracellular proteolysis, since the 31-kDa proIL-1 also remains intact in the presence of cultured monocytes. Furthermore, we have shown that when stringent measures are taken to prevent proteolysis during isolation of IL-1 polypeptides from monocytes by adding the serine protease inhibitor PMSF to the buffers, then the only intracellular form of IL-1β that can be detected is the 31-kDa precursor (48). This result is in direct contrast to previous work. Lepe-Zuniga et al. (40) identified IL-1 activity associated intracellularly with proteins of a variety of molecular weights. More recently Matsushima et al. (9) have concluded from detergent extraction of both cytosolic and membrane-bound IL-1 from monocytes, that proteolysis of the 31-kDa precursor takes place to a 23-kDa intermediate form within the cell and that final processing to the 17-kDa mature IL-1 is thereafter an extracellular event. The 23-kDa peptide can also be released from the monocyte membrane by digestion with plasmin or trypsin (9).

Not in dispute is the clear observation that maximal activity of the IL-1β polypeptide is achieved only upon proteolytic removal of the amino-terminal 116 amino acids from the 31-kDa precursor. Furthermore, the removal of approximately 70 amino-terminal residues necessary to generate a 23-kDA molecule may well be required to facilitate transport of the active peptide outside of the cell. It has been demonstrated, at least in vitro, that processing of the proIL-1β to the 17-kDa form can be achieved with high fidelity using serine proteases of the elastase type (41). As such, the achievement of total biological activity of IL-1 could be viewed as yet another example of proteolytic control of hormonal function. It is worth noting that cells of the human monocytic lineage are producers of substantial quantities of serine proteases and their corresponding inhibitors (42,43). The cosynthesis of both the enzyme required to process the IL-1 precursor to its most potent and/or transportable form, and also a specific inhibitor of that same processing enzyme certainly provides an elegant molecular control on the expression of this molecule.

Considering this, our recent isolation of a cDNA clone from an LPS-stimulated human monocyte library that codes for a 415 amino acid polypeptide that shows extremely high homology (35–40%) to members of the serine protease inhibitor (serpin) superfamily (44) has been of considerable interest. This monocyte-derived serpin is coded for by a 2.0 kb mRNA that, like IL-1β, is synthesized actively following LPS stimulation. It has an arginine residue at the active site (Arg-serpin) which makes it more closely related to antithrombin III and plasminogen activator inhibitor than α_1-antitrypsin (a Met-serpin). We are presently investigating the substrate specificity of this monocyte-derived Arg-serpin and its effect on both proIL-1β processing and LAF activity. Our working hypothesis is that the monocyte Arg-serpin clone may indeed be synonymous with the plasminogen activator inhibitor already identified in human monocytes and macrophages (42). With the demonstration that plasmin releases the active 23-kDa IL-1 polypeptide from stimulated monocytes (9) and that elastase cleaves pro IL-1β in vitro to the fully active 17-kDa, mature protein (41), it is possible that this monocyte-derived Arg-serpin represents a posttranslational level of monocyte control over expression of IL-1; namely preventing precursor processing to biologically active subpeptides.

SUMMARY AND CONCLUSION

Given the limited homology analysis that could be performed between the first two IL-1 cDNA sequences obtained in 1984 (6,7), we concluded that the two IL-1 genes subsequently referred to as IL-1α and IL-1β (5) are distantly related counterparts (15). This initial conclusion has been substantiated by a more detailed amino acid homology analysis now that the cDNAs for other human, murine, and rabbit IL-1s (5,19,47) have been isolated. More extensive alignment of the sequences has confirmed the high degree of structural conservation within six domains (referred to as A-E; Ref. 15), but an additional region of major homology D_2, located between domains D_1 and E at the carboxyl-terminus of the IL-1 polypeptides, has been identified. The hypothesis that these domains represent regions of functional significance has, to a large extent, stood the test of experimentation, at least for the C–D region relative to the LAF activity of IL-1 (23,24).

The degree of relatedness of the IL-1 genes has become even more apparent with the recent molecular cloning of genomic sequences for IL-1α (13) and IL-1β (12). These data strongly suggest that the IL-1β gene is an active retroposon derived by gene duplication from the ancestral IL-1α gene before divergence of the rodent and primate lineages. The two genes show a remarkable degree of conserved organization of their seven exons with respect to the number and position of intron/exon boundaries in relation to structural/functional domains within the polypeptides. The predominance of IL-1β gene expression over that of IL-1α in most cells may be accounted for by the presence of a more efficient set of typical eukaryotic promoter elements found in association with the IL-1β gene.

There is mounting evidence that multiple levels of control (transcriptional, posttranscriptional, and posttranslational) are exercised on the expression of the IL-1β gene. This stringent control on protein production may have evolved to curtail the biological activity of a very potent molecule. Although little is yet known about the molecular basis of monocyte stimulation, the kinetics of IL-1β mRNA induction in response to LPS and PMA stimulation of the human monocytic leukemia cell line (THP-1) are sufficiently different to suggest separate membrane receptor/transduction systems. The IL-1β gene promoter is extremely powerful and upmodulates several hundredfold within 2–3 hr following LPS stimulation. The IL-1β mRNA levels then fall rapidly to a stable plateau about 20 times background. This transient spike of IL-1β transcription is somewhat reminiscent of nuclear proto-oncogene expression (e.g., *c-myc, c-fos*) (45,28) and similarly was found to be superinducible under conditions of cycloheximide inhibition. Consistent with the observed data, we have proposed a model for the stringent transcriptional control of IL-1β gene expression based on two distinct protein factors, one activator and one repressor (27).

The evidence for posttranscriptional regulation of IL-1 gene expression via alternate splicing of mRNA is at the present only circumstantial. However the posttranslational control of both IL-1 precursor processing and active peptide transport through the cell membrane are clearly points at which the biological impact of IL-1 is regulated. The precise mechanism by which IL-1 leaves the monocyte is still poorly understood. Recent studies indicate that proteolytic processing of the 31-kDa proIL-1β molecule is probably coupled to transport (2,3), yielding a 23-kDa intermediate before release of bona fide 17-kDa IL-1β. The serine proteases elastase (41), and plasmin (9) have been implicated in this processing, and inhibitors of serine protease activity (e.g., PMSF) prevent this degradation (48). The human monocyte has been demonstrated to be a source of both elastase and plasminogen activator as well as their respective serpins (42,43). Our recent isolation of a novel Arg-serpin clone from a stimulated monocyte cDNA library has suggested that expression of biologically fully active IL-1 may be regulated at the level of posttranslational processing and transport by an elegant homeostatic mechanism involving cosynthesis of the required protease together with a specific inhibitor. Experiments currently in progress should serve to test this hypothesis.

ACKNOWLEDGMENTS

We are extremely grateful to Dr. Patrick Gray (Genentech, Inc.), Dr. Lee Gehrke, Dr. Stephen Jobling, and Dr. Matthew Fenton (MIT) for permission to relate some of their unpublished results. The indispensable contributions of Burton Clark, Melinda Gandy, Kathleen Collins, and Brian McDonald to the experiments performed in our laboratories are gratefully acknowledged. We also thank Dr. Charles Dinarello, Dr. Sheldon Wolff, and Dr. Alexander Rich for their assistance in carrying out this work. We thank Kay Leland for her photographic expertise. Our studies on IL-1 were supported by grants from Cistron Biotechnology, Inc., Pine Brook, New Jersey, the Whitaker Health Sciences Fund, Cambridge, Massachusetts, and the National Institutes of Health (AI00595).

REFERENCES

1. Dinarello, C. A. (1984). Interleukin-1. *Rev. Infect. Dis. 6*:51–95.
2. Auron, P. E. and Webb, A. C. (1987). Molecular biology of interleukin 1. *Lymphokines* (in press).
3. Oppenheim, J. J., Kovacs, E. J., Matsushima, K., and Durum, S. K. (1986). There is more than one interleukin 1. *Immunol. Today 7*:45–56.
4. Dinarello, C. A. (1986). Interleukin-1: Amino acid sequences, multiple biological activities, and comparison with tumor necrosis factor (cachectin). *Year Immunol. 2*:69–90.
5. March, C. J., Mosley, B., Larsen, A., Cerretti, P., Braedt, G., Price, V., Gillis, S., Henney, C. S., Kronheim, S. R., Grabstein, K., Conlon, P. J., Hopp, T. P., and Cosman, D. (1985). Cloning, sequence and expression of two distinct human interleukin-1 complementary DNAs. *Nature 315*: 641–647.
6. Auron, P. E., Webb, A. C., Rosenwasser, L. J., Mucci, S. F., Rich, A., Wolff, S. M., and Dinarello, C. A. (1984). Nucleotide sequence of human monocyte interleukin 1 precursor cDNA. *Proc. Natl. Acad. Sci. USA 81*:7907–7911.
7. Lomedico, P. T., Gubler, U., Hellman, C. P., Dukovich, M., Giri, J. G., Pan, Y. E., Collier, K., Semionow, R., Chua, A. O., and Mizel, S. B. (1984). Cloning and expression of murine interleukin-1 cDNA in *Escherichia coli. Nature 312*:458–462.
8. Gery, I. and Lepe-Zuniga, J. L. (1984). Interleukin 1: Uniqueness of its production and spectrum of activities. *Lymphokines 9*:109–125.
9. Matsushima, K., Taguchi, M., Kovacs, E. J., Young, H. A., and Oppenheim, J. J. (1986). Intracellular localization of human monocyte associated interleukin 1 (IL 1) activity and release of biologically active IL 1 from monocytes by trypsin and plasmin. *J. Immunol. 136*:2883–2891.
10. Matsushima, K., Durum, S. K., Kimball, E. S., and Oppenheim, J. J. (1985). Purification of human interleukin-1 from human monocyte culture supernatants and identity of thymocyte comitogenic factor, fibroblast proliferation factor, acute phase protein inducing factor, and endogenous pyrogen. *Cell. Immunol. 92*:290–301.
11. Mizel, S. B. (1982). Interleukin 1 and T cell activation. *Immunol. Rev. 63*:51–72.
12. Clark, B. D., Collins, K. L., Gandy, M. S., Webb, A. C., and Auron, P. E. (1986). Genomic sequence for human prointerleukin-1 beta: Possible evolution from a reverse transcribed prointerleukin-1 alpha gene. *Nucl. Acids Res. 14*:7897–7914.

13. Furutani, Y., Notake, M., Fukui, T., Ohue, M., Nomura, H., Yamada, M., and Nakamura, S. (1986). Complete nucleotide sequence of the gene for human interleukin 1 alpha. *Nucl. Acids Res. 14*:3167-3179.
14. Webb, A. C., Collins, K. L., Auron, P. E., Eddy, R. L., Nakai, H., Byers, M. G., Haley, L. L., Henry, W. M., and Shows, T. B. (1986). Interleukin-1 gene (IL1) assigned to long arm of human chromosome 2. *Lymphokine Res. 5*:77-85.
15. Auron, P. E., Rosenwasser, L. J., Matsushima, K., Copeland, T., Dinarello, C. A., Oppenheim, J. J., and Webb, A. C. (1985). Human and murine interleukin 1 possess sequence and structural similarities. *J. Mol. Cell. Immunol. 2*:169-177.
16. Soares, M. B., Schon, E., Henderson, A., Karathanasis, S. K., Cate, R., Zeitlin, S., Chirwin, J., and Efstradiatis, A. (1985). RNA-mediated gene duplication: The rat preproinsulin I gene is a functional retroposon. *Mol. Cell. Biol. 5*:2090-2103.
17. Weiner, A. M., Deininger, P. L., and Efstratiadis, A. (1986). Nonviral retroposons: Genes, pseudogenes, and transposable elements generated by the reverse flow of genetic information. *Ann. Rev. Biochem. 55*: 631-661.
18. Schaffner, W. (1985). In *Eukaryotic Transcription: The Role of cis and Transacting Elements in Initiation.* Edited by Y. Gluzman. Cold Spring Harbor Laboratory, New York, pp. 1-18.
19. Furutani, Y., Notake, M., Yamayoshi, M., Yamagishi, J., Nomura, H., Ohue, M., Furuta, R., Fukui, T., Yamada, M., and Nakamura, S. (1985). Cloning and characterization of the cDNAs for human and rabbit interleukin-1 precursor. *Nucl. Acids Res. 13*:5869-5882.
20. Dayhoff, M. O., ed. (1979). *Atlas of Protein Sequence and Structure*, Vol. 5, Suppl. 3, National Biomedical Research Foundation, Washington, D.C.
21. Dayhoff, M. O., Barker, W. C., and Hunt, L. T. (1983). Establishing homologies in protein sequences. *Methods Enzymol. 91*:524-545.
22. Toh, H., Hayashida, H., and Miyata, T. (1983). Sequence homology between retroviral reverse transcriptase and putative polymerases of hepatitis B virus and cauliflower mosaic virus. *Nature 305*:827-829.
23. Rosenwasser, L. J., Webb, A. C., Clark, B. D., Irie, S., Dinarello, C. A., Gehrke, L., Wolff, S. M., Rich, A., and Auron, P. E. (1986). Expression of biologically active IL-1 subpeptides by transfection of simian COS cells. *Proc. Natl. Acad. Sci. USA 83*:5243-5246.
24. Ghiara, P., Antoni, G., Perin, F., Presentini, R., Tagliabue, A., Censini, S., Volpini, G., and Boroschi, D. (1986). T cell activation induced by a synthetic peptide fragment of human interleukin-1. *Fed. Proc. 45*:849.
25. Jobling, S. A. and Gehrke, L. (1987). Enhanced translation of chimeric messenger RNAs containing a plant viral untranslated leader sequence. *Nature* (in press).

26. Krakauer, T. and Oppenheim, J. J. (1983). Interleukin 1 production by a human acute monocytic leukemia cell line. *Cell. Immunol. 80*: 223–229.
27. Fenton, M., Clark, B., Collins, K., Rich, A., Webb, A., and Auron, P. (1986). Expression of the human IL-1β gene in THP-1 cells following LPS stimulation. (Abstr.) Progress in Immunology IV, Sixth International Congress of Immunology, Toronto, Ontario, Canada.
28. Mitchell, R. L., Zokas, L., Schreiber, R. D., and Verma, I. M. (1985). Rapid induction of the expression of proto-oncogene *fos* during human monocytic differentiation. *Cell 40*:209–217.
29. Greenberg, M. E., Hermanowski, A. L., and Ziff, E. B. (1986). Effect of protein synthesis on growth factor activation of c-*fos*, c-*myc*, and actin gene transcription. *Mol. Cell. Biol. 6*:1050–1057.
30. Zullo, J. N., Cochran, B. H., Huang, A. S., and Styles, C. D. (1985). Platelet-derived growth factor and double-stranded ribonucleic acids stimulate expression of the same genes in 3T3 cells. *Cell 43*:793–800.
31. Parker, P. J., Coussens, L., Totty, N., Rhee, L., Young, S., Chen, E., Stabel, S., Waterfield, M. D., and Ullrich, A. (1986). The complete primary structure of protein kinase C—the major phorbol ester receptor. *Science 233*:853–859.
32. Leff, S. E., Rosenfeld, M. G., and Evans, R. M. (1986). Complex transcriptional units: Diversity in gene expression by alternative RNA processing. *Ann. Rev. Biochem. 55*:1091–1117.
33. Rosenwasser, L. J., Auron, P. E., Gehrke, L., Clark, B., McDonald, B., Bradley, B., Epstein, E., Collins, K., and Webb, A. (1986). In *Biologically Based Immunomodulators in the Therapy of Rheumatic Diseases.* Edited by S. Pincus, D. Pisetsky, and L. J. Rosenwasser. Elsevier Scientific Publishers, New York (in press).
34. Windt, M. R. and Rosenwasser, L. J. (1984). Human vascular endothelial cells produce interleukin-1. *Lymphokine Res. 3*:281.
35. Wagner, C. R., Vetto, R. M., and Burger, D. R. (1985). Expression of I-region associated antigen (Ia) and interleukin 1 by subcultured human endothelial cells. *Cell. Immunol. 93*:91–104.
36. Miossec, P., Cavender, D., and Ziff, M. (1986). Production of interleukin 1 by human endothelial cells. *J. Immunol. 136*:2486–2491.
37. Libby, P., Ordovas, J. M., Auger, K. R., Robbins, A. H., Birinyi, L. K., and Dinarello, C. A. (1986). Endotoxin and tumor necrosis factor induce interleukin-1 gene expression in adult human vascular endothelial cells. *Am. J. Pathol. 124*:179–186.
38. Le, J., Weinstein, D., Gubler, U., and Vilcek, J. (1986). Induction of membrane-associated interleukin 1 by tumor necrosis factor in human fibroblasts. (Abstr.) Congress on Research in Lymphokines and Other Cytokines, Basic Biology and Strategies for Clinical Application, Boston, Mass.

39. Blobel, G. and Dobberstein, B. (1975). Transfer of proteins across membranes. II. Reconstitution of functional rough microsomes from heterologous components. *J. Cell Biol.* *67*:852–861.
40. Lepe-Zuniga, J. L., Zigler, J. S., Zimmerman, M. L., and Gery, I. (1985). Differences between intra- and extracellular interleukin-1. *Mol. Immunol.* *22*:1387–1392.
41. Neblock, D. S., Dondero, R. S., Koch, G. A., Lavelli, T. J., Lisi, P. J., Malavarca, R. H., and Zivin, R. A. (1986). In *Biologically Based Immunomodulators in the Therapy of Rheumatic Diseases.* Edited by S. Pincus, D. Pisetsky, and L. J. Rosenwasser. Elsevier Scientific Publishers, New York (in press).
42. Vassalli, J.-D., Dayer, J.-M., Wohlwend, A., and Belin, D. (1984). Concomitant secretion of prourokinase and of a plasminogen activator-specific inhibitor by cultured human monocytes-macrophages. *J. Exp. Med.* *159*:1653–1668.
43. Remold-O'Donnell, E. (1985). A fast-acting elastase inhibitor in human monocytes. *J. Exp. Med.* *162*:2141–2155.
44. Carrell, R. and Travis, J. (1985). α_1-Antitrypsin and the serpins: Variation and countervariation. *Trends Biochem. Sci.* *10*:20–24.
45. Greenberg, M. E. and Ziff, E. B. (1984). Stimulation of 3T3 cells induces transcription of the c-*fos* proto-oncogene. *Nature* *311*:433–438.
46. White, B. A. and Bancroft, F. C. (1982). Cytoplasmic dot hybridization; a simple analysis of relative mRNA levels in multiple small cell and tissue samples. *J. Biol. Chem.* *257*:8569–8572.
47. Gray, P. W., Glaiser, D., Chen, E., Goeddel, D. V., and Pennica, D. (1986). Two interleukin 1 genes in the mouse: Cloning and expression of the cDNA for murine interleukin 1β. *J. Immunol.* *137*:3644–3648.
48. Auron, P. E., Warner, S. J. C., Webb, A. C., Cannon, J. G., Bernheim, H. A., McAdam, K. J. P. W., Rosenwasser, L. J., LoPresk, G., Mucci, S. F., and Dinarello, C. A. (1987). Studies on the molecular nature of human interleukin 1. *J. Immunol.* *138* (in press).

8

Characterization of the Plasma Membrane Interleukin-1 Receptor

STEVEN K. DOWER
Immunex Corporation, Seattle, Washington

Interleukin-1 (IL-1) is a term that has been applied to an activity, or group of activities, found in supernatants obtained from activated primary macrophages, or macrophage cell lines such as the murine cell line $P388D_1$ (1). The classic IL-1 biological activity, that of inducing thymocyte proliferation, is termed lymphocyte-activating factor, or LAF (2,3). Several other biological activities however, have been found to copurify with LAF activity, these include endogenous pyrogen (4), osteoclast-activating factor (5), catabolin (6), and a fibroblast growth factorlike activity (7). In addition, IL-1 has been implicated in upregulation of interleukin-2 (IL-2) production, antigen presentation, B-cell proliferation, acute-phase protein release from hepatocytes, release of prostaglandin from fibroblasts, and release of prostacyclins from vascular endothelial cells (8). Broadly, this spectrum of biological activities is consistent with a role for IL-1 as a soluble mediator of inflammatory responses. However the diversity of these activities raises the possibility that IL-1 may play a fundamental role in physiological homeostasis (9).

One unusual feature of IL-1 action is the wide range of cell types responsive to this hormone and the different types of response elicited from them (8). This has led to the suggestion that IL-1-like activity might be possessed by two or more different polypeptide hormones. This hypothesis has been confirmed in several laboratories, both by purification to homogeneity of proteins with IL-1 activity and by isolation of cDNA clones encoding such proteins (10–14). The available structural evidence indicates that IL-1 polypeptides fall into two families, termed IL-1α and IL-1β, and that in all species so far examined there exists both an α and a β form of the hormone. Both α and β IL-1s are initially synthesized as ca. 30,000-M_r polypeptides that are processed to 17,000-M_r polypeptides before, or during secretion from cells (10,13,29,41). Current efforts, using both natural and recombinant forms of IL-1α and IL-1β, are directed toward defining the relative contributions of these two hormones to the various biological activities previously associated with IL-1. Some functional dissociation between the two proteins is certainly possible because comparison between the cDNA sequences of the human IL-1s shows that they are only distantly related (13).

Both forms of IL-1 can elicit profound changes in cellular metabolism at very low concentrations (13). Furthermore, it has been demonstrated that IL-1-responsive cells can absorb IL-1 activity from IL-1-containing supernatants (15). Both of these considerations suggest that the IL-1s, as do other polypeptide hormones, exert effects on cells through specific plasma membrane receptor molecules. Our laboratory initially characterized such receptors on the murine T-lymphoma line LBRM-33-1A5 (16), using iodinated human IL-1β as a probe. More recently, we have compared the receptors on the LBRM-33-1A5 cell line with those on Balb/c 3T3 cells, and found them to be similar (17). We have also exolored the relationship between the binding of human IL-1α and human IL-1β to cells. These latter studies have shown that IL-1α and IL-1β bind to the same receptor on both murine and human cells (18). Finally, studies in progress show that IL-1α and IL-1β differ in their processing requirements for expression of biological activity; IL-1 can bind to the receptor and produce biological effects as the 30,000-M_r initial translation product, whereas IL-1β requires processing to the 17,500-M_r form to be active.

In this chapter we review and summarize our previous studies on plasma membrane IL-1 receptors and demonstrate that on all cell types yet examined, the biological actions of both forms of IL-1 appear to be mediated through an approximately 80,000-M_r cell surface receptor protein.

METHODS

Production, Purification, and Radiolabeling of Natural and Recombinant Human Interleukin-1

Natural interleukin-1β (nIL-1β) was purified from activated human peripheral blood monocyte supernatants by a series of three conventional column chromatography steps, as described by Kronheim et al. (19). The final preparation contained a single 17.5-kDa polypeptide, as determined by SDS-polyacrylamide gel electrophoresis (SDS-PAGE), amino acid analysis, and protein sequencing (13). This protein preparation was radiolabeled with ^{125}I using di-[^{125}I] iodo-Bolton-Hunter reagent (16).

Recombinant human interleukin-1α (rIL-1α) and interleukin-1β (rIL-1β) cDNAs were constructed to encode proteins corresponding to the secreted forms of the hormones, as described elsewhere (13). These cDNAs were placed in expression vectors and used to produce the recombinant proteins in *Escherichia coli*, as described previously (13).

The rIL-1α and rIL-1β were purified from *E. coli* cultures, as described elsewhere (20). Purified rIL-1β was labeled with di-[^{125}I] iodo-Bolton-Hunter reagent. Purified rIL-1α was labeled with sodium [^{125}I] iodide using a chloramine-T method (18). The SDS-PAGE analysis of iodinated nIL-1β, rIL-1β, and rIL-1α, showed that each of the three ligand preparations contained a single 17,500-M_r radiolabeled polypeptide (Fig. 1).

Assays of Interleukin-1 Biological Activity

Interleukin-1 biological activity was measured in two types of biological assay. The first, the 1A5 conversion assay (21) measures the capacity of IL-1, in combination with 0.1% phytohemaglutinin (PHA), to elicit IL-2 production from mitomycin C-treated LBRM-33-1A5 cells (a mouse T-lymphoma cell line). The IL-2 produced is assayed by its capacity to maintain proliferation of CTLL-2, a murine T cell line that requires this hormone for growth. The second assay measured the fibroblast growth factorlike activity of IL-1, using Balb/c 3T3 cells, a mouse fibroblast line. The assay used was based on that described by Schmidt et al. (7).

Binding Assays and Data Analysis

Assays for quantitation of site numbers and affinities of IL-2 binding to cells were carried out by mixing suspension of cells with radiolabeled IL-1 in 150 μl of RPMI 1640 containing 1% bovine serum albumin (BSA), 0.1% sodium azide, and 20 mM HEPES pH 7.4 (binding medium). Incubations were done for 2 hr at 9°C in 96-well, round-bottomed microtiter plates on a rocker platform. Nonspecific binding was measured in parallel using samples containing cells, ^{125}I-labeled IL-1, and a 100-fold molar excess of unlabeled IL-1. Kinetic experiments were carried out in the same fashion, except that 15-ml centrifuge tubes were used for the incubations: time zero was defined as the time when cells were added. At the end of the incubation period, cells and bound ligand were separated from unbound

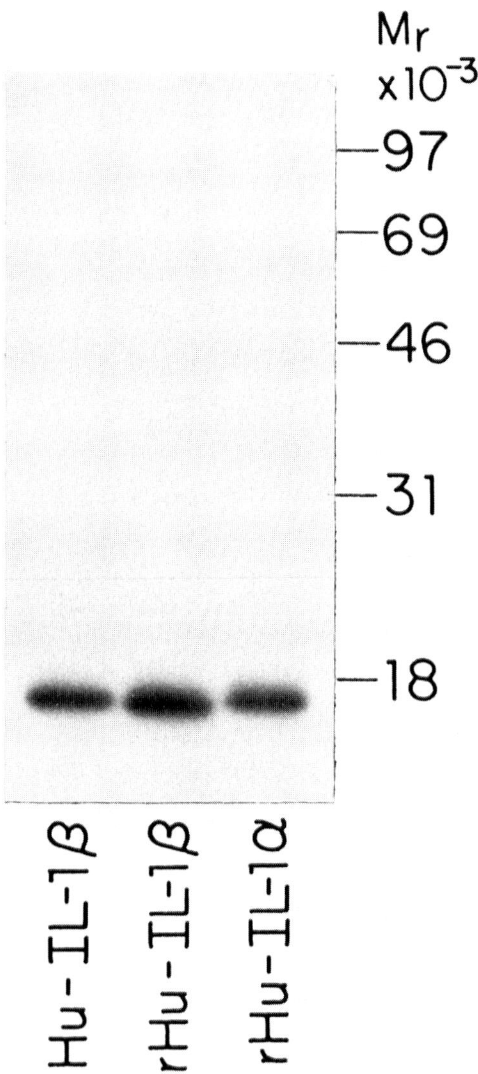

Figure 1 SDS-PAGE of radiolabeled IL-1 preparations: The ^{125}I-labeled IL-1 preparations were boiled for 3 min in sample buffer containing 5% 2-mercaptoethanol and subjected to electrophoresis on a 10–20% gradient polyacrylamide gel as described previously (16). The positions of various molecular-weight markers are indicated at the left.

ligand by a phthalate oil centrifugation method, as described previously (22,23).

Binding and kinetic data were expressed as bound (molecules of IL-1/cell) and free (IL-1, molar) calculated from the cell concentration used and the specific activity of the ligand (cpm/mmole).

All mathematical modeling was done using RS/1 (Bolt, Barenak, and Newman) a scientific data management package running on a VAX 1170 under VMS. Parameter values were estimated by nonlinear least-squares fitting of kinetic or equilibrium-binding models, described elsewhere (23), to the appropriate data sets. When it was necessary for the purpose of illustration to convert direct-binding data into the Scatchard coordinate system, the best-fit line or curve was calculated from the parameter values estimated by analyzing the data in the form of bound versus free IL-1.

Estimation of the Size of the Interleukin-1 Receptor by Affinity Cross-linking

Details of the method used for affinity cross-linking human ^{125}I-labeled nIL-1β to LBRM-33-1A5 cells have been given elsewhere (16). Briefly, cells were incubated with ^{125}I-labeled nIL-1β in the presence or absence of unlabeled nIL-1β, washed and treated with disuccinimidyl suberate (DSS), dithiobissuccinimidyl propionate (DSP), or disuccinimidyl tartate (DST). After a 1 hr cross-linking treatment, the cells were washed, extracted with phosphate-buffered saline (0.15) pH 7.4 containing Triton X-100 (1%) and protease inhibitors, and the extracts analyzed by SDS-PAGE in 8% slab gels (24,25).

CHARACTERIZATION OF THE INTERLEUKIN-1 RECEPTOR ON MURINE T CELLS

For the initial characterization of the plasma membrane IL-1 receptor, we chose to use the murine T-lymphoma cell line LBRM-33-1A5, because these cells had been extensively studied for IL-1 responsiveness in our laboratory (15,21).

Figure 2 illustrates the association kinetics of ^{125}I-labeled rIL-1α (panel A) and ^{125}I-labeled nIL-1β (panel B) with LBRM-33-1A5 cells. In panel C, the rate constants derived by fitting an exponential association model (23) to the data are plotted against the IL-1 concentration for both forms of IL-1. The exchange kinetics of α and β IL-1 with the cells are very similar, as shown by the similar slopes and intercepts of the rate plots in

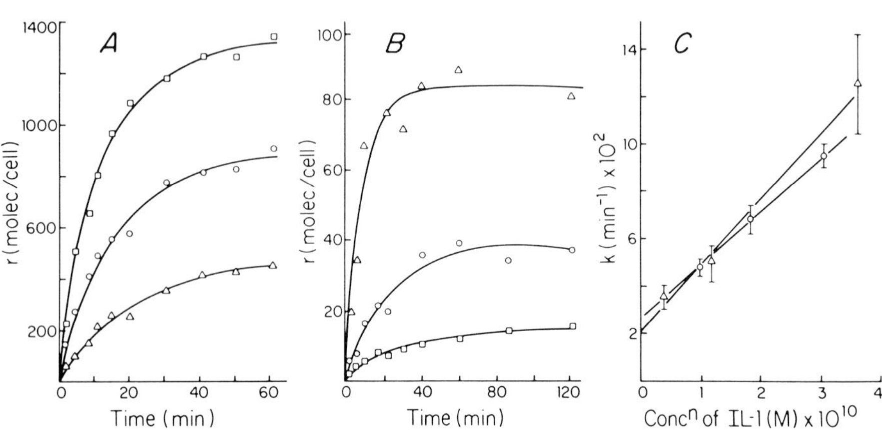

Figure 2 Association kinetics of IL-1α and IL-1β with LBRM-33-1A5 cells: (A) Cells (6.7×10^7 cells/ml) were incubated with 3.1×10^{-10} M (open squares), 1.8×10^{-10} M (open circles), or 9.8×10^{-11} M (open triangles) rIL-1α at 8°C for the indicated times. Nonspecific binding measured in the presence of 1.6×10^{-6} M unlabeled rIL-1α was 2.0×10^{12} molecules/cell/M. (B) Cells (5.3×10^7 cells/ml) were incubated with 3.6×10^{-10} M (open triangles), 1.2×10^{-10} M (open circles), or 3.54×10^{-11} M (open squares) nIL-1β for the indicated times. Nonspecific binding measured in the presence of 6×10^{-9} M unlabeled nIL-1β was 1.15×10^{11} molecules/cell/M. (C) Plot of the association rate constant k_r, against the molar concentration of ^{125}I-labeled IL-1 initially present in the medium for nIL-1β (open triangles) and rIL-1α (open circles).

panel C. The linearity of the plots, plus the close agreement between the theoretical best-fit curves and the experimental data shown in panels A and B, suggest that both forms of IL-1 are interacting with a single class of sites on the cell surface (26). The differences in the Y axes in panels A and B are because the experiments for IL-1α and IL-1β were done with different preparations of LBRM-33-1A5 cells. Parameter values estimated from fitting an exponential association model to the data in panel C are given in Table 1. The ratios for the forward and reverse rate constants yield an approximate estimate of the affinity of the ligand for its receptor and suggest that the K values of IL-1α and IL-1β for the LBRM-33-1A5 cells are similar.

Table 1 Kinetic Parameters[a] for Interaction of rIL-1α and nIL-1β with LBRM-33-1A5

	rIL-1α	nIL-1β
k_+ (M^{-1} min^{-1})	$2.32 \pm 0.01 \times 10^8$	$2.8 \pm 0.3 \times 10^8$
k_- (min^{-1})	$2.5 \pm 0.2 \times 10^{-2}$	$2.1 \pm 0.6 \times 10^{-2}$
k (M^{-1})	$0.9 - 1.0 \times 10^{10}$	$0.9 - 2.0 \times 10^{10}$

[a]Parameters were derived by analyzing the data in Fig. 2 as described in Materials and Methods.

A practical use of the results of the association kinetics experiment is to estimate how long it is necessary to incubate IL-1 with these cells for the system to become close to equilibrium. The reaction rate becomes slower as the concentration of ligand is decreased but cannot be less than k_- (23). Here, one can estimate that for the reaction to reach 95% of the infinite-time-bound value for either form of IL-1 at 8°C should take no longer than 110–140 min. For convenience we have chosen to use an incubation time of 2 hr. The results of such an equilibrium-binding experiment, in which three radiolabeled IL-1 preparations (nIL-1β, rIL-1β, and rIL-1α) were compared for binding to the same LBRM-33-1A5 cell preparation, is shown in Fig. 3. The data were fit with a simple equilibrium-binding model and the parameter values given in Table 2 were thus estimated. These values were used to calculate the continuous curves passing through the data in both panels of Fig. 3. The data reveal that while the three ligand preparations bind to the cells with differing affinities, the order being rIL-1α > nIL-1β > rIL-1β, all three forms of IL-1 detect similar numbers of high-affinity sites. While this is to be expected for nIL-1β and rIL-1β, it raises the possibility that α and β IL-1 bind to the same receptor on murine T cells. As a final comment on the binding data; the number of receptors for the IL-1s on the LBRM-33-1A5 cells in this experiment (approximately 3×10^3) is relatively low for a polypeptide hormone. However in an extensive series of binding assays with these cells, the average number of receptors was found to be even lower (approximately 500 sites per cell) and the numbers measured in different experiments fluctuated considerably (16,18). It is reasonable to suppose that the instability of the IL-1 receptor number on these cells is related to the

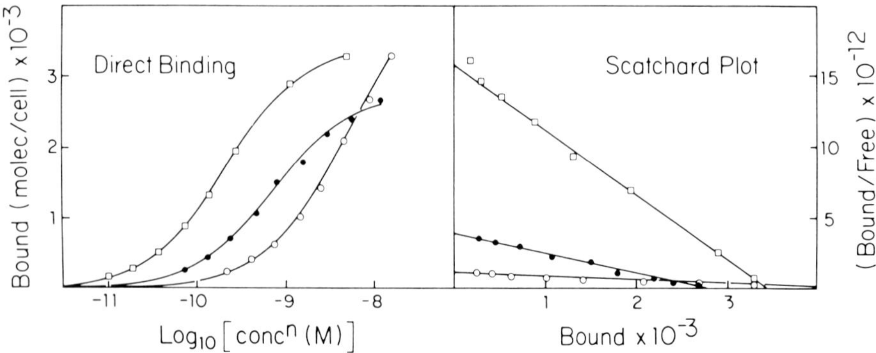

Figure 3 Comparison between the binding of nIL-1β (closed circles), rIL-1β (open circles), and rIL-1α (open squares) to LBRM-33-1A5 cells: Cells (1.8×10^7/ml) were incubated with various concentrations of radiolabeled IL-1s as described in the methods section. Nonspecific binding was measured in the presence of 5.7×10^{-7} M unlabeled homologous IL-1 in each case. The continuous curves passing through the data were calculated from the best-fit parameter values given in Table 2.

fact that its expression is not required for continued proliferation. Indeed, the cells can be maintained indefinitely in media that contain no detectable IL-1 activity, nor do we have any evidence that these cells produce endogenous IL-1.

The similarity in site numbers on LBRM-33-1A5 cells (see Fig. 3) raised the possibility that α and β IL-1 interact with the same receptor. To examine this directly, the cross-competition experiment on LBRM-33-1A5 cells shown in Fig. 4 was conducted. In this experiment each form of IL-1 (nIL-1β, rIL-1β, and rIL-1α) in turn was used as an ^{125}I-labeled probe. For each labeled IL-1, all three forms of the unlabeled hormone were used as competitors. The data were fit with a competitive inhibition model (26), using the K values from Table 2, and hence the values for maximal inhibition and K_I for each labeled IL-1/unlabeled IL-1 pair were estimated. The values of M, K and K_I obtained for each were used to calculate the curves passing through the data. Several features of the data in Fig. 4 are consistent with the hypothesis that there is a single class of IL-1 receptors on the LBRM-33-1A5 cells that binds both α and β IL-1. First, regardless of which form of the hormone is radiolabeled, all three forms of the unlabeled competitor produce close to 100% inhibition of binding. Second,

Table 2 Equilibrium Binding Parameters[a] for the Interaction of nIL-1β, rIL-1β, and rIL-1α with LBRM-33-1A5 Cells

From binding of ^{125}I-labeled IL-1s

Ligand	Sites/cell × 10^{-3}	$K(M^{-1}) \times 10^{-9}$	Nonspecific binding (molec./cell/M) × 10^{-10}
nIL-1β	2.8 ± 0.1	1.4 ± 0.1	13 ± 1
rIL-1β	3.2 ± 0.2	0.3 ± 0.02	12 ± 4
rIL-1α	3.43 ± 0.02	4.6 ± 0.7	13 ± 2

From cross-competition experiments

Inhibitor		^{125}I-labeled IL-1			
		nIL-1β	rIL-1β	rIL-1α	Average
nIL-1β	$K_I(M^{-1}) \times 10^{-9}$	2.8 ± 0.3	5.9 ± 0.6	3.4 ± 0.4	4.0 ± 1.8
Maximum inhibition	(%)	98 ± 3	82 ± 2	97 ± 3	92 ± 9
rIL-1β	$K_I(M^{-1}) \times 10^{-9}$	1.2 ± 0.1	2.2 ± 0.3	2.0 ± 0.4	1.8 ± 0.3
Maximum inhibition	(%)	97 ± 2	94 ± 1	96 ± 4	96 ± 2
rIL-1α	$K_I(M^{-1}) \times 10^{-9}$	9.9 ± 0.5	14.3 ± 0.8	9.7 ± 0.2	11.3 ± 2.1
Maximum inhibition	(%)	108 ± 2	97 ± 1	104 ± 5	103 ± 6

[a]Parameter values were obtained by nonlinear least-squares fitting as described elsewhere (18,23).

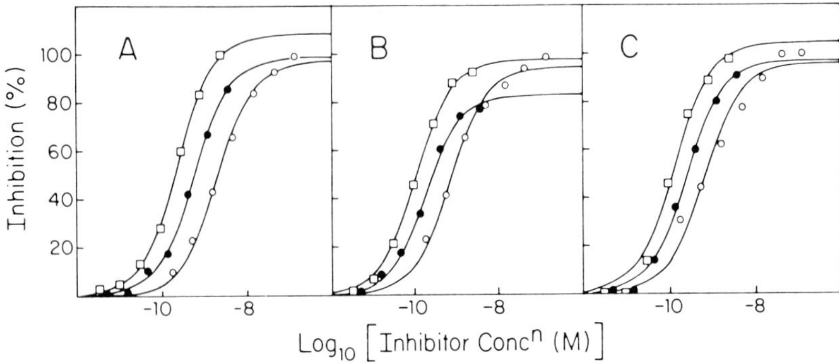

Figure 4 Cross-competition between IL-1α and IL-1β for the IL-1 receptor on LBRM-33-1A5 cells: Cells (3.1×10^7/ml) were incubated with mixtures of labeled and unlabeled IL-1s. Concentration of labeled IL-1s used were (A) nIL-1β 3.9×10^{-10} M, (B) rIL-1β 1.9×10^{-9} M, and (C) rIL-1α 9.2×10^{-10} M. All data are corrected for nonspecific binding measured in the presence of 5.6×10^{-7} unlabeled homologous IL-1 in each case. Dose-response curves in each panel are for unlabeled nIL-1β (closed circles), rIL-1β (open circles), and rIL-1α (open squares). Continuous curves are calculated using the best-fit parameter values given in Table 2.

in all cases the model produces a good fit to the data, as judged by the fact that the curves in Fig. 4 pass through the data. This shows that a model based on one class of noncooperative sites is an adequate description of the system. Third, irrespective of which IL-1 preparation is labeled the relationship between the midpoints of the inhibition dose-response curves remains the same, i.e., the K_I values are in the order rIL-1α > nIL-1β > rIL-1β (see Table 2), showing that there is no detectable subpopulation of receptors capable of preferentially binding one form of the hormone. Finally, the relationship between the inhibition dose-response curves for the unlabeled IL-1s in Fig. 4 is the same as that for the radiolabeled preparations (Fig. 3). Taken together, the data in Figs. 3 and 4 clearly show that there is a single type of IL-1 receptor on the LBRM-33-1A5 cells and that it binds both α and β IL-1.

We have extended this type of analysis to human B cells (18), to murine and human fibroblasts, and in a more limited study to both in vitro-propagated human T-cell lines and activated human peripheral blood mononuclear cells. The data are always consistent with the hypothesis that the cells bear a single type of IL-1 receptor that binds both α and β IL-1.

The IL-1 receptor on LBRM-33-1A5 cells is specific for IL-1 as indicated by the experiment summarized in Table 3. The data show, using ^{125}I-labeled human nIL-1β as a probe, that unlabeled nIL-1β will inhibit probe binding to cells, but that a series of other hormones, including IL-2, IL-3, platelet-derived growth factor (PDGF), and fibroblast growth factor (FGF), do not.

To further characterize the molecular basis of IL-1 specific binding by murine T cells, we performed the affinity cross-linking experiment illustrated in Fig. 5. The basis for such an experiment is the notion that if a labeled polypeptide hormone is avidly bound to cells via a surface receptor polypeptide, then treatment of those cells with a bivalent cross-linking reagent will form covalent complexes from some of the noncovalent complexes, and that this species will migrate with the sum of the molecular weights of hormone and receptor on denaturing SDS gels. The method has the advantage, as compared with affinity precipitations from surface or biosynthetically labeled cells that the only labeled species in the system is the ligand. Hence there is no background in the analysis. This method however, has been found to give rise to rather variable results, different laboratories working in the same system obtaining different molecular weight ratio (M_r) values for the same receptor (27). To increase our confidence in the results, we performed the cross-linking experiment shown in Fig. 5 with three different cross-linkers (DSS, DSP, DST) and analyzed the cell extracts using SDS-PAGE both under reducing (B) and nonreducing (A) conditions. In five of the six conditions, a prominent band appeared at an M_r of 97,000, in addition to that at 17,500 resulting from noncovalently cell-bound nIL-1β. This species was not detected when unlabeled nIL-1β was added as competitor, nor was it present if no cross-linker was used (lanes 1 and 2). It was also not detected when DSP cross-linked extracts were analyzed under reducing conditions, showing that it resulted from attachment of the ^{125}I-labeled nIL-1β via cross-linker to a second protein, because DSP contains a disulfide bond and is cleaved by reduction. This species was detected whether or not protease inhibitors were included in the extraction buffer and within 10 min after addition of cross-linker; it presumably represents ^{125}I-labeled nIL-1β cross-linked to an M_r 79,500 cell surface protein. In addition to this species, DSS-treated samples analyzed under reducing conditions showed a second species of M_r 133,000. We do not know whether this is a ternary complex of IL-1β with p 79.5 and a 36,000 M_r protein, or a complex of IL-1β with an M_r 115,000 protein. This species is also present, albeit to a lesser extent, in the extracts of DST-treated cells, analyzed under reducing conditions. There are

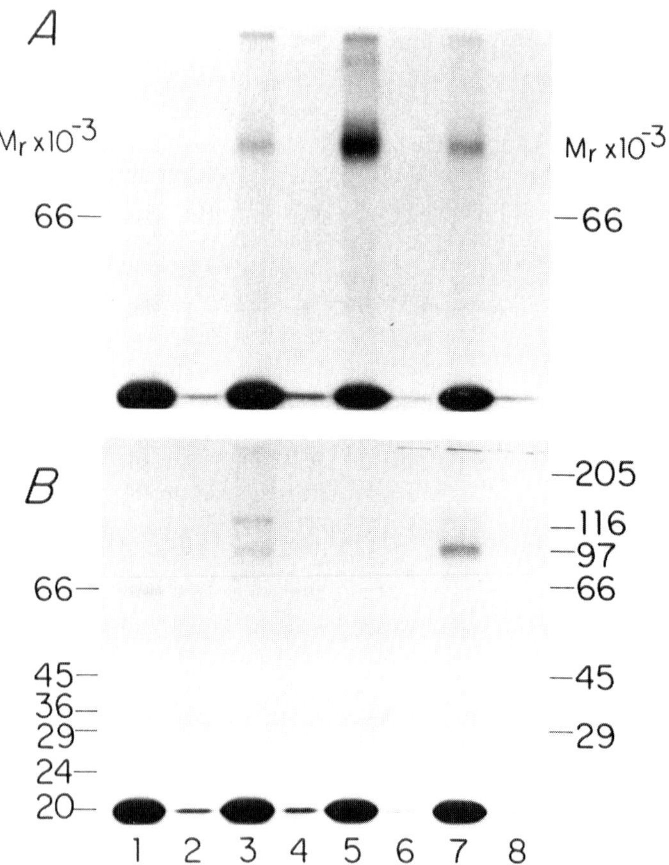

Figure 5 Determination of the molecular size of IL-1 receptor by affinity cross-linking: (A) Samples were denatured in the absence of reducing agent. (B) Samples were denatured in the presence of mercaptoethanol. The LBRM-33-1A5 cells (6.7×10^7/ml) were incubated with 5.5×10^{-10} ^{125}I-labeled nIL-1β alone (lanes 1, 3, 5, and 7) or with 5.5×10^{-10} ^{125}I-labeled nIL-1β and 1.8×10^{-8} M nIL-1β (lanes 2, 4, 6, and 8). Cells were then washed and treated with PBS (lanes 1 and 2), or 1 mg/ml DSS in PBS (lanes 3 and 4), or 1 mg/ml DSP in PBS (lanes 5 and 6), or 1 mg/ml DST in PBS (lanes 7 and 8). Finally, all samples were washed and extracted with PBS containing 1% Triton X-100 and the extracts analyzed by SDS-PAGE. The molecular size positions were estimated using standards run in a parallel track.

Table 3 Specificity of IL-1 Receptors on LBRM-33-1A5 Cells

Inhibitor	Conc^n (M)	^{125}I-labeled IL-1β (M)	I (%)
IL-1β	2×10^{-8}	3.6×10^{-10}	100 ± 1
IL-1β	2×10^{-9}	3.6×10^{-10}	87 ± 4
TSH	1.2×10^{-7}	3.6×10^{-10}	17 ± 4
PDGF	1.2×10^{-7}	3.6×10^{-10}	15 ± 2
EGF	6×10^{-7}	3.6×10^{-10}	11 ± 10
hu LH	3 μg/ml[a]	3.6×10^{-10}	15 ± 10
hu GH	1.7×10^{-7}	3.6×10^{-10}	9 ± 14
Porcine insulin	6×10^{-7}	3.6×10^{-10}	15 ± 13
NGF	7×10^{-8}	3.6×10^{-10}	9 ± 5
FSH	3 μg/ml[a]	3.6×10^{-10}	5 ± 19
hu IL-2	2.4×10^{-7}	3.6×10^{-10}	6 ± 0
mu IL-3	3.0×10^{-9}	3.6×10^{-10}	15 ± 3
FGF	6×10^{-7}	3.6×10^{-10}	5 ± 3

[a]All incubations were performed at 8°C for 2 hr. Some hormone preparations were only partially pure; concentrations of these are given in μg/ml of total protein.

also higher molecular weight species present in the extracts, these are due to highly cross-linked material accumulating in sample wells or at the interface between the stacking gel and the running gel. In summary, the affinity cross-linking data are consistent with a minimal model for the IL-1 receptor as a single polypeptide chain of M_r 79,500. However it is clear from the data that the receptor may be a more complex structure.

CELLULAR DISTRIBUTION OF INTERLEUKIN-1 RECEPTORS

We have surveyed a variety of primary cells and cell lines for expression of specific interleukin-1 receptors, using human ^{125}I-labeled nIL-1β as a probe. Table 4 summarizes the results of these studies. For some cells (see Table 4, footnote) a complete binding analysis was done; however usually, measurements were done at a single ^{125}I-labeled nIL-1β concentration. This suffices to establish the presence of receptors and to give an approximate estimate of their abundance.

Table 4 Cellular Distribution of IL-1 Receptors

Primary cells

Species	Cell type	IL-1 (M)[b]	(Molecules/cell) bound
mouse	thymocytes	4×10^{-10}	<10
mouse	thymocytes PNA^+ fraction	4×10^{-10}	<10
mouse	thymocytes PNA^- fraction	4×10^{-10}	27 ± 5
mouse	spleen cells	4×10^{-10}	<10
mouse	lymph node cells	4×10^{-10}	<10
human	peripheral blood mononuclear cells	4×10^{-10}	27 ± 1
human	T-cell line	4×10^{-10}	100 ± 0
human	gingival fibroblasts	–	4.9×10^3 [a]

In vitro cell lines

Species	Cell type	Designation	IL-1 (M)[b]	(Molecules/cell) bound
mouse	T-lymphoma	LBRM-33-1A5	–	550 ± 570[a]
mouse	T-lymphoma	LBRM-33-5A4	4×10^{-10}	<10
mouse	T-lymphoma	EL-4	5×10^{-10}	185 ± 81
mouse	fibroblast	L929	10^{-9}	144 ± 28
mouse	fibroblast	SC-1	5×10^{-10}	1850 ± 112

human	T-lymphoma	Jurkat-FHCRC	4×10^{-10}	<10
human	T-lymphoma	HSB-2	4×10^{-10}	79 ± 5
human	T-leukemia	PEER	5×10^{-10}	<10
human	monocyte	U937	4×10^{-10}	<10
human	myelogenous leukemia	KG-1	4×10^{-10}	<10
human	erythroleukemia	K562	4×10^{-10}	<10
human	promyelocyte	HL-60	4×10^{-10}	<10
human	myeloma	ARH77	5×10^{-10}	330 ± 3
human	B-lymphoma	BMB	5×10^{-10}	540 ± 0
human	melanoma	A375	–	465 ± 25[a]
human	hepatoma	HEP-2	–	540[a]
rat	fibroblast	XC	5×10^{-10}	450 ± 22
rat	hepatoma	HEP-2	–	540[a]
rat	epithelial cell	HTC	–	510[a]
bovine	endothelial cell	CPAE	–	750[a]

[a]Binding was tested with a complete ^{125}I-labeled nIL-1β dose-response curve.
[b]Concentration of ^{125}I-labeled nIL-1β used to test for the presence of receptors. All data are corrected for nonspecific binding of radiolabeled ligand measured in the presence of at least 1×10^{-8} M unlabeled IL-1.

The data show that the IL-1 receptor is a widely distributed cell surface protein, being found on cells from differing lineages; in general, fibroblasts, both primary diploid fibroblasts and cell lines, show the highest level of expression. Further, the pattern of receptor expression matches that previously reported for interleukin-1 biological action, i.e., the cells that express receptors are those previously reported to be IL-1 responsive.

In the particular case of murine lymphoid cells, it is striking that the only population that we have examined that shows detectable levels of IL-1 receptors is the PNA$^-$ fraction of thymocytes. It is this subpopulation of thymocytes that has previously been shown to respond to IL-1 (28). It is curious, given the role as an early signal previously ascribed to interleukin-1 in peripheral blood T-cell activation, that murine spleen cells appear to bear no detectable receptors. However this apparent discrepancy may be resolved by some preliminary data from our laboratory, which suggest that IL-1 receptor expression on murine spleen cells increases markedly upon activation with concanavalin A (S. K. Dower and P. J. Morrissey, unpublished data). If IL-1 receptor expression, as is IL-2 receptor expression, is an activation-driven phenomenon, this would also account for why receptors are easily detectable on some T-cell lines maintained in vitro by repeated stimulation with antigen.

COMPARISON BETWEEN THE INTERLEUKIN-1 RECEPTOR ON MURINE T CELLS AND MURINE FIBROBLASTS

Given the wide distribution of cell surface IL-1-binding sites on different types of cells, it was of interest to conduct a more detailed comparison between the receptors on two or more cell types. As two representative, but very different cell types, we chose to compare the receptors on LBRM-33-1A5 T-lymphoma cells with those on Balb/c 3T3, a murine fibroblast line. Figure 6 shows a comparison of direct binding of ^{125}I-labeled natural human IL-1β to these two cell lines (panel A), and inhibition of binding of this ligand by unlabeled nIL-1β and fibroblast growth factor (panel B), and finally a comparison of the sizes of the two receptors by affinity cross-linking with DSP (panel C). The results of analysis of these data are summarized in Table 5.

The data show that while the 3T3 cells bind ^{125}I-labeled nIL-1β with a similar affinity to that for LBRM-33-1A5 cells, these fibroblasts express more receptors than the T-lymphoma cells. Because IL-1 exhibits fibroblast growth factor-like activity, we compared inhibition of ^{125}I-labeled

Table 5 Comparison of IL-1 Receptors and Biological Action of nIL-1β on LBRM-33-1A5 Cells and Balb/c 3T3 Cells

Parameter[a]	LBRM-33-1A5	Balb/c 3T3
IL-1 receptors/cell	238 ± 16	4800 ± 500
K (M^{-1}) of ^{125}I-labeled nIL-1β	3.6 ± 0.4 × 10^9	2.1 ± 0.6 × 10^9
K_I for unlabeled nIL-1β (M[%])	7 ± 1 × 10^9 (99 ± 3)	2.6 ± 0.5 × 10^9 (98 ± 4)
Concentration of nIL-1β at half-maximal biological activity (M)	ca 5 × 10^{-14}	ca 5 × 10^{-11}
M_r of IL-1 receptor	ca 79,500	ca 78,000

[a]Parameter values were estimated from the data in Fig. 6 as described elsewhere (17).

nIL-1β binding by unlabeled nIL-1β with that by unlabeled purified fibroblast growth factor. The data show that although unlabeled IL-1β completely blocks binding of labeled IL-1, fibroblast growth factor shows little inhibition on either cell type (B) (see Table 3). The data suggest that the receptor on the fibroblasts, as is that on the T-lymphoma cells, is IL-1 specific. Finally, the affinity cross-linking experiment shown in panel C reveals that an approximately M_r 97,000 species is detected on both cells, although the M_r of the 3T3 cell receptor appears to be slightly less; subtraction of the M_r for nIL-1β suggests that the IL-1 receptor on 3T3 cells is about 78,000.

The results of the comparison show that the receptors for IL-1 on Balb/c 3T3 and LBRM-33-1A5 cells bind nIL-1β with similar affinities whether labeled or unlabeled hormone is used (see Table 5), and that the receptors have similar molecular weights. However when the biological response curves for the two types of cells are compared with the receptor-binding curves, as shown in Fig. 7, it can be seen that the former are quite different. It takes a far lower concentration of nIL-1β to drive the production of IL-2 by the T cells than to drive proliferation of the fibroblasts. This observation may not be surprising for two reasons. First, the types of response elicited from the two types of cell are quite different. Minimally with T cells the only consequence of IL-1 binding is activation of IL-2 gene transcription, whereas presumably a complex array of events must be brought into play in the fibroblasts to effect enhanced

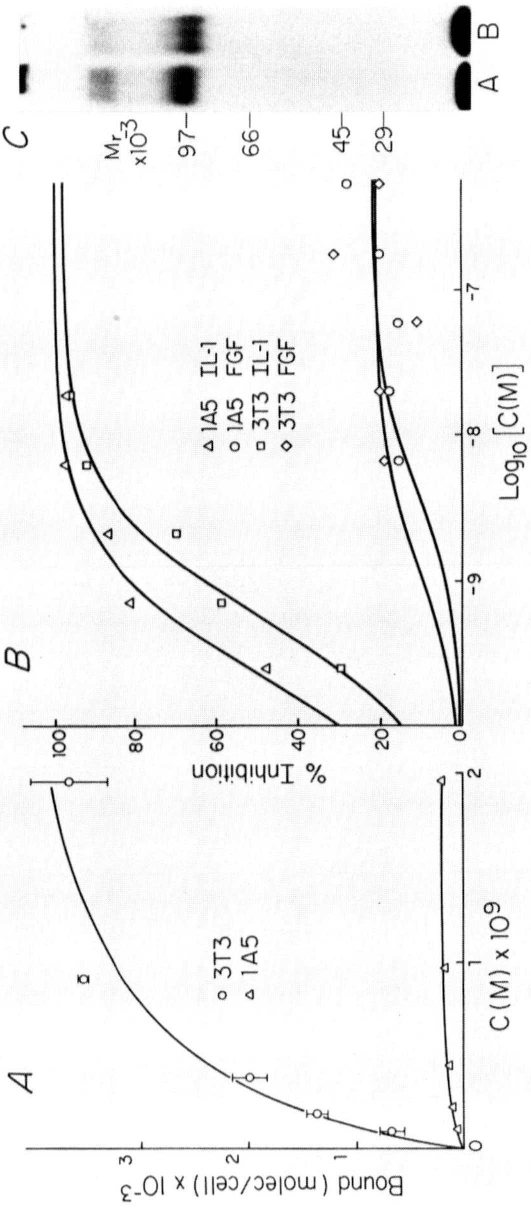
A
Bound (molec/cell) x 10-3
3
2
1
0
○ 3T3
△ 1A5
1
2
C (M) x 10^9
B
% Inhibition
100
80
60
40
20
0
△ 1A5 IL-1
○ 1A5 FGF
□ 3T3 IL-1
◇ 3T3 FGF
-9
-8
-7
Log10 [C(M)]
C
Mr x10-3
97—
66—
45—
29—
A
B

Figure 6 Comparison of the IL-1 receptors on murine T cells and murine fibroblasts: (A) Binding of ^{125}I-labeled nIL-1β to LBRM-33-1A5 cells and Balb/c 3T3 cells. LBRM-33-1A5 cells (open triangles) (7.3×10^7 cells/ml) or Balb/c 3T3 cells (open circles) (8.7×10^6 cells/ml) were incubated with various concentrations of ^{125}I-labeled nIL-1β. Nonspecific binding, measured in the presence of 1.9×10^{-8} M unlabeled nIL-1β was 1.7×10^{11} molecules/cell/M for the LBRM-33-1A5 cells and 2.7×10^{12} molecules/cell/M for the BALB/c 3T3 cells. All data shown have been corrected for these background values, by subtraction. The continuous curves passing through the data were generated from Eq. 3 with the best-fit parameter values given in Table 3. The error bars on the data points, given where error values exceed the symbol size, are calculated from duplicate measurements. (B) Specificity of nIL-1β binding to LBRM-33-1A5 and BALB/c 3T3 cells. LBRM-33-1A5 cells (open triangles and circles) (7.3×10^7 cells/ml) and BALB/c 3T3 cells (open squares and diamonds) (8.7×10^6 cells/ml) were incubated in the presence of 2.1×10^{-10} M ^{125}I-labeled nIL-1β and various concentrations of either unlabeled IL-1β (open triangles and squares) or fibroblast growth factor (open diamonds and circles). The continuous curves were calculated from the best-fit parameter values given in Table 3 using Eq. 4. Maximal binding for the 3T3 cells was 2050 molecules/cell, background was 564 molecules/cell; for the 1A5 cells maximal binding was 146 molecules/cell and the background was 35 molecules/cell. (C) Characterization of the IL-1 receptors on LBRM-33-1A5 cells and BALB/c 3T3 cells by affinity cross-linking: LBRM-33-1A5 cells (A) (1×10^7 cells) or BALB/c 3T3 cells (B) (2×10^7 cells) were incubated with ^{125}I-labeled nIL-1β (3.7×10^{-10} M) for 2 hr at 8°C. Cells were then washed, treated with DSP, extracted and analyzed by SDS-PAGE under nonreducing conditions as described in *Materials and Methods*. The molecular weight positions indicated in the right margin were estimated from standards run in a parallel track.

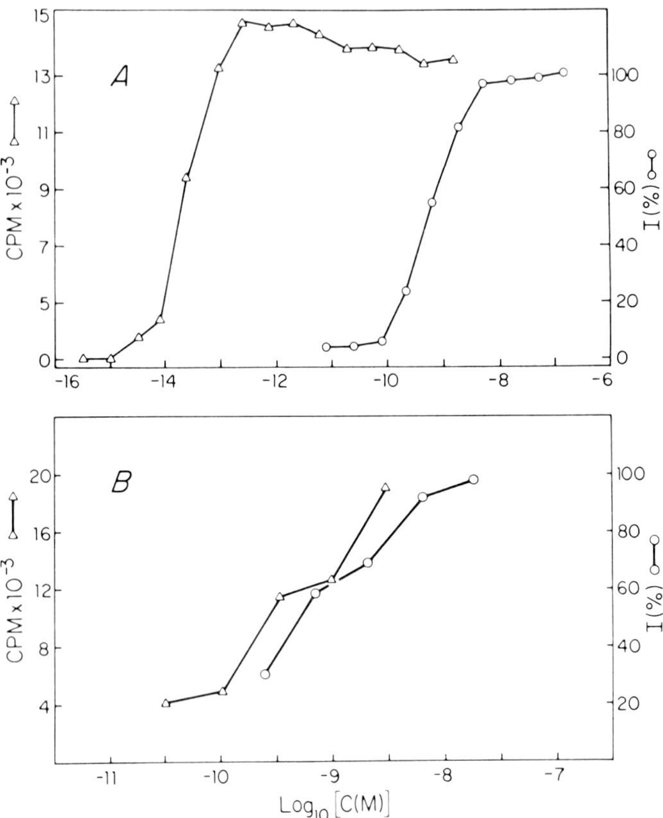

Figure 7 Comparison of the concentration dependence of nIL-1β activity and receptor binding on (A) LBRM-33-1A5 cells and (B) BALB/c 3T3 cells: (A) The IL-1-driven IL-2 production (open triangles) was measured in the standard IL-1 conversion assay as described elsewhere (21). Inhibition of binding of ^{125}I-labeled nIL-1β (open circles) was measured using 2.7×10^{-10} M ^{125}I-labeled nIL-1β and 1.1×10^{8} cells/ml. Maximum binding was 39 molecules ^{125}I-labeled nIL-1β per cell and background was 11 molecules/cell. (B) Proliferation of BALB/c 3T3 cells (open triangle) was measured as described in *Materials and Methods*, background in the presence of serum alone, has been subtracted from the data, and was 1.26×10^{4} cpm/well. The points are averages of duplicate cultures. The inhibition data (open circles) are taken from the experiment illustrated in Fig. 6B.

proliferation. Second, when IL-1 drives T-cell IL-2 production, e.g., the thymocyte proliferation assay, it takes 10^2–10^3 times higher levels to produce the effect than those for the LBRM-33-1A5 cells. The low level of IL-1 needed to elicit a response from the LBRM-33-1A5 is probably not representative of T cells because the LBRM-33-1A5 conversion assay was constructed to produce maximum sensitivity (21). Nevertheless, the data indicate that under appropriate conditions some mouse T cells can respond to IL-1 at about 10 molecules of hormone bound per cell. To understand the mechanism of signaling by the IL-1/IL-1 receptor complex and to establish the degree of homology between the IL-1 receptors expressed on different cell types (where they transmit apparently different signals), it will be necessary to obtain cDNA clones for the receptors from these various cell types.

RELATIONSHIP BETWEEN BINDING AND BIOLOGICAL ACTIVITY FOR THE INITIAL TRANSLATION PRODUCTS AND THE PROCESSED FORMS OF INTERLEUKIN-1α AND INTERLEUKIN-1β

Both IL-1α and IL-1β are encoded by mRNAs that specify initial translation products of about M_r 30,000 (10–13). There is also direct evidence that the primary translation product of the murine IL-1α gene produced in $P388D_1$ cells is M_r 30,000 (11). During release from cells, these proteins seem to be processed to yield the forms of about M_r 17,000 found in culture supernatants. Protein sequence data derived from the secreted forms of murine IL-1α (11,29) and human IL-1β (13) show that the NH_2-terminus of the α form of IL-1 lies at Ser-113, while that of the β form lies at Ala-117.

The biological activity of the β form of human IL-1 appears to be only expressed after the protein has been partially degraded to the M_r 17,000 form. Thus both Auron et al. (10) and March et al. (13) found little or no detectable biological activity encoded by the full-length IL-1β cDNA. Interleukin-1α, on the other hand, appears capable of being biologically active as the full-length protein of 271 amino acids, as in vitro translation of pA^+ mRNA from activated human monocytes yielded IL-1 activity and this was shown by cDNA cloning and sequencing to be due to IL-1α (13).

The data shown in Fig. 8 provide a mechanistic explanation for these observations. In this experiment, cDNAs encoding both the complete IL-1α and IL-1β proteins and truncated forms corresponding to the natural

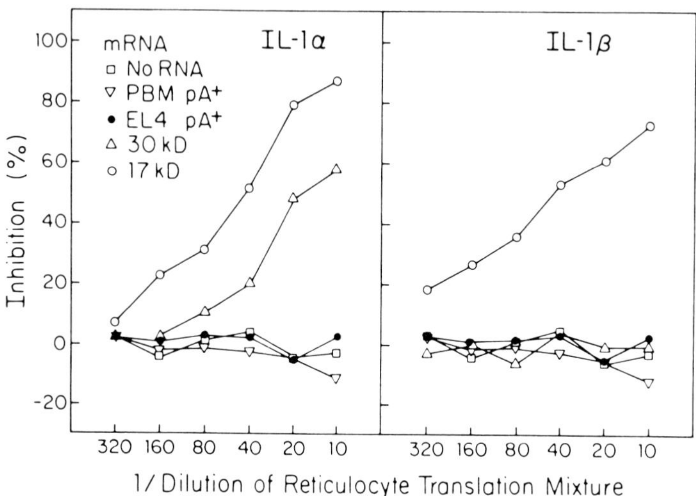

Figure 8 Inhibition of the binding of ^{125}I-labeled rIL-1α to LBRM-33-1A5 cells by reticulocyte translation mixtures containing IL-1 mRNAs: Reticulocyte translations were performed from the indicated RNA species as described elsewhere (40). The LBRM-33-1A5 cells (6×10^7/ml) were incubated with the indicated dilutions of translation mixtures and 1.8×10^{-9} M ^{125}I-labeled rIL-1α for 2 hr at 8°C. Nonspecific binding was measured in the presence of 10 μg/ml (5.7×10^{-7} M) unlabeled rIL-1α.

secreted proteins of approximately 17,000 M_r were used to make mRNAs in the SP6 in vitro transcription system. These mRNAs were then used to generate IL-1 proteins by in vitro translation, and translation mixtures were tested for IL-1 receptor-binding activity by the capacity to inhibit ^{125}I-labeled IL-1α binding to LBRM-33-1A5 cells. The data show that while both the full-length protein and the truncated 17,000-M_r form of IL-1α can bind to the interleukin-1 receptor on these cells, IL-1β only binds to receptors if it is truncated to about 17,000 M_r. In further experiments (39), it was found that the pattern of expression of biological activity matched that for receptor binding when the four IL-1 species were compared. Finally, we have eliminated the trivial explanation that the 271-residue initial translation product of the IL-1α gene is exquisitely protease-sensitive and breaks down to form the 17,000 M_r protein that is responsible for the binding and biological activity detected, by showing that in murine T cells exposed to the 30,000-M_r IL-1α translation mix labeled with [^{35}S]methionine, there is a prominent approximately 30,000 M_r IL-1 receptor-bound species cell-associated after extensive washing (39).

There have been many reports of forms of IL-1 with M_r values in the range of 30,000–40,000 (40). Our data indicate that the presence of the initial translation product of the IL-1α gene in culture supernatants may account for such observations.

CONCLUDING REMARKS

The interleukin-1 family of hormones exerts a wide range of biological activities on a diverse range of cell types, including T and B lymphocytes, hepatocytes, synovial cells, and fibroblasts (8). Current evidence indicates that the interleukin-1 family includes two molecules, IL-1α and IL-1β (10–14). These proteins share in common certain overall structural features, they are both initially translated as approximately 30,000 M_r polypeptides that are processed to polypeptides of approximately 17,000 M_r before, or during secretion from cells (13,31). Comparison of their primary sequences shows that human IL-1α and IL-1β are only distantly related, having 26% homology (13).

With this background, two features of the receptor component of this system are striking. First, on cells where the receptor has been characterized, it appears to be rather similar. While the structural information on the IL-1 receptor is at this point scanty, the data we have suggest that similar or even identical receptor molecules transduce IL-1 signals leading to quite different metabolic effects on different cell types (16–18). Second, the two forms of interleukin-1 both interact with the same receptor molecule with similar affinities (18). Structurally, this is surprising, given that the two IL-1 polypeptides are quite dissimilar at the primary sequence level. It is also curious from a biological standpoint, both because it runs contrary to the notion that different biological activities could be associated with the two forms of IL-1 and also because it raises the question of why the two forms of IL-1 are both produced in vivo. It would seem that if both IL-1s act via the same receptor, they must, of necessity, act on the same target cells. It may be however that cell types other than those we have examined possess receptors that are selective for one form of IL-1. Alternatively, the in vivo pharmacokinetic properties of the IL-1s may, for example, divide their roles between local and long-range actions or perhaps between homeostatis and more acute inflammatory responses.

At this point, we do not have the evidence to discriminate between these alternatives.

One feature of the IL-1α/IL-1β receptor system that we have noted on several occasions is the low levels of IL-1 receptors on all cells so far examined. The system shares this property in common with several others recently described, including tumor necrosis factor (30,31), interleukin-3 (32,33), GM colony-stimulating factor (34–37), and γ-interferon (38). It may be that by using recombinant DNA technology to characterize hormones present in the natural setting at very low concentrations, we are also finding a group of systems in which the receptors are present at low concentrations. This would seem to be logical, particularly for a hormone like interleukin-1 that has such a widespread distribution of biological effects and hence receptor-bearing cells among different tissues in the body and for which there is no specific organ capable of producing large quantities of the molecule. One would conclude, with hindsight, that for interleukin(s)-1 to exert systemic effects in the body after release from an area of damaged tissue it would be necessary for the many different IL-1-responsive cells to all bear low numbers of receptors.

ACKNOWLEDGMENTS

I would like to thank my colleagues at Immunex, many of whom have been involved in the characterization of the interleukin-1s and their receptor.

REFERENCES

1. Mizel, S. B. (1982). Interleukin-1 and T-cell activation. *Immunol. Rev. 63*:51.
2. Oppenheim, J. J. and Gery, I. (1982). Interleukin-1 is more than an interleukin. *Immunol. Today 3*:113.
3. Gery, I. and Waksman, B. H. (1972). Potentiation of T-lymphocyte response to mitogens. II. The cellular source of potentiating mediators. *J. Exp. Med. 136*:143.
4. Dinarello, C. A., Goldin, N. P., and Wolff, S. M. (1974). Demonstration and characterization of two distinct human leukocytic pyrogens. *J. Exp. Med. 139*:1369.
5. Dewhirst, F. E., Stashenko, P. P., Mole, J. E., and Tsurumachi, T. (1985). Purification and partial sequence of human osteoclast activating factor: Identity with interleukin-1β. *J. Immunol. 135*:2562.

6. Saklatvala, J., Sarsfield, S. J., and Townsend, Y. (1985). Pig Interleukin-1: Purification of two immunologically distinct leukocyte proteins that cause cartilage resorption, lymphocyte activation, and fever. *J. Exp. Med. 162*:1208.
7. Schmidt, J. A., Mizel, S. B., Cohen, D., and Green, I. (1982). Interleukin-1: A potential regulator of fibroblast proliferation. *J. Immunol. 128*:2177.
8. Dinarello, C. A. (1984). Interleukin-1. *Rev. Infect. Dis. 6*:51.
9. Powanda, M. C. (1985). The role of interleukin-1 in homeostatis. In *Progress in Leukocyte Biology Vol. 2, The Physiological, Metabolic, and Immunologic Action of Interleukin-1.* Edited by M. J. Kluger, J. J. Oppenheim and M. C. Powanda, Alan R. Liss, New York, p. 535.
10. Auron, P. E., Webb, A. C., Rosenwasser, L. J., Mucci, S. F., Rich, A., Wolff, S. M., and Dinarello, C. A. (1984). Nucleotide sequence of human monocyte interleukin-1 precursor cDNA. *Proc. Natl. Acad. Sci. USA 81*:7907.
11. Lomedico, P. T., Gubler, U., Hellman, C. P., Dukovich, M., Giri, J. G., Pan, Y.-C. E., Collier, K., Semionow, R., Chua, A. O., and Mizel, S. B. (1984). Cloning and expression of murine interleukin-1 cDNA in *Escherchia coli. Nature 312*:458.
12. Furukani, Y., Notake, M., Yamayoshi, M., Yamagishi, J., Nomura, H., Ohue, M., Furata, R., Fukui, T., Yamada, M., and Nakamura, S. (1985). Cloning and characterization of the cDNA's for human and rabbit interleukin-1 precursor. *Nucl. Acids Res. 13*:5869.
13. March, C. J., Mosley, B., Larsen, A., Cerretti, D. P., Braedt, G., Price, V., Gillis, S., Henney, C. S., Kronheim, S. R., Grabstein, K., Conlon, P. J., Hopp, T. P., and Cosman, D. (1985). Cloning, sequence and expression of two distinct human interleukin-1 complementary DNAs. *Nature 315*:641.
14. Van Damme, J., DeLey, M., Opdenakker, G., Billiau, A., DeSomer, P., and Van Beeumen, J. (1985). Homogenous interferon inducing 22 K factor is related to endogenous pyrogen and interleukin-1. *Nature 316*: 266.
15. Gillis, S. and Mizel, S. B. (1981). T-cell lymphoma model for the analysis of interleukin-1-mediated T-cell activation. *Proc. Natl. Acad. Sci. USA 78*:1133.
16. Dower, S. K., Kronheim, S. R., March, C. J., Conlon, P. J., Hopp, T. P., Gillis, S., and Urdal, D. L. (1985). Detection and characterization of high affinity plasma membrane receptors for interleukin-1. *J. Exp. Med. 162*:501.
17. Dower, S. K., Call, S. M., Gillis, S., and Urdal, D. L. (1986). Similarity between the interleukin-1 receptors on a murine T-lymphoma cell line and on a murine fibroblast cell line. *Proc. Natl. Acad. Sci. USA 83*:1060.

18. Dower, S. K., Kronheim, S. R., Cantrell, M., Deeley, M., Gillis, S., Henney, C. S., and Urdal, D. L. (1986). The cell surface receptors for interleukin-1α and interleukin-1β are identical. *Nature (London) 324*:266.
19. Kronheim, S. R., March, C. J., Erb, S. K., Conlon, P. J., Mochizuki, D. Y., and Hopp, T. P. (1985). Human interleukin-1: Purification to homogeneity. *J. Exp. Med. 161*:490.
20. Kronheim, S. R., unpublished observations.
21. Conlon, P. J. (1983). A rapid biologic assay for the detection of interleukin-1. *J. Immunol. 131*:1280.
22. Segal, D. M. and Hurwitz, E. (1977). Binding of affinity crosslinked IgG to cells bearing Fc receptors. *J. Immunol. 118*:1338.
23. Dower, S. K., Ozato, K., and Segal, D. M. (1984). The interaction of monoclonal antibodies with MHC class I antigens on mouse spleen cells. I. Analysis of the mechanism of binding. *J. Immunol. 132*:751.
24. Laemelli, V. K. (1970). Determination of protein molecular weight in polyacrylamide gels. *Nature 277*:680.
25. Urdal, D. L., Kawase, I., and Henney, C. S. (1982). NK cell-target interactions: Approaches towards definition of recognition structures. *Cancer Metast. Rev. 1*:65.
26. Dower, S. K., Titus, J. A., and Segal, D. M. (1984). The binding of multivalent ligands to cell surface receptors. In *Cell Surface Dynamics: Concepts and Models.* Edited by H. S. Perelson, C. DeLisi, and F. Weigel, Marcel Dekker, New York and Basel, p. 277.
27. Kunos, G., Kan, W. H., Greguski, R., and Venter, J. C. (1983). Selective affinity labelling and molecular characterization of hepatic α-adrenergic receptors with (^{3}H)-phenoxybenzanine. *J. Biol. Chem. 58*:326.
28. Conlon, P. J., Henney, C. S., and Gillis, S. (1982). Cytokine dependent thymocyte responses: Characterization of IL-1 and IL-2 target subpopulations and mechanism of action. *J. Immunol. 128*:797.
29. Giri, J. G., Lomedico, P. T., and Mizel, S. B. (1985). Studies on the synthesis and secretion of interleukin-1. I. A 33,000 molecular weight precursor for interleukin-1. *J. Immunol. 134*:343.
30. Kull, F. C., Jacobs, S., and Cuatrecasas, P. (1985). Cellular receptor for ^{125}I-labelled tumor necrosis factor: Specific binding, affinity labelling and relationship to sensitivity. *Proc. Natl. Acad. Sci. USA 82*:5756.
31. Rubin, B. Y., Anderson, S. L., Sullivan, S. A., Williamson, B. D., Carswell, E. A., and Old, L. J. (1985). High affinity binding of ^{125}I-labelled human tumor necrosis factor (LuK II) to specific cell surface receptors. *J. Exp. Med. 162*:1099.
32. Palaszynski, E. W. and Ihle, J. N. (1984). Evidence for specific receptors for interleukin-3 on lymphokine-dependent cell lines established from long-term bone marrow culture. *J. Immunol. 132*:1872.

33. Park, L. S., Friend, D., Gillis, S., and Urdal, D. L. (1986). Characterization of the cell surface receptor for a multi-lineage colony stimulating factor (CSF-2α). *J. Biol. Chem. 261*:205.
34. Walker, F. and Burgess, A. W. (1985). Specific binding of radioiodinated granulocyte-macrophage colony stimulating factor to hemopoetic cells. *EMBO J. 4*:933.
35. Gasson, J. C., Kaufman, S. E., Weisbaut, R. H., Tomonaga, M., and Golde, D. W. (1986). High affinity binding of granulocyte-macrophage colony stimulating factor to normal and leukemic human myeloid cells. *Proc. Natl. Acad. Sci. USA 83*:669.
36. Park, L. S., Friend, D., Gillis, S., and Urdal, D. L. (1986). Characterization of the cell surface receptor for granulocyte-macrophage colony stimulating factor. *J. Biol. Chem. 261*:4177.
37. Walker, F., Nicola, N. A., Metcalf, D., and Burgess, A. W. (1985). Hierarchical down-modulation of hemopoetic growth factor receptors. *Cell 43*:269.
38. Sarkar, F. H. and Gupta, S. L. (1984). Receptors for human γ-interferon: Binding and crosslinking of ^{125}I-labelled recombinant human γ-interferon to receptors on WISH cells. *Proc. Natl. Acad. Sci. USA 81*:5160.
39. Mosley, B., Urdal, D., Prickett, K. S., Larsen, A., Cosman, D., Conlon, P. J., Gillis, S., and Dower, S. K. (1986). The IL-1 receptor binds the human IL-1α precursor but not the IL-1β precursor. *J. Biol. Chem.* (in press).
40. Oppenheim, J. J., Kovacs, E. J., Matsushima, K., and Durum, S. K. (1986). There is more than one interleukin-1. *Immunol. Today 7*:45.
41. Cosman, D., Deeley, M. C., Kronheim, S. R., Hopp, T. P., Conlon, P. J., Gillis, S., and Mosley, B. (1987). Interleukin-1α: Cloning, expression, and biological activities. In *Recombinant Lymphokines and Their Receptors.* Edited by S. Gillis. Marcel Dekker, New York and Basel, p. 125.

9

cDNA Cloning, Expression, and Activity of Human Granulocyte-Macrophage Colony-Stimulating Factor

MICHAEL A. CANTRELL, DIRK M. ANDERSON, VIRGINIA L. PRICE, MICHAEL C. DEELEY, RANDELL T. LIBBY, KENNETH GRABSTEIN, DOUGLAS PAT CERRETTI, DIANE Y. MOCHIZUKI, ROBERT J. TUSHINSKI, and DAVID J. COSMAN
Immunex Corporation, Seattle, Washington

Granulocyte-macrophage colony-stimulating factor (GM-CSF) is a glycoprotein that is required for the growth and differentiation of hematopoietic progenitor cells into granulocytes and macrophages (1–3). There has been great interest in studying this protein both to determine more about its biological function and to ascertain its possible value as a therapeutic agent for antitumor therapy and control of immune system deficiencies.

The difficulty of isolating sufficient quantities of purified GM-CSF has led to interest in isolating the GM-CSF gene. Our group and others have now isolated and expressed cDNAs encoding GM-CSF (4–6). Use of recombinant GM-CSF (rGM-CSF) has aided in determining that this protein has neutrophil migration inhibition factor (NIF-T) activity (7), that in the presence of erythropoietin 1 it has burst-promoting activity for erythroid burst-forming units, and that it can stimulate the formation of multipotent colonies containing granulocytes, monocytes, erythroid cells, and megakaryocytes (8).

We here discuss the strategies we have used for isolation of the gene and its expression in yeast and *Escherichia coli.* Additionally, we describe a new activity of recombinant GM-CSF, namely its ability to stimulate macrophage-mediated killing of tumor cells.

MATERIALS AND METHODS

Construction of Yeast Expression Plasmids

A DNA fragment containing the coding sequence of mature GM-CSF was obtained by digesting (pHG23) (Fig. 1 and Ref. 4) with SfaNI, which cleaves near the mature NH_2-terminus, and NcoI, which cleaves in the 3′ noncoding region of the cDNA. This fragment was then engineered into the expression vectors (pαADH2HuGM) and (pYαfHuGM) (Fig. 2), designed for the synthesis and secretion of GM-CSF in yeast. All restriction enzyme, polymerase, and ligase reactions were performed according to manufacturer's procedures. DNA fragment purifications (ELUTIP-Schleicher and Schuell) and *E. coli* transformations were performed according to established procedures (9).

These vectors contain DNA sequences from (pBR322) for selection and replication in *E. coli* (the Ap^r gene and origin of replication) and yeast (the TRP-1 gene and 2-μ origin of replication). Expression of foreign genes is under control of the glucose repressible ADH2 promoter (10,11), obtained through the Washington Research Foundation, or the α-factor promoter (12,13). Adjacent to the promoter in both plasmids is the α-factor leader sequence sufficient to direct the secretion of heterologous proteins (13,14). The α-factor leader sequence had been modified by the addition of a second KEX2-processing site to allow complete processing of secreted protein (13). The SfaNI/NcoI human GM-CSF fragment was inserted in-frame with the α-factor leader peptide by means of a synthetic oligonucleotide recreating the amino-terminal coding region to the SfaNI site.

Growth of Yeast Strains

Saccharomyces cerevisiae strain 79 (α, *trp*1, *leu*2) was grown in either selective medium [YNB–trp, consisting of 0.67% yeast nitrogen base (Difco), 0.5% casamino acids, 2% glucose, 10 μg/ml adenine, and 20 μg/ml uracil] or rich medium (YPD, consisting of 1% yeast extract, 2% peptone, and 1% glucose supplemented with 80 μg/ml adenine and 80 μg/ml uracil). Yeast transformations were performed as described by Hinnen (15) selecting for Trp^+ transformants.

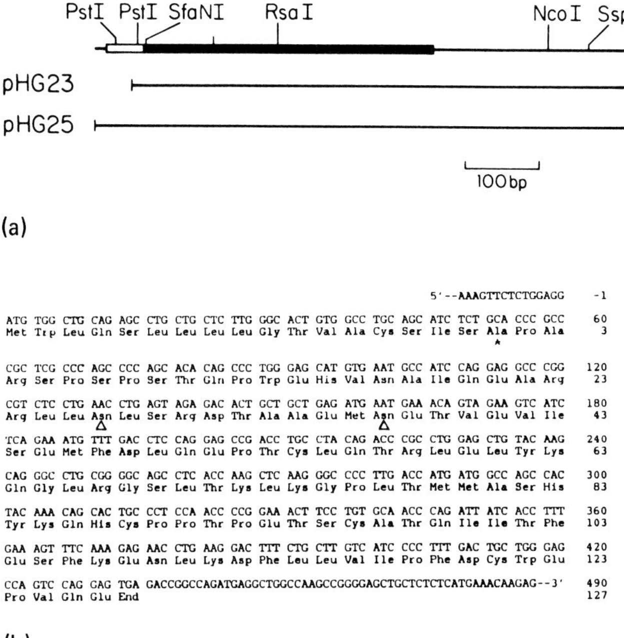

Figure 1 (a) Partial restriction map of human GM-CSF cDNA. Coding sequences are boxed: the open box represents the signal sequence and the shaded box represents the coding region for mature protein. The sizes of the cDNA inserts in (pHG23) and (pHG25) are indicated. (b) The nucleotide sequence and the predicted amino acid sequence for human GM-CSF. The cDNA sequence of the complete 5′ and 3′ untranslated regions is not shown. The nucleotides are numbered from the presumed initiator methionine codon. The amino acids are numbered from the amino-terminus of the mature protein (star; Ref. 5). Triangles indicate possible N-linked glycosylation sites.

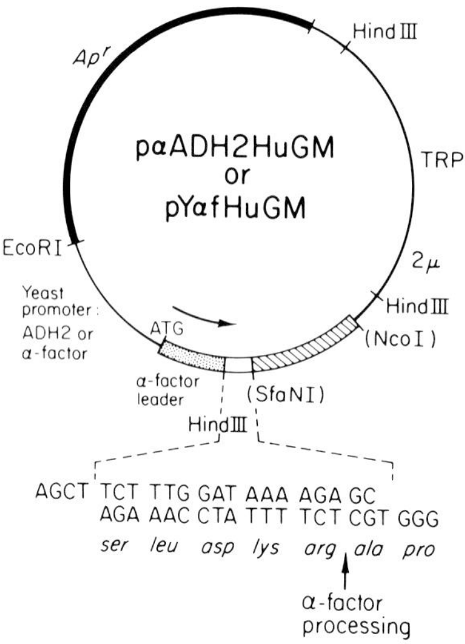

Figure 2 Structure of the yeast expression vectors (pαADH2HuGM) and (pYαfHuGM). The yeast-*E. coli* shuttle vector contains sequences from (pBR322) that allow selection (Ap^r) and replication in *E. coli* (thick lines), the yeast *TRP*-1 gene, and the 2 μ origin of replication for selection and autonomous replication in a trp1 yeast strain (thin lines). The small EcoRI to HindIII fragment includes the yeast α-factor promoter adjacent to the α-factor leader sequence, or alternatively, the ADH2 promoter adjacent to the α-factor leader. The synthetic oligonucleotides shown are used to fuse the α-factor sequences with GM-CSF sequences (hatched box). Restriction sites shown in parentheses were lost during construction.

Cultures were prepared for biological assay by inoculating 20–50 ml of rich medium with the appropriate strains and growing them at 30°C to the stationary phase. Cells were then removed by centrifugation, the medium was filtered through a 0.45 μm cellulose acetate filter, and phenylmethylsulfonyl fluoride was added (to 1 mM) to control proteolysis. Sterile supernatants were stored at 4°C.

Larger-scale fermentations were done in a 10 L New Brunswick Microferm fermentor. Cells were removed from the medium using a Millipore Pellicon filtration system.

Construction of *Escherichia coli* Expression Plasmids

A 525-bp fragment containing the GM-CSF-coding region was produced by NcoI digestion of (pHG23) followed by blunting with T4 polymerase and digestion with SfaNI. A vector fragment from (pLNIL2) (16) was produced by digestion with XbaI and StuI. This vector fragment was ligated with the GM-CSF-coding fragment and with synthetic oligonucleotides that have XbaI and SfaNI-compatible ends and that recreate the translation initiation sequence of (pLNIL2) and the first two codons of GM-CSF (Fig. 3). The resultant plasmid, (pLNGM), was transformed into *E. coli* strain RR1 (ATCC No. 31343) harboring the plasmid (pRK248cIts) (ATCC No. 33766, Ref. 17), a plasmid that is compatible for coexistence with (pLNGM) in *E. coli* and contains the bacteriophage lambda cI857 temperature-sensitive repressor of P_L. (pLNGM) was transferred into strain MM294 (pRK248cIts), which is $hsdR^-$, $hsdM^+$ (ATCC No. 33625) prior to transfer into CAG629(pACYC184cIts), which is $hsdR^+$ $HsdM^+$. CAG629 (a generous gift from Carol A. Gross, University of Wisconsin) is a derivative of *E. coli* strain SC122 (18) and has the genotype *lacZam trpam phoam* $supC^{ts}$ *malrpsL phe rel* lon^- $htpR^-$ tet^r. (pACYC184cIts) was constructed by inserting the 2.4-kb BglII DNA fragment containing the cI857 gene from bacteriophage lambda into (pACYC184) at the BamH1 site (19).

The construction of plasmids (pLB5001) and (pLB5001-4) is described in detail elsewhere (Libby et al., manuscript in preparation). Plasmid (pIN-III-ompA-3) (20) was received from Masoyori Inouye (SUNY, Stony Brook). A fragment from (pIN-III-ompA-3) was generated by BamHI digestion followed by treatment with AMV reverse transcriptase (Boehringer Mannheim) and EcoRI digestion. The vector fragment was ligated to the GM-CSF-coding region generated by SfaNI and SspI digestion of (pHG23), and to short synthetic oligonucleotides bearing EcoRI and SfaNI cohesive ends. The JM107 transformants containing the resultant plasmid, (pLB5001), expressed human GM-CSF with four additional amino-terminal amino acids. (pLB5001-4) (Fig. 4) producing the mature form of GM-CSF beginning with alanine-1 (see Fig. 1) was generated from (pLB5001) by in vitro mutagenesis (21) using an oligonucleotide 24 residues in length directing the deletion of 12 bp at the junction of *ompA* and GM-CSF-coding sequences. The nucleotide sequence in this region of (pLB5001-4) was confirmed using dideoxy sequencing (22).

The plasmid (pLNompGM) (see Fig. 3) was constructed by using the 625-bp fragment obtained from (pLB5001-4) by NcoI digestion, blunting

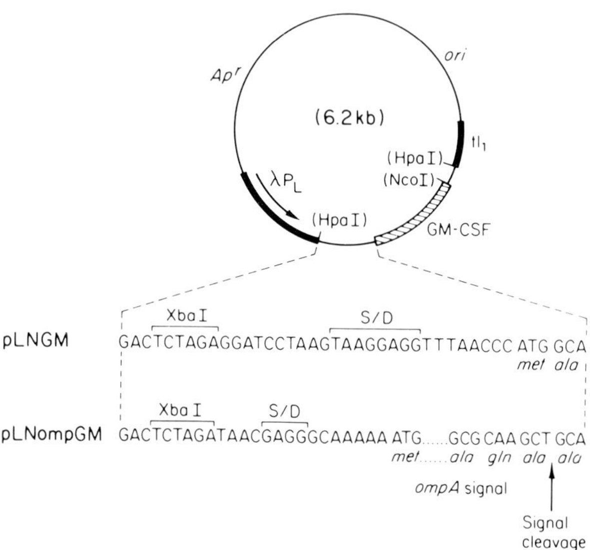

Figure 3 Structure of *E. coli* expression vectors using the P_L promoter. The plasmids differ only in the region between the P_L promoter and the transcription terminator (t11). The ampicillin resistance gene (Ap^r) and the origin of replication (*ori*) are derived from (pBR322). SD denotes the Shine-Dalgarno sequences. The alanine listed at the end of each oligonucleotide is the first alanine of mature GM-CSF. The dotted line in the (pLNompGM) oligonucleotide represents 51 nucleotides encoding the internal portion of the *ompA* signal (20).

with the Klenow fragment of *E. coli* polymerase I (Boehringer Mannheim) and XbaI digestion. This fragment was ligated to the XbaI and StuI-digested (pLNIL2) vector fragment described previously to produce (pLNompGM).

Expression of rGM-CSF in *E. coli*

The strains RR1(pRK248cIts) or CAG629(pACIC84cIts) containing (pLNGM) were propagated in LB (10 g yeast extract, 5 g tryptone, 5 g NaCl) or superinduction medium (SIM; 23) at 30°C using ampicillin, and tetracycline or chloramphenicol, respectively (9). Overnight cultures grown in SIM plus antibiotics were diluted 100-fold into the same medium and vigorously shaken until the A_{600} was 0.4–0.5.

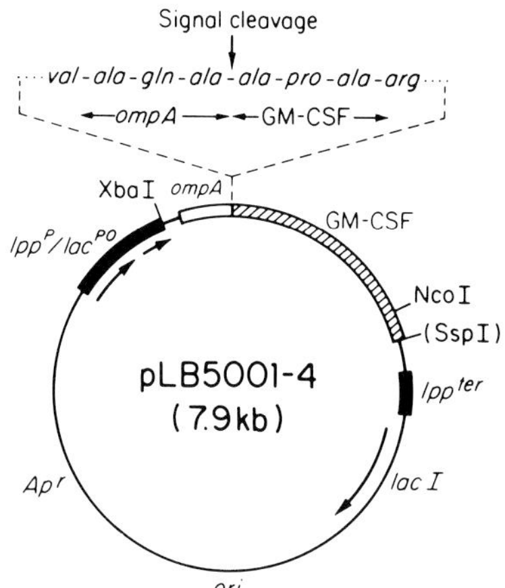

Figure 4 Structure of the *E. coli* expression vector (pLB5001-4). This plasmid is identical with the (pIN-III-ompA-3) vector (20), except for the region downstream of the *ompA* signal (clear box) that contains GM-CSF cDNA (hatched box). Abbreviations: ampicillin resistance (Ap^r), origin of replication (*ori*), hybrid *lpp* promoter and *lac* promoter-operator (lpp^{P}/lac^{PO}), *lpp* transcriptional terminator (lpp^{ter}) and *lac* repressor gene (*lacI*).

The cultures were then induced by temperature shift to 42°C and 1-ml samples were removed at various times, centrifuged, and frozen as previously described (24). Cell pellets were resuspended for sodium dodecyl sulfate-polyacryamide gel electrophoresis (SDS-PAGE) and immunological analysis in SDS sample buffer containing β-mercaptoethanol (25) and visualized by either silver (26) or Coomassie blue R-250 staining (25). Duplicate cell pellets to be tested for biological activity were resuspended in 30 mM Tris (pH 7.5), 10 mM EDTA and frozen and thawed for three cycles in dry ice/methanol. Lysozyme (Sigma) was then added to 200 μg/ml, the samples were incubated at 4°C or 37°C for 30 min, sonicated briefly to reduce viscosity and filter sterilized before biological assay.

Strains JM107(pLB5001-4) and JM107(pRK248cIts)(pLNompGM), which contain secretion vectors, were propagated and induced in M9MAM medium [M9 medium (9) with 0.4% glucose, 22 μg/ml methionine, 0.02X methionine assay medium (Difco), and 5 μg/ml thiamine] plus appropriate antibiotics. The strain containing (pLNompGM) was induced and harvested as described for (pLNGM). The strain containing (pLB5001-4) was prepared for induction as described previously with the exception that all growth was at 37°C and induction was begun by the addition of 2 mM IPTG (Bethesda Research Laboratories).

All *E. coli* samples discussed were harvested under growth conditions and at times after induction that maximized production of GM-CSF for that particular strain and expression plasmid.

Generation of Rabbit Antihuman GM-CSF Antiserum

New Zealand adult, female rabbits were immunized subcutaneously with 250 μg of yeast-produced rGM-CSF protein emulsified in Freund's complete adjuvant, subcutaneously (SC) in two sites. Approximately 1 month later, the animals were boosted with 200 μg of GM-CSF emulsified in Freund's incomplete adjuvant (FIA), SC in two sites. The animals were then bled every 2 weeks and the serum tested for GM-CSF antibodies by dot blot analysis. One rabbit demonstrated a modest titer to GM-CSF beginning at week 6, following the primary immunization. This animal was subsequently injected with an additional 100 μg of GM-CSF protein in FIA at week 12. Serum titers to GM-CSF were monitored over the course of immunization and for 8 weeks after (through week 20). Titers were consistently higher than 1:2500 against GM-CSF protein as assayed by dot blot analysis.

Generation of Monoclonal Antibody to GM-CSF

Balb/c female mice (8–12 weeks of age) were immunized with 50 μg of yeast-produced rGM-CSF protein emulsified in Freund's complete adjuvant subcutaneously, in the hind footpads. Approximately 3 weeks later an animal, showing reactivity to GM-CSF protein by dot blot (detailed later), was boosted with 100 μg of GM-CSF protein intravenously. Four days after the intravenous injection with GM-CSF, the animal was exsanguinated and the spleen cells fused to the myeloma cell line NS-1. Ten to fourteen days later, culture supernatants were tested for reactivity to human GM-CSF protein by the dot blot asday. Of approximately 600 wells tested, one hybridoma supernatant, designated 3G11, was consistently reactive to GM-CSF protein. Following cloning by limiting dilution, this cell line was further characterized and ascites produced. The resulting antibody preparation was then purified from ascites as described previously by Dower et al. (27).

Immunological Detection of rGM-CSF

The amount of rGM-CSF in conditioned yeast medium and *E. coli* extracts was determined quantitatively by enzyme-linked immunoabsorbent assay (ELISA) using the dot blot procedure described by Urdal et al. (28) and Conlon et al. (29) with the following variations. One-microliter aliquots of serially diluted yeast supernatants in phosphate-buffered saline (PBS) were spotted onto a nitrocellulose filter (Schleicher and Schuell BA85) alongside serial dilutions of homogeneous preparations of purified rGM-CSF. *Escherichia coli* extracts prepared by SDS lysis [2% SDS, 62.5 mM Tris (pH 6.8), 1% β-mercaptoethanol] were serially diluted in PBS containing 2% SDS. The filter was air dried and placed in "blocking" suffer consisting of 3% bovine serum albumin (BSA) in PBS for 1 hr. The filter was then sequentially exposed (30) to antihuman GM-CSF antibody 3G11, goat antimouse IgG conjugated to horseradish peroxidase, and color-developing solution according to the manufacturer's specifications (BioRad). Western blot analysis of total cellular protein of *E. coli* extracted with SDS lysis buffer containing 10% glycerol, boiled for 5 min and separated by SDS-PAGE was performed as described earlier following electrophoretic transfer (Hoeffer) to nitrocellulose sheets by methods supplied by the manufacturer. Quantitation of rGM-CSF content in *E. coli* extracts was also performed by Western blot analysis in which serial dilutions of samples were electrophoresed alongside dilutions of purified rGM-CSF standards. A single species of 3G11 reactive material of the predicted molecular mass was evident in the *E. coli* extracts. Control samples of either yeast supernatants or *E. coli* extracts prepared from non–rGM-CSF-producing cultures did not produce a 3G11-dependent signal in either immunological procedure.

Assay of Tumoricidal Activity

Human peripheral blood monocytes were prepared from Ficoll-Hypaque-purified peripheral blood leukocytes by Percoll density gradient centrifugation (31). These cells were then allowed to adhere in 96-well culture plates for 1 hr in RPMI with 5% fetal bovine serum. Nonadherent cells were removed by three washings. The adherent population was found to be greater than 95% monocytes as judged by Wright-Giemsa stain. Adherent cells were treated for 24 hr with the indicated additive, at which time the culture medium was replaced and [^{125}I] iododeoxyuridine-labeled A375 target cells were added. After an additional 72 hr, residual adherent A375 cells were harvested and counted. Earlier studies (32) showed that more than 90% of the ^{125}I present in the supernatants of these cultures is in soluble form and the rest is associated with dead cells and debris. Percentage cytotoxicity was calculated as: 100 × [1-(cpm in target cells cultured with activated monocytes/cpm in target cells cultured with control monocytes)].

RESULTS AND DISCUSSION

Complementary DNA Cloning and Analysis of the GM-CSF Gene

The procedures used for isolation and analysis of the human GM-CSF gene have been described (4). A DNA fragment from the coding region of a mouse GM-CSF cDNA was used to probe a human cDNA library. Clones were isolated that contained the entire coding region and most of the noncoding regions for human GM-CSF mRNA (see Fig. 1).

Ribonucleic acid from HUT-102 cells (an HTLV-I-transformed T-cell lymphoma) and from T lymphocytes activated with mitogen plus concanavalin A was analyzed by Northern blot using an SP6-derived GM-CSF-specific probe. A single size of mRNA of approximately 900 nucleotides was found. Analysis of genomic DNA by Southern hybridizations indicated that the GM-CSF gene is probably a single copy gene (4).

Expression of Recombinant GM-CSF in Yeast

GM-CSF has been synthesized and secreted by the yeast *S. cerevisiae* under control of either the α-factor promoter or the alcohol dehydrogenase 2 (ADH2) promoter and the α-factor leader peptide (see Fig. 2). The α-factor leader is a peptide of 84 amino acids capable of directing the secretion of foreign proteins (13,14). The yeast expression vector shown in Fig. 2 also contains sequences necessary for selection and replication in both *E. coli* and *S. cerevisiae.*

Appropriate yeast strains (*trp*$^-$) containing either (pYαfHuGM) or (pαADH2HuGM) (see Fig. 2) secrete mature, biologically active GM-CSF into the culture medium in very low amounts (Table 1, columns A and C). However significantly higher levels of cross-reacting material (CRM) are detected serologically by ELISA (see Table 1, columns B and D). Little or no GM-CSF activity could be demonstrated intracellularly.

It was thought that proteolytic degradation of the GM-CSF, perhaps during the secretory process, was a major factor limiting yields. During

Table 1 Production of Recombinant GM-CSF by Yeast

	μg Secreted GM-CSF/ml of medium			
	α-factor promoter		ADH2 promoter	
	A[a]	B[b]	C[a]	D[b]
GM-CSF (wild type)	0.05–0.07	4–6	0.5–1.0	20–30
GM-CSF (Leu-23)	0.5–1.0	2–3	5–13	25–35

[a]Fluorescamine assay of HPLC-purified, biologically active GM-CSF.
[b]Cross-reacting material detected by ELISA.

the secretory process, the α-factor leader is removed proteolytically by the KEX2 gene product after the dibasic residues Lys-Arg (33,34). At least one other yeast protease capable of recognizing dibasic residues has also been identified (35). The presence of a dibasic Arg-Arg, which can also serve as a KEX2 substrate (34), at amino acids 23 and 24 of mature GM-CSF suggested that this protein might be sensitive to one of the yeast proteases. To test this possibility, the arginine at position 23 was changed to a leucine by in vitro mutagenesis (21). This change makes human GM-CSF homologous to murine GM-CSF at the altered position. The loss of the dibasic residues resulted in approximately a tenfold increase in secreted, biologically active GM-CSF (see Table 1, column A).

Table 1 also compares the expression of GM-CSF under control of the constitutive α-factor promoter and the glucose-repressible ADH2 promoter (10,11). Increased expression of both the wild-type and mutant (Leu-23) GM-CSF was obtained with the ADH2 promoter by a factor of 5 to 10. This could be due to differences in the promoter strengths, the availability of positive regulatory elements (both promoters require positive activation by factors provided by single-copy chromosomal genes), or the interaction of the specific promoter with the foreign gene.

Secretion of proteins from yeast, including the glycosylation process, takes place by a mechanism similar to that found in mammalian cells (36). The predicted molecular mass of the unglycosylated, mature GM-CSF is 14,476. Analysis of secreted GM-CSF from yeast by SDS-PAGE and

Western blots revealed GM-CSF of heterogeneous molecular mass with major species at M_r 17,000 and M_r 25,000, indicative of glycosylated protein. Some hyperglycosylated material M_r 35,000–40,000 was also observed. The high-molecular-weight forms of GM-CSF have been shown to be susceptible to glycanase, an enzyme similar to endoglycosidase F that hydrolyzes both high mannose and complex asparagine-linked sugars. Glycanase treatment of secreted GM-CSF resulted in biologically active material with a molecular mass of 14,500–17,000, demonstrating N-linked glycosylation.

Amino acid sequence analysis of purified, secreted GM-CSF from yeast revealed two forms of the protein. Approximately 60% of the GM-CSF had the expected amino-terminal sequence for mature GM-CSF of Ala-Pro-Ala-Arg-Ser-Pro, while 40% was missing the amino-terminal Ala-Pro pair. Proteolytic cleavage of the Ala-Pro amino acid pair from the NH_2-terminus of this protein is consistent with the report by Achstetter et al. (37) of a class of dipeptidyl aminopeptidases in yeast. They have demonstrated both the presence of a cytoplasmic dipeptidyl aminopeptidase II, which has been shown to be active on Ala-Pro-containing artificial substrates, and an aminopeptidase P from membrane fractions that is active on the Ala-Pro artificial substrate. We are currently investigating the use of an aminopeptidase P-minus strain to alleviate NH_2-terminal proteolysis.

Expression of Recombinant GM-CSF in *E. coli*

Expression of GM-CSF in *E. coli* was initially performed by inserting the coding sequence into an expression vector that had given high-level expression of the human lymphokine IL-1β (Kronheim et al., in preparation) and of bovine IL-2 (16). The vector, designated (pLNGM), utilizes the strong leftward promoter, P_L, of bacteriophage lambda and a synthetic consensus sequence for initiation of translation followed by the GM-CSF-coding sequence, and terminating with the bacteriophage lambda transcription terminator, t11 (see Fig. 3). Induction of the P_L promoter in *E. coli* strain RR1(pRK248cIts) resulted in production of GM-CSF. Analysis of extracts from induced *E. coli* cultures showed production of approximately 1×10^4 units of GM-CSF activity (CFU-C) per milliliter of culture medium as measured in a human bone marrow colony formation assay (4). However the level of production of GM-CSF was too low to allow visualization of the protein on SDS-PAGE analysis of total *E. coli* proteins.

A number of additional plasmids were constructed utilizing alternative translation initiation regions, but none of these gave increased expression of GM-CSF. Use of alternative codons for a substantial portion of the coding region also resulted in no increase in the level of production of GM-CSF. These results led to the suggestion that poor production was caused by instability of rGM-CSF protein in *E. coli* because of endogenous proteases. To explore this possibility the plasmid (pLNGM) was transferred into the *E. coli* strain CAG629 which is a *lon*$^-$, *htpR*$^-$ double mutant conferring reduced levels of one or more proteases (18). The strain was transformed initially with the plasmid (pACYC184cIts), which encodes a bacteriophage lambda temperature-sensitive cI repressor of the P_L promoter. Transfer of (pLNGM) into this strain followed by induction by temperature shift resulted in GM-CSF activity at a tenfold higher level (approximately 1×10^5 CFU-C/ml) than with strain RR1. Total *E. coli* cellular protein was analyzed by SDS-PAGE and silver staining as described previously (16). Protein profiles from induced cultures harboring (pLNGM) contained a band of the predicted molecular mass for nonglycosylated GM-CSF (M_r 14,476), whereas this peptide species was absent from control cultures in which (pLNGM) was substituted with a control plasmid (pPL-λ). The level of GM-CSF was determined by quantitative Western blots using the monoclonal antibody 3G11. The induced *E. coli* cultures contained approximately 5–10 μg GM-CSF/ml of culture. Determination of the total protein content of these cultures showed that the GM-CSF corresponds to 0.15–0.3% of the *E. coli* cellular protein.

If sensitivity to cytoplasmic proteases is a major factor limiting production of GM-CSF in *E. coli*, then secretion of the protein out of the cytoplasm and into the periplasmic space by use of a signal sequence should increase the level of the protein. We therefore inserted the coding sequence for GM-CSF into a secretion expression vector developed by Ghrayeb et al. (20). This vector, (pIN-III-*omp*-a3), allows expression of inserted genes under the control of both the *E. coli* lipoprotein promoter (*lpp*) and the *lac* promoter-operator. Expression is regulated by the *lac* repressor which is also produced by the vector. Translation initiation and secretion are controlled by sequences from the *E. coli ompA* gene, which codes for a major outer membrane protein. The sequence of the vector (pLB5001-4) (see Fig. 4) upstream of the coding sequence for mature GM-CSF was altered by in vitro mutagenesis to remove four extra codons at the junction of *ompA* and GM-CSF sequences to allow proper proteolysis of the *ompA* signal peptide from mature GM-CSF (Libby et al., in preparation). Induction with IPTG of *E. coli* JM107 containing (pLB5001-4) and analysis of cellular protein on SDS-PAGE showed production of rGM-CSF.

Immunological detection by dot blots and quantitative Western blots revealed one band of the predicted molecular mass at the level of 5–10 μg rGM-CSF/ml of culture medium which corresponded to 0.25–0.5% of the total cellular protein. This level of production of GM-CSF is similar to the level of GM-CSF produced by (pLNGM) in the protease-deficient strain but is much greater than the level of GM-CSF found after induction of (pLNGM) in strains such as RR1, containing wild-type levels of cytoplasmic proteases.

To determine whether the increased level of GM-CSF produced by (pLB5001-4) was primarily due to secretion or to the use of the *lpp* promoter, we constructed an additional secretion vector, (pLNompGM), which used the P_L promoter and transcription terminator as in (pLNGM) but contains the modified DNA sequence for the *ompA* signal sequence and translation initiation region (see Fig. 3). Induction of *E. coli* strain JM107 (pRK248cIts) containing (pLNompGM) and analysis as before showed expression of GM-CSF at a level of approximately 4–8 μg/ml of culture, which corresponded to 0.13–0.25% of cellular protein.

Therefore it is probable that secretion of GM-CSF out of the *E. coli* cytoplasm was the primary factor increasing GM-CSF production in (pLB5001-4). We have not eliminated the possibility that differences in the translation initiation regions of the constructs affected the levels of GM-CSF.

Amino acid sequence analysis of rGM-CSF produced by (pLB5001-4) and purified to homogeneity has shown the material to be completely processed at the predicted alanine (see Fig. 4; Libby et al., in preparation).

Effect of GM-CSF on Macrophage Tumoricidal Activity

It was traditionally thought that the primary function of CSFs was to promote the growth and differentiation of hematopoietic precursor cells. It is now becoming increasingly clear that CSFs can also affect survival and activation of cells of hematopoietic origin. Previous studies have indicated that GM-CSF can induce antibody-dependent cellular cytotoxicity (38), the killing of schistosomula by neutrophils and eosinophils (39), and the intracellular killing of *Leishmania* spp. by macrophages (40). We have recently shown that rGM-CSF can also stimulate nonspecific tumoricidal activity of monocytes in vitro (41).

Purified, rGM-CSF produced by yeast induced peripheral blood monocytes to express tumoricidal activity against the malignant melanoma cell line A375 (Table 2). Lipopolysaccharide (LPS) was not required for the function of GM-CSF in this assay, and added LPS had no stimulatory effect.

Table 2 Activation of Peripheral Blood Monocytes for Tumor Cytotoxicity in vitro by GM-CSF and IFNγ

	% Cytotoxicity				
	Level of LPS (ng/ml)				
Lymphokine	None	10.0	1.0	0.1	0.01
None	0	83	79	39	0
GM-CSF, 500 CFU-C/ml	36			36	36
IFNγ, 100 U/ml	8			82	15

Purified peripheral blood monocytes were prepared and cultured as described in Materials and Methods in the presence of lipopolysaccharide, purified natural IFNγ or purified GM-CSF as indicated. After 24 hr, the culture medium was replaced and ^{125}I-labeled A375 target cells were added. After an additional 72 hr, residual adherent A375 cells were harvested and counted. Units of IFNγ were determined with a virus plaque-reduction assay and comparison with an NIH international IFNγ standard.

This is in marked contrast to the requirement for suboptimal levels of LPS for stimulation by γ-interferon (IFN-γ) of monocyte killing of tumor cells (see Table 2; Ref. 42). Preparations of rGM-CSF used in these tests were shown to be free of endotoxin (less than 1 pg/μg rGM-CSF). The GM-CSF-activated monocytes were also able to lyse several other tumor targets including a murine melanoma and a human bladder carcinoma.

This regulation of monocyte activity by GM-CSF may provide a mechanism whereby T lymphocytes, in response to antigen, may regulate a nonspecific cytotoxic reaction by macrophages against tumors.

SUMMARY

Isolation of cDNAs for GM-CSF has allowed analysis of the gene and its expression in various human cell populations. Initially, low-level expression in yeast was increased by manipulation of the coding sequence and the specific promoter used. Increased expression in *E. coli* was obtained by use of a protease-deficient strain or by addition of a signal sequence for secretion of the protein out of the cytoplasm. Availability of the recombinant protein permits more definitive studies of its structure and function than could be performed with naturally occurring material. An example of such studies is our recent analysis of the stimulatory effect of the recombinant protein on monocyte killing of tumor cells. Such regulation of macrophage activation by GM-CSF may represent an important pathway of antitumor defense.

ACKNOWLEDGMENTS

We thank Judy Reaveley for preparation of the manuscript. For excellent technical help, we are indebted to Noel Balantac, Terri Chiaverotti, Billy Clevenger, Steve Gimpel, Toby Hemenway, and Ralph Klinke. This work was made possible by an ongoing collaboration between Immunex Corporation, Hoechst A. G., and Behringwerke A. G.

REFERENCES

1. Burgess, A. W., Camakaris, J., and Metcalf, D. (1977). Purification and properties of colony-stimulating factor from mouse lung-conditioned medium. *J. Biol. Chem. 252*:1998–2003.
2. Metcalf, D. (1986). The molecular biology and functions of the granulocyte-macrophage colony-stimulating factors. *Blood 67*:257–267.
3. Metcalf, D. and Burgess, A. W. (1982). Clonal analysis of progenitor cell commitment to granulocyte or macrophage production. *J. Cell. Physiol. 111*:275–283.
4. Cantrell, M. A., Anderson, D., Cerretti, D. P., Price, V., McKereghan, K., Tushinski, R. J., Mochizuki, D. Y., Larsen, A., Grabstein, K., Gillis, S., and Cosman, D. (1985). Cloning, sequence, and expression of a human granulocyte/macrophage colony-stimulating factor. *Proc. Natl. Acad. Sci. USA 82*:6250–6254.
5. Wong, G. G., Witek, J. W., Temple, P. A., Wilkens, K. M., Leary, A. C., Luxenberg, D. P., Jones, S. S., Brown, E. L., Kay, R. M., Orr, E. C., Shoemaker, C., Golde, D. W., Kaufman, R. J., Hewick, R. M., Wang, E. A., and Clark, S. C. (1985). Human GM-CSF: Molecular cloning of the complementary DNA and purification of the natural and recombinant proteins. *Science 228*:810–815.
6. Lee, T., Yokota, T., Otsuka, T., Gemmell. L., Larson, N., Luk, J., Arai, K., and Rennick, D. (1985). Isolation of cDNA for a human granulocyte-macrophage colony-stimulating factor by functional expression in mammalian cells. *Proc. Natl. Acad. Sci. USA 82*:4360–4364.
7. Gasson, J. C., Weisbart, R. H., Kaufman, S. E., Clark, S. C., Hewick, R. M., Wong, G. G., and Golde, D. W. (1984). Purified human granulocyte-macrophage colony-stimulating factor: Direct action on neutrophils. *Science 226*:1339–1342.

8. Sieff, C. A., Emerson, S. G., Donahue, R. E., Nathan, D. G., Wang, E. A., Wong, G. G., and Clark, S. G. (1985). Human recombinant granulocyte-macrophage colony-stimulating factor: A multilineage hematopoietin. *Science 230*:1171–1173.
9. Maniatis, T., Fritsch, E. F., and Sambrook, J. (1982). *Molecular Cloning, A Laboratory Manual.* Cold Spring Harbor Publications, Cold Spring Harbor, N.Y.
10. Russell, D. W., Smith, M., Williamson, V. M., and Young, E. T. (1982). Nucleotide sequence of the yeast alcohol dehydrogenase II gene. *J. Biol. Chem. 258*:2674–2682.
11. Beier, D. R. and Young, E. T. (1982). Characterization of a regulatory region upstream of the ADR2 locus of *S. cerevisiae. Nature 300*:724–728.
12. Kurjan, J. and Herskowitz, I. (1982). Structure of a yeast pheromone gene (*MFα*): A putative α-factor precursor contains four tandem copies of mature α-factor. *Cell 30*:933–943.
13. Brake, A. J., Merryweather, J. P., Cort, D. G., Heberlein, U. A., Masiary, T. P., Mullenback, G. T., Urdea, M. S., Valenzuela, P., and Barr, P. J. (1984). α-Factor-directed synthesis and secretion of mature foreign proteins in *Saccharomyces cerevisiae. Proc. Natl. Acad. Sci. USA 81*: 4642–4646.
14. Bitter, G. A., Chen, K., Banks, A., and Lai, R.-H. (1984). Secretion of foreign proteins from *Saccharomyces cerevisiae* directed by α-factor gene fusion. *Proc. Natl. Acad. Sci. USA 81*:5330–5334.
15. Hinne, A., Hicks, J. B., and Fink, G. R. (1978). Transformation of yeast. *Proc. Natl. Acad. Sci. USA 75*:1929–1933.
16. Cerretti, D. P., McKereghan, K., Larsen, A., Cantrell, M. A., Anderson, D., Gillis, S., Cosman, D., and Baker, P. E. (1986). Cloning, sequence and expression of bovine interleukin-2. *Proc. Natl. Acad. Sci. USA 83*:3223–3227.
17. Bernard, H. U., Remaut, E., Hershfield, M. V., Das, H. K., Helinski, D. R., Yanofsky, C., and Franklin, N. (1979). Construction of plasmid cloning vehicles that promote gene expression from the bacteriophage lambda P_L promoter. *Gene 5*:59–76.
18. Baker, T. A., Grossman, A. D., and Gross, C. A. (1984). A gene regulating the heat shock response in *Escherichia coli* also affects proteolysis. *Proc. Natl. Acad. Sci. USA 81*:6779–6783.
19. Chang, A. C. Y. and Cohen, S. N. (1978). Construction and characterization of amplifiable multicopy DNA cloning vehicles derived from the P15A cryptic miniplasmid. *J. Bacteriol. 134*:1141–1156.
20. Ghrayeb, J., Kimura, H., Takahara, M., Hsiung, H., Masin, Y., and Inouye, M. (1984). Secretion cloning vectors in *E. coli. EMBO J. 3*:2437–2442.

21. Bauer, C. E., Hesse, S. D., Yaechter-Brulla, D. A., Lynn, S. P., Gumport, R. I., and Gardner, J. F. (1985). A genetic enrichment for mutations constructed by oligonucleotide-directed mutagenesis. *Gene 37*:73–81.
22. Biggin, M. D., Gibson, T. J., and Hong, G. F. (1983). Buffer gradient gels and ^{35}S label as an aid to rapid DNA sequencing. *Proc. Natl. Acad. Sci. USA 80*:3963–3965.
23. Mott, J. E., Grant, R. A., Hoo, Y., and Platt, T. (1985). Maximizing gene expression from plasmid vectors containing the λ P_L promoter: Strategies for overproducing transcription termination factor p. *Proc. Natl. Acad. Sci. USA 82*:88–92.
24. March, C. J., Mosley, B., Larsen, A., Cerretti, D. P., Braedt, G., Price, V., Gillis, S., Henney, C. S., Kronheim, S. R., Grabstein, K., Conlon, P. J., Hopp, T. P., and Cosman, D. (1985). Cloning, sequences and expression of two distinct human interleukin-1 complementary DNAs. *Nature 315*:641–647.
25. Laemmli, U. K. (1970). Cleavage of structural proteins during the assembly of the head of bacteriophage T4. *Nature 227*:680–685.
26. Oakley, B. R., Kirsch, D. R., and Morris, N. R. (1980). A simple ultrasensitive silver stain for detecting proteins in polyacrylamide gels. *Anal. Biochem. 105*:361–363.
27. Dower, S. K., Hefeneider, S. H., Alpert, A. R., and Urdal, D. L. (1985). Quantitative measurement of human IL-2 receptor levels with intact and detergent solubilized human T-cells. *Mol. Immunol. 22*:937–947.
28. Urdal, D. L., March, C. J., Gillis, S., Larsen, A., and Dower, S. K. (1984). Purification and chemical characterization of the receptor for interleukin-2 from activated human T lymphocytes and from a human T-cell lymphoma cell line. *Proc. Natl. Acad. Sci. USA 81*:6481–6485.
29. Conlon, P. J., Luk, F. H., Park, L. S., Hopp, T. P., and Urdal, D. L. (1985). Generation of anti-peptide monoclonal antibodies which recognize mature CSF-2α (IL-3) protein. *J. Immunol. 135*:328–332.
30. Burnette, W. N. (1981). "Western blotting": Electrophoretic transfer of proteins from sodium dodecyl sulfate-polyacrylamide gels to unmodified nitrocellulose and radioactive detection with antibody and radioiodinated protein A. *Anal. Biochem. 112*:195–203.
31. Gmelig-Meyling, F. and Waldmann, T. A. (1980). Separation of human blood monocytes and lymphocytes on a continuous Percoll gradient. *J. Immunol. Methods 33*:1–9.
32. Kleinerman, E. S., Schost, A. J., Fogler, W. E., and Fidler, I. J. (1983). Tumoricidal activity of human monocytes activated in vitro by free and liposome encapsulated human lymphokines. *J. Clin. Invest. 72*:304–315.
33. Julius, D., Schekman, R., and Thorner, J. (1984). Glycosylation and processing of prepro-α-factor through the yeast secretory pathway. *Cell 36*:309–318.

34. Achstetter, T. and Wolf, D. (1985). Hormone processing and membrane-bound proteins in yeast. *EMBO J. 4*:173–177.
35. Mizuno, K. and Matsuo, H. (1984). A novel protease from yeast with specificity towards paired basic residues. *Nature 309*:558–560.
36. Schekman, R. and Novick, P. (1982). The secretory process and yeast cell-surface assmebly. In *The Molecular Biology of the Yeast Saccharomyces.* Edited by J. Strathern, E. Jones, and J. Broach. Cold Spring Harbor Laboratory, Cold Spring Harbor, N.Y., pp. 361–393.
37. Achstetter, T., Ehmann, C., and Wolf, D. H. (1983). Proteolysis in eucaryotic cells: Aminopeptidases and dipeptidyl aminopeptidases of yeast revisited. *Arch. Bioch. Biophys. 226*:292–305.
38. Lopez, A. F., Nicola, N. A., Burgess, A. W., Metcalf, D., Battye, F. L., Sewell, W. A., and Vadas, M. (1983). Activation of granulocyte cytotoxic function by purified mouse colony-stimulating factors. *J. Immunol. 131*:2983–2988.
39. Dessein, A. J., Vadas, M. A., Nicola, N. A., Metcalf, D., David, J. R. (1982). Enhancement of human blood eosinophil cytotoxicity by semi-purified eosinophil colony-stimulating factor(s). *J. Exp. Med. 156*:90–103.
40. Handman, E. and Burgess, A. W. (1979). Stimulation by granulocyte-macrophage colony-stimulating factor of *Leishmania tropica* killing by macrophages. *J. Immunol. 122*:1134–1137.
41. Grabstein, K. H., Urdal, D. L., Tushinski, R. J., Mochizuki, D. Y., Price, V. L., Cantrell, M. A., Gillis, S., and Conlon, P. J. (1986). Induction of macrophage tumoricidal activity by granulocyte-macrophage colony stimulating factor. *Science 232*:506–508.
42. Pace, J. L. and Russell, S. W. (1981). Activation of mouse macrophages for tumor cell killing. *J. Immunol. 126*:1863–1867.

10
Human Erythroid-Potentiating Activity

BELINDA R. AVALOS, DAVID W. GOLDE, and JUDITH C. GASSON
UCLA School of Medicine, Los Angeles, California

STEVEN C. CLARK
Genetics Institute, Cambridge, Massachusetts

The survival, proliferation, and differentiation of hematopoietic progenitor cells in vitro is dependent upon the presence of specific glycoprotein hormones (1); at least two classes of mediators important in the regulation of erythropoiesis have been identified. Erythropoietin, the primary regulator of erythropoiesis, exerts its action upon relatively mature erythroid precursors, CFU-E (colony-forming units, erythroid), and morphologically recognizable progenitors that ultimately give rise to fully hemoglobinized erythrocytes. The growth of more primitive erythroid precursors, BFU-E (burst-forming units, erythroid), is primarily modulated by another class of hormones referred to as burst-promoting activities (BPA).

In the mouse, burst-promoting activities may be lineage-independent and support the growth of pluripotent hematopoietic stem cells and early committed precursors of all lineages (2). Interleukin-3 (IL-3), isolated from EL-4 lymphocytic and WEHI-3 myelomonocytic murine cell lines, has potent burst-promoting activity, and also stimulates growth and differentiation of pluripotent stem cells; hence the alternative term *multi-colony-stimulating factor* (*CSF*) (3). The human counterpart of murine IL-3 or multi-CSF has recently been characterized (4).

In the human, burst-promoting activity has been found in medium conditioned by activated T lymphocytes, monocytes, and human T-lymphotropic virus (HTLV)-infected T-lymphoblast cell lines (5–7). Recently, a burst-promoting activity was purified from the HTLV-II-infected Mo T-lymphoblast cell line (8,9). This hormone is also capable of stimulating the growth of CFU-E, and therefore is referred to as erythroid-potentiating activity (EPA). Complementary DNA (cDNA) clones encoding EPA have been isolated and expressed in mammalian cells to produce biologically active biosynthetic (recombinant) EPA (10). The availability of sufficient quantities of biosynthetic EPA protein makes it possible to study both in vivo and in vitro activities of this important human burst-promoting activity.

PURIFICATION AND CHARACTERIZATION OF ERYTHROID-POTENTIATING ACTIVITY

Human EPA was purified to homogeneity from medium conditioned by the Mo T-lymphoblast cell line using sequential lectin affinity chromatography, gel filtration, and reverse-phase high-performance liquid chromatography (RP-HPLC) (8). This highly reproducible procedure yields 10–25 μg of purified protein from an initial volume of 10 L of serum-free conditioned medium. Purified EPA is a heat-stable glycoprotein with a molecular mass (M_r) of 28,000, that appears as a single band when analyzed by sodium dodecyl sulfate-polyacrylamide gel electrophoresis (SDS-PAGE) under both reducing and nonreducing conditions. Removal of carbohydrate from EPA by digestion with endoglycosidase F generates a protein with an apparent M_r of 18,000 (9).

Purified EPA stimulates the growth of both human and murine BFU-E and CFU-E in vitro (9,11,12) in a dose-dependent fashion. Stimulation of erythroid burst formation occurs at concentrations of 100–200 pM. Erythroid-potentiating activity does not stimulate the growth of myeloid or mixed colonies, and thus differs in its biological activity from IL-3 (3,4).

Additionally, purified EPA enhances colony formation by the K562 erythroleukemia and KG-1 human myeloid leukemia cell lines established from patients with chronic and acute myeloid leukemias, respectively (7,13). This observation is significant, because it demonstrates direct action of EPA on the colony-forming cells of the K562 and KG-1 cell lines. The availability of these responsive cell lines makes them convenient homogeneous target cell populations for studying EPA action.

MOLECULAR CLONING AND EXPRESSION OF ERYTHROID-POTENTIATING ACTIVITY

Until recently, it has not been possible to study the precise physiological roles of growth factors in the regulation of hematopoiesis owing to the lack of sufficient quantities of the purified proteins. The availability of molecular clones for human hemopoietins such as granulocyte-macrophage colony-stimulating factor (GM-CSF), erythropoietin, and EPA, has substantially contributed to our understanding of their molecular structures and expression. In addition, it has been possible to produce large quantities of biosynthetic protein for further investigation.

Using Edman degradation and analysis by a gas phase sequenator, partial NH_2-terminal amino acid sequence was obtained from purified EPA (10). This partial amino acid sequence (Fig. 1) was used to construct three pools of overlapping oligonucleotide probes. A cDNA library prepared from Mo mRNA was enriched for sequences specific to mature T cells by hybridizing the single-stranded cDNA to mRNA from cells of the human B-cell line, Daudi, and the immature T-cell line, CEM. The pooled oligonucleotide probes were hybridized to replicate filters containing the recombinant plasmids. Potential EPA clones were identified by colony hybridization and subsequently verified by restriction analysis and hybridization to each of the three pools of oligonucleotide probes.

The pool of eight strongly hybridizing 14-mers corresponding to amino acid residues 21–25 was used as a primer for sequencing the putative EPA cDNA clones. The resulting DNA sequence predicted the amino acid sequence of residues 1–19, confirming that these cDNA clones encoded the EPA protein.

The complete nucleotide sequence of the cDNAs encoding EPA was determined by dideoxy sequencing of M13 subclones (Fig. 2). The cDNA encodes a protein of 207 amino acids. Based on the NH_2-terminal sequence of the mature protein, a signal peptide of 23 amino acids is predicted by the nucleotide sequence. This region is rich in hydrophobic amino acids similar to other signal peptides. The predicted relative molecular mass of the mature protein is in good agreement with the apparent 18,000 M_r observed following digestion with endoglycosidase F (9). The presence of twelve cysteine residues in the deduced amino acid sequence predicts a protein structure that could account for the marked heat stability of EPA.

```
1         5              10              15              20              25
(A) T C V P P H ? Q T A F C N S D L V I R A K F V G T
```

Figure 1 Partial NH_2-terminal amino acid sequence of purified EPA.

Further confirmation that these clones encode EPA was obtained by Northern blot analysis of mRNA prepared from cells previously found to produce burst-promoting activity. A 0.9-kb transcript that hybridized to the EPA cDNA probe was found in Mo cells, UCD-144-MLA cells derived from a gibbon lymphosarcoma cell line, U-937 monocytic cells, mature T-lymphoblast cell lines, and peripheral blood lymphocytes (10). Dexamethasone treatment of U-937 and Mo cells decreased EPA mRNA twofold. Similar results have been seen with other T-cell-derived growth factors such as interleukin-2 (IL-2) and GM-CSF (14). Treatment of Mo cells with phytohemagglutinin and phorbol myristate acetate failed to significantly increase EPA mRNA despite a two- to tenfold increase in GM-CSF mRNA under similar conditions (14).

Definitive evidence that the cDNA clone encoded EPA was obtained by expression of the protein in mammalian cells (10). The EPA cDNA clone was inserted into the p91023 (B) mammalian expression vector and transiently expressed in COS monkey kidney cells. Efficient expression of the cDNA clone, as determined by radioimmunoassay (>1 μg/ml) of unfractionated COS cell supernatants, occurred within 72 hr after transfection (unpublished data).

Supernatants from COS cells transfected with either the 91023 (B) vector alone or the vector containing the EPA coding region were assayed for stimulation of human peripheral blood BFU-E growth. Biological activity of the biosynthetic EPA transiently expressed in COS cells was observed at concentrations as low as 5 pM (as estimated by radioimmunoassay). Stimulation of erythroid bursts to greater than 130% of control occurred at these concentrations. Minimal stimulation above control of BFU-E growth was observed with supernatants from mock-infected or uninfected COS cells, suggesting constitutive production by COS cells of a factor that stimulates human erythroid precursors.

In addition to transient expression of EPA in COS cells, Chinese hamster ovary (CHO) cells have been stably transfected with the EPA cDNA clone. The CHO cells containing integrated copies of the 91023 (B) vector with the EPA-coding region, as well as the dihydrofolate reductase gene, were selected in methotrexate (10). After approximately 2 months of selection,

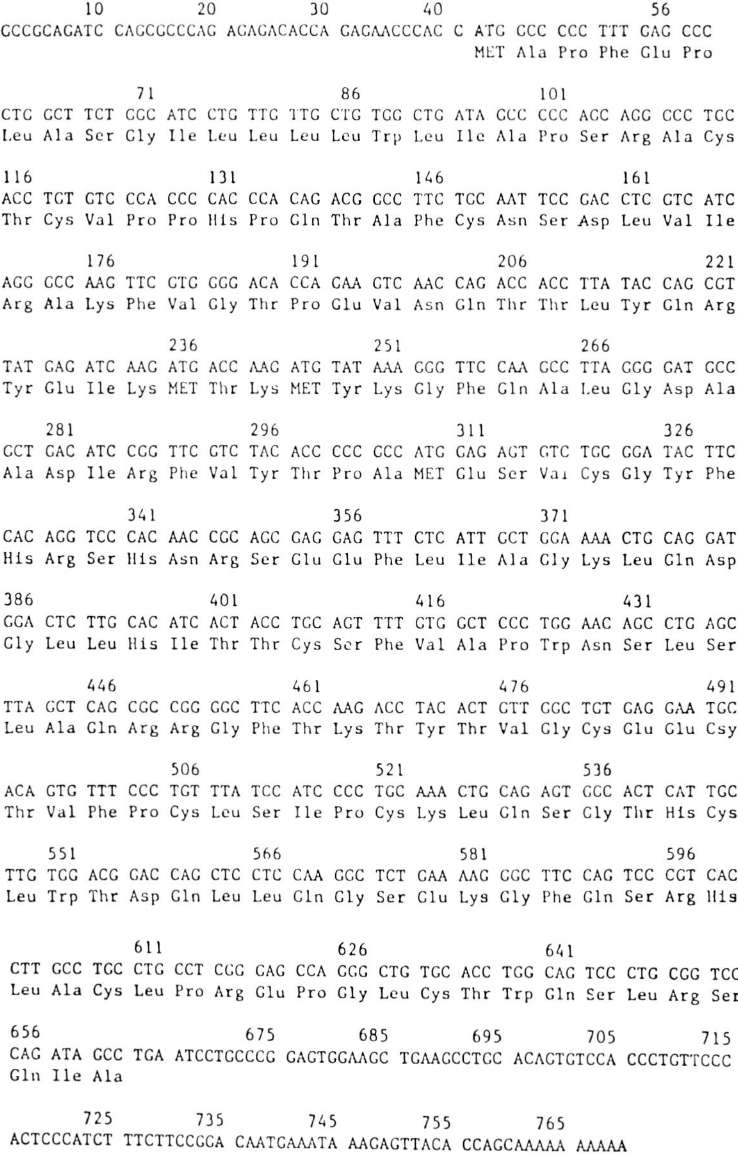

Figure 2 Nucleotide and deduced amino acid sequence of the cDNA clone encoding EPA.

one CHO cell clone was found to constitutively produce levels of biosynthetic EPA similar to those obtained by transient expression in COS cells. Biological activity of biosynthetic EPA in the medium conditioned by this CHO cell clone was observed in the picomolar range of concentrations similar to the activity of the purified protein from Mo-conditioned medium. No endogenous burst-promoting activity was seen in supernatants from CHO cells not producing biosynthetic EPA.

Purified biosynthetic EPA retains all the biological activities attributed to the purified natural protein (see section on biological activities). Large quantities of biosynthetic EPA have been purified to further investigate the biological activities of this protein both in vitro and in vivo.

STRUCTURE OF THE GENE ENCODING ERYTHROID-POTENTIATING ACTIVITY

The EPA cDNA clone was used to study the molecular organization of the human EPA gene (10). A human genomic library was constructed using DNA from the HTLV-II-infected cell line, J-LB-III and Charon 30 phage. Using the EPA cDNA clone as a probe, three overlapping genomic clones were isolated. A 5.2 kb HindIII fragment that hybridized to the cDNA

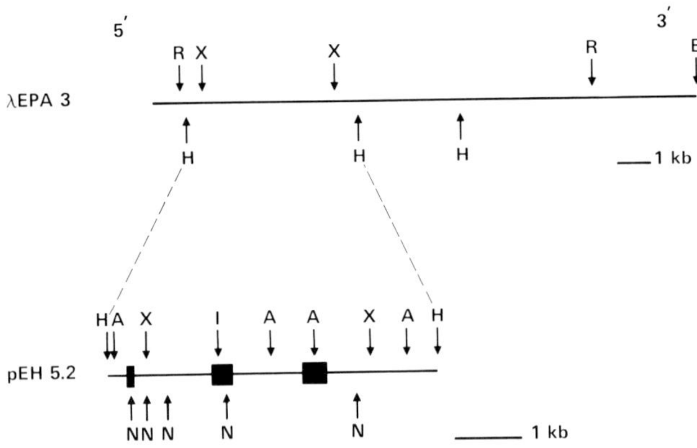

Figure 3 Genomic organization of human EPA. Restriction map of an EPA genomic clone in Charon 30 (λ EPA 3) and subcloned into pBR 322 (pEH 5.2) are shown. Restriction sites are: R, EcoRI; X, Xba I; H, HindIII; A, AvaI; N, NcoI; I, HindII.

probe was subcloned and further characterized by restriction enzyme analysis. In every case, the restriction pattern agreed with that observed by Southern analysis of several human DNA samples. The EPA appears to be encoded by a single gene of approximately 3 kbp in length, with at least two intervening sequences (Fig. 3). The chromosomal localization of the EPA gene is currently under investigation.

BIOLOGICAL ACTIVITIES OF BIOSYNTHETIC ERYTHROID-POTENTIATING ACTIVITY

Purified biosynthetic EPA exhibits all of the biological activities of the purified natural protein. Biosynthetic EPA stimulates the growth of both human and murine BFU-E and CFU-E at concentrations ranging from 10 pM to 10 nM (Fig. 4). Additionally, purified biosynthetic EPA enhances colony formation by the K562 erythroleukemia and KG-1 human myeloid leukemia cell lines. No enhancement in colony formation by EPA however has been observed with the HL-60 myeloid cell line.

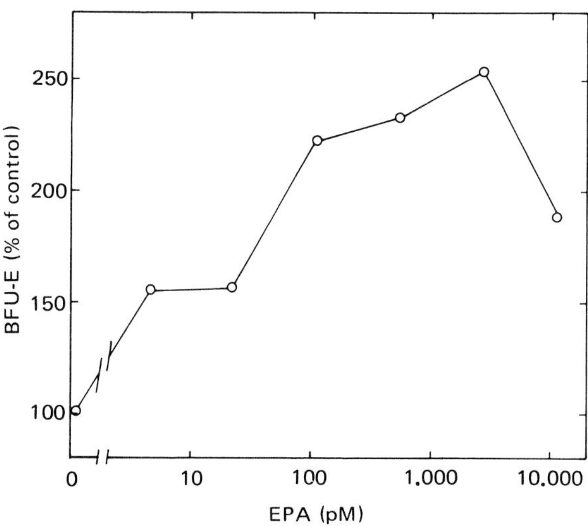

Figure 4 Dose-response curve for purified biosynthetic EPA. Purified biosynthetic EPA was assayed at various concentrations for stimulation of erythroid bursts.

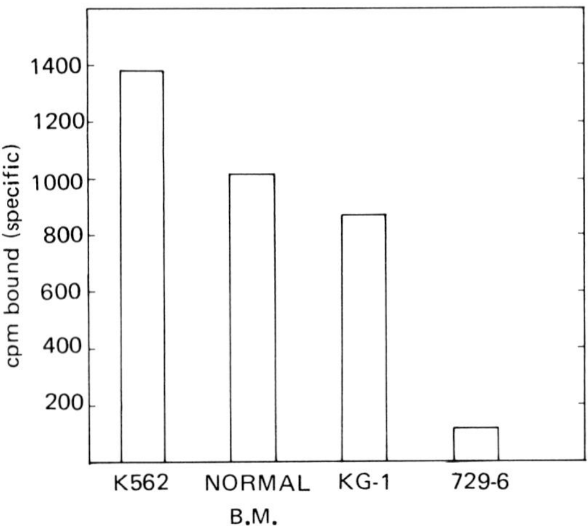

Figure 5 Specific binding of ^{125}I-labeled EPA. Radiolabeled ^{125}I EPA (100,000 cpm) was added to 4.0 × 10^6 cells and specific binding was measured after 2 hr incubation; 100-fold excess unlabeled EPA was added. Nonspecific binding was that which was not completed by excess unlabeled EPA.

The development of a specific-binding assay for human EPA is necessary to study its mechanism of action on responsive target cells. Using a modification of the chloramine-T method (15), radiolabeling of purified biosynthetic EPA with ^{125}I was accomplished without apparent damage to the protein. Binding of radiolabeled EPA to the responsive cell line, K562, was investigated as a function of time and temperature using 4.0 × 10^6 cells and 100,000 cpm of ^{125}I-labeled EPA. At 37°C, EPA appears to be rapidly internalized and degraded, similar to other peptide hormones. At 0 and 23°C, equilibrium binding is reached after approximately 2 hr.

Specific binding by various cells and cell lines was studied at 0°C following incubation with ^{125}I-labeled EPA for 2 hr. Specific binding was observed by the responsive cell lines, K562 and KG-1, as well as by bone marrow cells obtained from a normal donor (Fig. 5). No significant specific binding however was seen by normal granulocytes, normal fibroblasts, or the B-lymphocyte-derived cell line, 729-6. Further studies are in progress to assess equilibrium binding by ^{125}I-labeled EPA; however preliminary studies suggest the existence of more than one class of binding sites.

CONCLUSIONS

Burst-promoting activity is an important mediator of early erythropoiesis. Human erythroid-potentiating activity is a recently characterized hematopoietic growth factor that stimulates the growth of primitive and more mature erythroid precursors. This 28,000 M_r glycoprotein has been purified to homogeneity from medium conditioned by the HTLV-II-infected Mo-T lymphoblast cell line. Complementary DNA clones encoding EPA have been isolated and protein expressed in mammalian cells. Purified biosynthetic EPA has all the biological properties attributed to the purified natural protein. Erythroid-potentiating activity stimulates the growth of both human and murine BFU-E and CFU-E. Additionally, EPA enhances colony formation by the two human leukemic cell lines K562 and KG-1.

The observation that EPA stimulates the growth of normal erythroid precursors, as well as leukemic cell lines in the picomolar concentration range, suggests that the first step in the mechanism of action of this glycoprotein hormone is likely to be interaction with a specific cell surface receptor protein. Preliminary equilibrium binding studies suggest the existence of more than one class of binding sites. However further characterization of the mechanism of action of EPA awaits the purification and molecular cloning of the EPA receptor protein.

Recently, identity in the amino acid sequence has been reported for EPA and the human collagenase inhibitor, tissue inhibitor of metalloproteinases (TIMP) (16). The ascribed dual functionality of EPA as a glycoprotein hormone and enzyme inhibitor makes it a most interesting molecule that warrants further characterization.

REFERENCES

1. Burgess, A. W. and Metcalf, D. (1980). *Blood 56*:947–958.
2. Iscove, N. N. (1977). *Cell Tissue Kinet. 10*:323–334.
3. Ihle, J. N., Heller, J., Oroszlan, S., Henderson, L. E., Copeland, T. D., Fitch, F., Prystowsky, M. G., Goldwasser, E., Schrader, J. W., Palaszynski, E., Dy, M., and Lebel, B. (1983). *J. Immunol. 131*:282–287.
4. Yang, Y.-C., Ciarletta, A. B., Temple, P. A., Chung, M. P., Kovacic, S., Witek-Giannotti, J. S., Leary, A. C., Kriz, R., Donahue, R. E., Wong, G., and Clark, S. (1986). *Cell 47*:3–10.
5. Abboud, C. N., Brennan, J. K., Barlow, G. H., and Lichtman, M. A. (1981). *Blood 58*:1148–1154.
6. Ascensao, J. L., Kay, N. E., Earenfight-Engler, T., Koren, H. S., and Zanjani, E. D. (1981). *Blood 57*:170–173.

7. Gasson, J. C., Chen, I. S. Y., Westbrook, C. A., and Golde, D. W. (1983). In *Normal and Neoplastic Hematopoiesis.* Edited by D. W. Golde and P. A. Marks. Alan R. Liss, New York, pp. 129-139.
8. Westbrook, C. A., Gasson, J. C., Gerber, S. E., Selsted, M. E., and Golde, D. W. (1984). *J. Biol. Chem. 259*:9992-9996.
9. Gasson, J. C., Bersch, N., and Golde, D. W. (1985). In *Stem Cell Physiology.* Edited by J. Palek. Alan R. Liss, New York, pp. 95-104.
10. Gasson, J. C., Golde, D. W., Kaufman, S. E., Westbrook, C. A., Hewick, R. M., Kaufman, R. J., Wong, G. G., Temple, P. A., Leary, A. C., Brown, E. L., Orr, E. C., and Clark, S. C. (1985). *Nature 316*:768-771.
11. Golde, D. W., Bersch, N., Quan, S. G., and Lusis, A. J. (1980). *Proc. Natl. Acad. Sci. USA 77*:593-596.
12. Golde, D. W., Westbrook, C. A., and Lusis, A. J. (1984). In *Growth and Maturation Factors*, Vol. 2. Edited by G. Guroff. John Wiley & Sons, New York, pp. 37-54.
13. Gauewerky, C. E., Lusis, A. J., and Golde, D. W. (1982). *Blood 59*: 300-305.
14. Wong, G. G., Witek, J. S., Temple, P. A., Wilkens, K. M., Leary, A. C., Luxenberg, D. P., Jones, S. S., Brown, E. L., Kay, R. M., Orr, E., Shoemaker, C., Golde, D. W., Kaufman, R. J., Hewick, R. M., Wang, E. A., and Clark, S. C. (1985). *Science 228*:810-815.
15. Hunter, W. M. and Greenwood, F. C. (1982). *Nature 194*:495-496.
16. Docherty, A. J. P., Lyons, A., Smith, B. J., Wright, E. M., Stephens, P. E., Harris, T. J. R., Murphy, G., and Reynolds, J. J. (1985). *Nature 318*:66-69.

11

Mouse Interleukin-3
Recombinant cDNA Cloning, Expression, and Characterization

TIM R. MOSMANN, JOHN S. ABRAMS, KEN-ICHI ARAI, NAOKO ARAI, MARTHA W. BOND, FRANK D. LEE, ATSUSHI MIYAJIMA, SHOICHIRO MIYATAKE, DONNA M. RENNICK, JOLANDA SCHREURS, CRAIG A. SMITH, YUTAKA TAKEBE, TAKASHI YOKOTA, GERARD ZURAWSKI, and SANDRA M. ZURAWSKI
DNAX Research Institute of Molecular and Cellular Biology, Palo Alto, California

A number of biological activities in induced T-cell supernatants and WEHI-3-conditioned medium were initially described under several names. Later, it became clear that all of these activities were mediated by the same molecule. Because a functionally significant name is difficult to assign to this variety of activities, the name interleukin-3 (IL-3, originally proposed for the α-steroid dehydrogenase-inducing activity, Ref. 1) appears to be most useful, as no single function is emphasized by this choice. The biological activities mediated by IL-3 include the induction of 20-α-steroid dehydrogenase (20-αSDH) in nu/nu splenic lymphocytes (1); the stimulation of growth of mast cell lines (2–4), P cells (5), and histamine-producing cells (6); the induction of Thy1 antigen on bone marrow cells (1); and the stimulation of multilineage colonies in vitro (containing granulocytes, macrophages, erythroid and mast cells) from bone marrow cells (7).

The major source of IL-3 appears to be T lymphocytes, predominantly of the helper ($Ly1^+Ly2^-$) phenotype (8). Induction of IL-3 synthesis requires activation by either antigen plus antigen-presenting cells, or by concanavalin A (Con A). In addition, the tumor cell line WEHI-3 constitutively produces low levels of IL-3 (9), possibly the result of an aberrant rearrangement of DNA in the region of the IL-3 gene (10).

Purification of IL-3 to homogeneity was reported in 1982 (11), and the purified material was active in all the assays just described (12), suggesting that the various activities were all mediated by a single molecule. Final proof came in 1984, when we and others reported the cDNA cloning of mouse IL-3 (13,14). The lymphokine expressed by the cDNA clone possessed the full range of described activities (13,15). The cDNA cloning of IL-3 has resulted in ready availability of DNA probes for analyzing the regulation of expression of the IL-3 gene, and recombinant IL-3 protein for analyzing the functions of IL-3. In this chapter we describe the isolation of IL-3 cDNA clones, the expression of mouse IL-3 in monkey COS cells, the subsequent expression in mammalian, yeast, and bacterial cells, and the biological activity of the expressed products.

ISOLATION OF A COMPLEMENTARY DNA CLONE ENCODING MOUSE INTERLEUKIN-3

The cDNA-cloning vector that we chose for cDNA cloning of mouse lymphokines was the (pcD) vector developed by Okayama and Berg (16; Fig. 1). This vector contains the (pBR322) replication origin to allow propagation in *Escherichia coli* and also contains the simian virus 40 (SV40) replication origin that allows transient replication in mammalian cells expressing the SV40 T antigen (e.g., the COS monkey cell line). The cDNA is inserted at a site downstream from the early region promoter of SV40, so that any full-length cDNA insert will, in principle, be expressed from this promoter. During construction of the cDNA library, the cDNA is synthesized directly onto one strand of the vector, using an oligo-dT tail on the other vector strand as primer. This ensures that the cDNA is correctly oriented. The final construction step of closing the plasmid is selective for full-length cDNA transcripts, so that the final cDNA library contains a high proportion of long, correctly oriented cDNA inserts (16).

When cDNA clones produced in this vector are transfected into COS cells, the plasmids replicate extensively in the transfected cells, reaching numbers of up to several thousand copies per cell in a few days. The cDNA inserts are transcribed under the control of the SV40 early promoter, and the resulting mRNAs transcribed from full-length or nearly full-length clones should be translated and the protein processed normally,

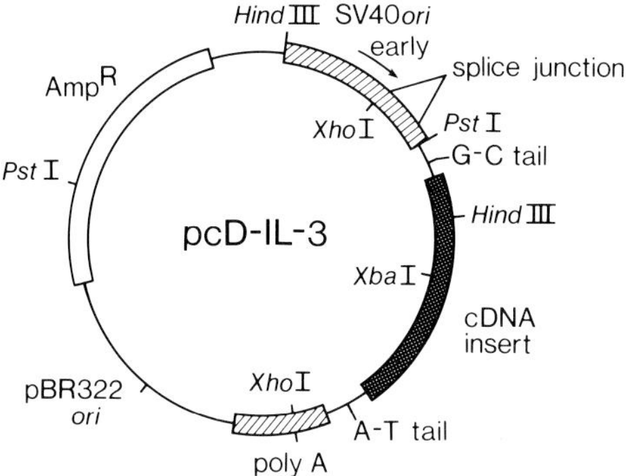

Figure 1 The (pcD) expression vector containing the mouse IL-3 cDNA insert (*Source*: modified from Ref. 13.)

unless cell type-specific posttranslational modifications are necessary. All lymphokine cDNA clones that we have studied to date are expressed in a functional form by COS cells, including mouse IL-2, IL-3, granulocyte-macrophage colony-stimulating factor (GM-CSF), interferon-γ (IFN-γ), and B-cell-stimulating factor (BSF-1), and human IL-2, GM-CSF, and IFN-γ.

We initially evaluated T-cell lines for the production of lymphokines in two ways: by bioassay of induced T-cell supernatants, and by preparation of mRNA from induced T cells, injection into *Xenopus laevis* oocytes, and bioassay of lymphokines in the supernatants. An inducer T-cell clone, Cl.Ly1/9 (17), was identified as a strong producer of several lymphokine activities, and a cDNA library was prepared from mRNA of Con A-induced Cl.Ly1/9 T cells. The cDNA library was screened by a combination of methods, including size selection, screening for cDNA clones representing induced mRNAs, and hybrid selection followed by oocyte translation. In the last method, poly-A^+ RNA containing IL-3 mRNA was incubated with filters containing bound DNA from pools of clones from the cDNA library. The RNA that hybridized to the DNA on the filter was eluted, injected into oocytes, and IL-3 activity measured in the supernatants. Positive pools of clones were subdivided and the procedure repeated. Finally, a single clone was isolated, which proved to be a partial clone of IL-3, lacking part of the 5′ sequence. This clone was used to screen the library for full-length copies. Several longer cDNA clones were transfected into COS cells, and IL-3 activity was detected in the supernatants (13).

After the functional IL-3 cDNA clones were isolated, reconstruction experiments were performed to determine the sensitivity of detection of cDNA clones in the library by direct expression. We found that one positive clone could be detected in the presence of 100 negative clones. This sensitivity has allowed us to replace the laborious hybrid selection and oocyte injection procedures with direct screening of transfection supernatants for biological activity. We have subsequently used such direct expression screening to isolate cDNA clones for mouse IL-2 (18), human GM-CSF (19), and mouse BSF-1 (20).

EXPRESSION OF RECOMBINANT MOUSE INTERLEUKIN-3

Expression in Mammalian Cells

As described in the previous section, transient expression in COS cells provided a convenient source for evaluating the expression of lymphokine cDNA clone pools and for providing small quantities of recombinant material for analysis of function. To obtain larger amounts of lymphokines from mammalian sources for biochemical and structural characterization, we have produced stable cell lines secreting IL-3. Initially, we selected for long-term stable transfectants of L cells containing either the cDNA clone in the (pcD) vector (see earlier discussion), or a genomic clone of IL-3 (10) in the λ Charon 4A vector. In both cases, the IL-3 transfectant was isolated by cotransfection of the IL-3 DNA clone with the (pSV2neo) plasmid (21), followed by selection for G418 resistance and screening for high-level IL-3 secretion (10). Stable transfectants were isolated from both sources and produced variable levels of IL-3 activity in the supernatant. The best of the cDNA transfectants produced levels of IL-3 comparable with, or greater than, the levels produced by cloned T cell lines, and the genomic transfectants produced somewhat lower levels.

We have also inserted lymphokine cDNA or genomic DNA into the bovine papilloma virus (BPV) expression vector system. Bovine papilloma virus is a small DNA virus that can replicate as stable multicopy (20–100 copies per cell) extrachromosomal elements in transformed cells (22). Several vector systems based on BPV have been used to generate cell lines that produce large quantities of a number of secretory or membrane proteins, e.g., α_5- and γ-interferon (23), human growth hormone (24), and influenza virus hemagglutinin (25). We constructed plasmids containing mouse IL-3 genomic DNA (10) or cDNA (Fig. 2) placed downstream of the SV40 early region promoter into the [pdBPV-MMT neo(342-12)]

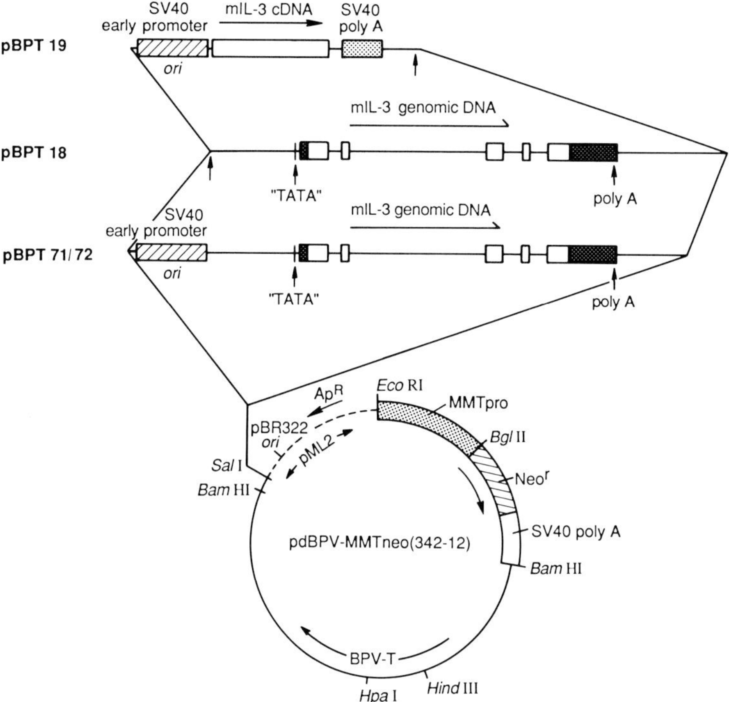

Figure 2 BPV vectors containing IL-3 cDNA and genomic inserts.

vector (26), which is composed of the entire BPV genome, a G418 resistance gene cassette, and (pML2d) [a derivative of (pBR322) lacking the "poison" sequence (27) that reduces the efficiency of transfection of mammalian cells] (Y. Takebe et al., in preparation). Recombinant DNAs were transfected into mouse C127 cells by the calcium phosphate method (28), and stable transformants were selected by G418 resistance or focus formation. The transformed mouse cells secreted high levels of IL-3 into the medium.

In contrast to the original properties of the vector, the recombinant DNAs were found as head-to-tail tandem arrays of approximately 50-100 copies, possibly integrated into the cellular DNA. Regardless of the state of the DNA, the stable cell lines carry many copies of the gene of interest. This high copy number state seems to be the reason for the efficient expression of the foreign gene. Among such cell lines, the highest IL-3 production was obtained from cell lines transformed with the BPV vector carrying a mouse IL-3 genomic DNA insert placed downstream of the SV40 early region promoter-enhancer, (pBPT71) and (pBPT72), containing the genomic insert in opposite orientations; both produced levels of IL-3 activity similar to or higher than those in activated T-cell clone supernatants. From these stable sources, we have purified recombinant mouse IL-3 protein to homogeneity: 0.2 mg of purified protein was recovered per liter of culture medium, with about 40% recovery (see later discussion).

Expression in Yeast

Expression of a lymphokine gene in mammalian host/vector systems has some advantages for the expression of authentic lymphokine molecules. No additional regulatory signals are normally required beyond the provision of an effective promoter, and the synthesized protein may reasonably be expected to undergo correct processing and cleavage of the signal peptide, addition of carbohydrate, and secretion. However microorganisms have the advantage of rapid and convenient growth and are suitable for large-scale production of expressed proteins. Yeast has the additional advantage of glycosylating the expressed proteins, although the carbohydrate added may not have the same structure as that added by mammalian cells.

Some mammalian cDNA clones, such as human IFNγ (29), can be expressed in the yeast *Saccharomyces cerevisiae* simply by promoting transcription and relying on the translational signals of the mammalian cDNA to function for translation in the yeast cells. As a first attempt to express IL-3 in yeast, we constructed yeast plasmids in such a way that the entire IL-3 cDNA was transcribed from the strong yeast promoter (ADC1) and terminated by the yeast TRP5 terminator. The yeast cells carrying these plasmids produced reasonably high levels of IL-3 mRNA with the expected size, but the level of IL-3 activity was very low, suggesting that low-level production of IL-3 might be due to inefficient translation, inefficient processing of IL-3, instability of IL-3 protein in yeast cells, or a combination of these. To avoid these potential problems, especially inefficient processing and instability of heterologous proteins, we have constructed a general secretion vector (pMFα8) employing the secretory sequences of the mating pheromone α-factor of *S. cerevisiae* (30). The α-factor is an oligopeptide secreted by MATα cells. It is initially synthesized as a large precursor molecule and cleaved at specific sites. The secretion vector (pMFα8) contains the DNA fragment of the α-factor gene (*MFα1*) carrying its own promoter, the secretory sequences, and the first processing site of the α-factor precursor. As shown in Fig. 3, the nucleotide sequence of the first processing site has been modified to provide a unique StuI site immediately after the codons specifying the Lys-Arg dipeptide, which is the recognition and cleavage site of the processing enzyme that is the product of the *KEX2* gene (31). Therefore by inserting the mature protein coding sequence into the StuI site of (pMFα8), α-factor precursor-mature protein fusions can be made. By using this system we have shown earlier that correctly processed, mature mouse IL-2 was produced and secreted into the yeast culture medium (32). We have also produced large quantities of active mouse and human GM-CSF using the same vector (Miyajima et al., manuscript in preparation).

Two different amino-terminal sequences of IL-3 have been reported; one starts at amino acid 27 (Ala) (12) and the other starts at residue 33 (Asp) (33). The DNA fragments starting at either codon 27 or 33 were prepared and inserted into the StuI site of the secretion vector (pMFα8) (see Fig. 3). The recombinant plasmids (pMG19) and (pMG23) have IL-3 cDNA starting at codons 27 and 33 respectively (30).

The yeast cells carrying (pMG19) or (pMG23) produced reasonably high levels of IL-3 activity measured by the proliferation assays on the MC/9 mast cell line (Fig. 4). The mast cell growth factor (MCGF) activity in cell extracts (cytoplasm plus periplasm) as well as culture fluid increased as the cells grew. Although the activity in cell extracts was decreased in stationary cultures, the activity in the culture medium gradually increased even in the stationary phase. There was no significant difference in MCGF activity between (pMG19) and (pMG23). This agrees with the results obtained with synthetic IL-3 starting at codons 27 and 33 (34). The CSF activity of IL-3 produced by yeast is described later.

We purified biologically active IL-3 from cell extracts and culture medium of yeast cells carrying (pMG19), and determined the NH_2-terminal sequence. The IL-3 purified from cell extracts and medium started from alanine, as expected, but an additional component isolated from the medium retained the leader sequence of the α-factor precursor. Western (protein) blotting analysis of the culture medium showed that a monoclonal antibody specific for IL-3 (see following discussion) reacted with heterogeneous molecules, suggesting that unprocessed fusion proteins with different degrees of glycosylation were secreted into the medium (Fig. 5). In addition, a component at an apparent molecular weight of about 10,000 was recognized by the antibody. This polypeptide probably results

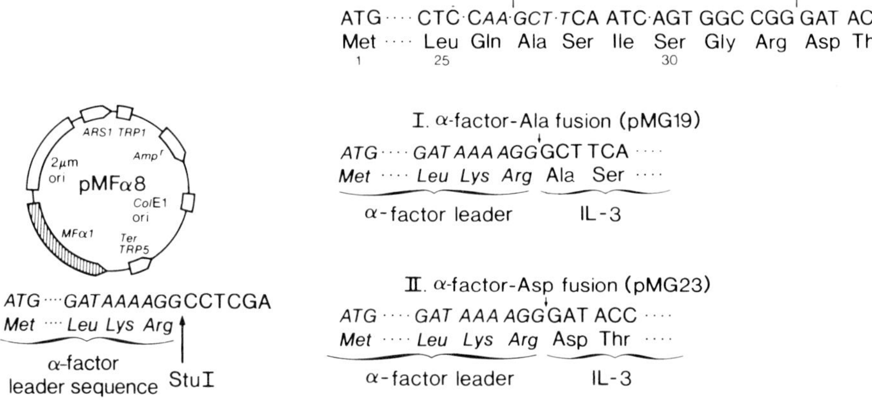

Figure 3 Yeast expression plasmids containing mouse IL-3 cDNA inserts in the α-factor secretion vector.

from the cleavage of IL-3 at an internal Arg-Arg site (residues 74 and 75) that may be recognized by the KEX2 enzyme. In the case of mouse GM-CSF expressed in yeast cells, the normal sequence contains two potential N-glycosylation sites. Removal of these sites by in vitro mutagenesis resulted in a more homogeneous product as assessed by SDS-PAGE (A. Miyajima, manuscript in preparation). It is possible that removal of the Arg-Arg site and some or all of the four potential glycosylation sites in mouse IL-3 could result in higher activities and a more homogeneous product.

Expression in *Escherichia coli*

Expression in *E. coli* can be used to provide large quantities of expressed protein, because expression levels of several percent can be achieved for some proteins. A possible disadvantage of expression in *E. coli* is that proteins will not be glycosylated. Although this may potentially affect the stability, antigenicity, or biological activity of the expressed lymphokine, we have expressed several lymphokines in *E. coli* with retention of biological activity, including human IL-2, human and mouse GM-CSF (R. Kastelein, personal communication), mouse IL-2, mouse IL-3, and human αIL-1 (G. Zurawski, unpublished results).

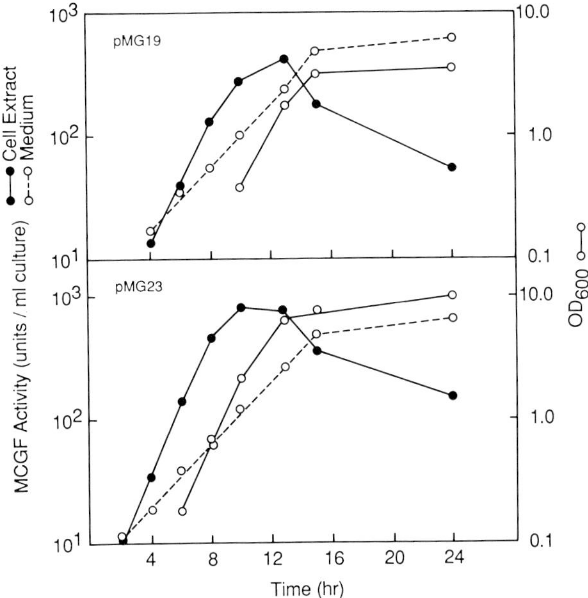

Figure 4 Expression of IL-3 in yeast as a function of cell growth: IL-3 activity in cell extracts or culture medium was assayed by a proliferation assay using MC/9 cells as indicators. Yeast cell growth was monitored by measuring the OD_{600} of the culture.

Because *E. coli* does not normally recognize mammalian translation control sequences or cleave the mammalian secretion precursor, several modifications to the cDNA are required for expression in *E. coli.* We have constructed a general cDNA expression vector, (pTAC-RBS), that contains a TAC promoter (35) and a ribosome-binding site upstream of a Sst1 restriction site used for insertion of the cDNA sequence. The lymphokine cDNA insert must be modified to remove the leader sequence and fuse the mature coding sequence to the vector so that the sequence starts with an ATG codon followed immediately by the mature lymphokine sequence.

A schematic representation of the final expression construction is shown in Fig. 6. The ~400 bp NH_2-terminal-encoding BamHI fragment from the

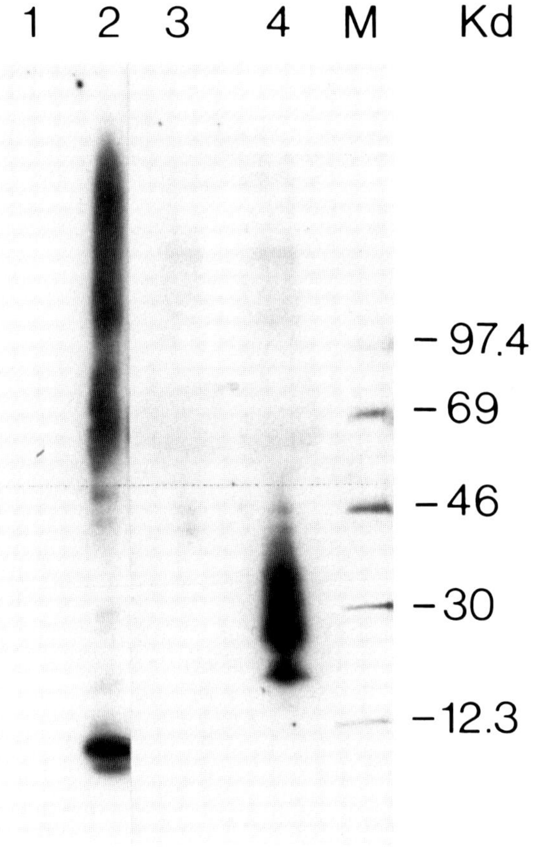

Figure 5 Western (protein) blotting of yeast-expressed and mammalian IL-3, detected with a rat monoclonal antibody. A sample volume corresponding to 25 μl of 16-fold concentrated yeast control medium (lane 1), yeast-expressed IL-3-containing medium from pMG19 (lane 2), sample volumes corresponding to 80 μl of tenfold concentrated control medium (lane 3), or Con A-induced Cl.Ly1/9 medium, were loaded on an SDS, 5–15% continuous gradient polyacrylamide gel. After transfer to nitrocellulose, the proteins were detected with the CB1 10F4 rat monoclonal antiIL-3 antibody, followed by radioiodinated antirat Ig.

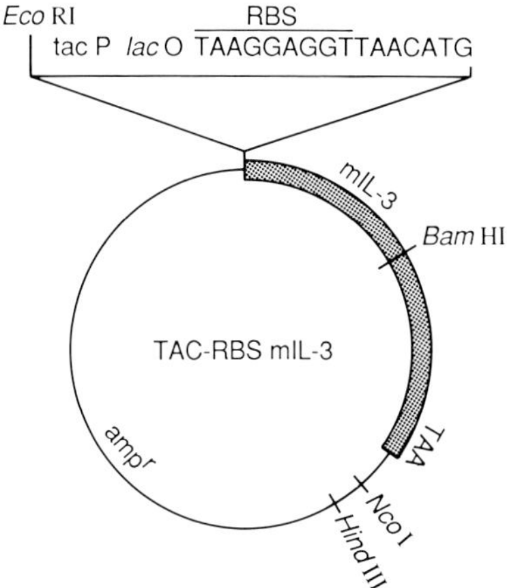

Figure 6 (pTAC-RBS) vector containing IL-3 for expression in *E. coli.*

IL-3 cDNA clone (13) was recloned into BamHI-cleaved M13mp8 RF DNA. Single-stranded DNA from the appropriate clone was used as a template for dsDNA synthesis using a synthetic DNA primer complementary to residues 124–138 (13). After S1 digestion and BamHI cleavage, the 168 bp dsDNA fragment was cloned into the (pTAC-RBS) vector DNA. In-phase fusion of the initiator ATG to the appropriate mature NH_2-terminal coding region (using the NH_2-terminal sequence (13) starting at amino acid 33) was verified by DNA sequence analysis. A BamHI-HindIII fragment (containing COOH-terminal mIL-3 sequences from the BamHI site within the coding region to the NcoI site 46 residues distal to the stop codon; Ref. 13) was then inserted to complete the construction.

The (pTAC-RBS mIL-3) expression plasmid was grown in the host JM101 and cell extracts were assayed by sodium dodecyl sulfate polyacrylamide gel electrophoresis (SDS-PAGE) and Western blotting (S. Zurawski et al., in preparation), using the monoclonal anti-IL-3 antibody CB1-10F4 (described later). Figure 7 shows an autoradiogram of a Western blot analysis containing expressed proteins from the (pTAC-RBS-mIL-3) plasmid, as well as three mutant forms of this plasmid, (pTAC-RBS mIL-3 Cys$^-$), (pTAC-RBS mIL-3 del2), and (pTAC-RBS mIL-3 Pro7). These plasmids encode proteins with, respectively, the COOH-terminal cysteinyl residue altered to serine, the six COOH-terminal residues replaced with a

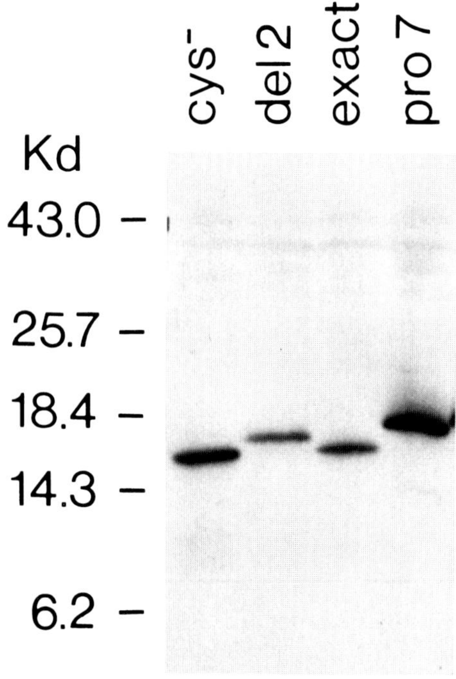

Figure 7 Analysis of mutants of IL-3 in *E. coli* by Western blotting.

peptide of 18 amino acids, and an additional seven prolyl residues at the COOH-terminus (Fig. 8).

Despite the detection of expressed mIL-3 by Western blotting, identical gels stained for protein failed to reveal abundant accumulation of the protein. Figure 9 shows that if protein synthesis in the JM101 (pTAC-RBS mIL-3) strain was inhibited by the addition of chloramphenicol (100 μg/ml), then all accumulated mIL-3 was degraded within 30 min. In contrast, mIL-2 expressed in a similar expression vector in the JM101 host was not labile over the same period. The lability of expressed mIL-3 in the bacteria can be substantially reduced in a lon$^-$ *E. coli* host (P. Liebowitz, personal communication). In such a system, expression levels of up to 1.6×10^8 U/ml culture can be achieved, representing 13–16% total protein.

The expression of biologically active mIL-3 was tested by sonication lysis of cells expressing mIL-3, followed by fractionation by centrifugation.

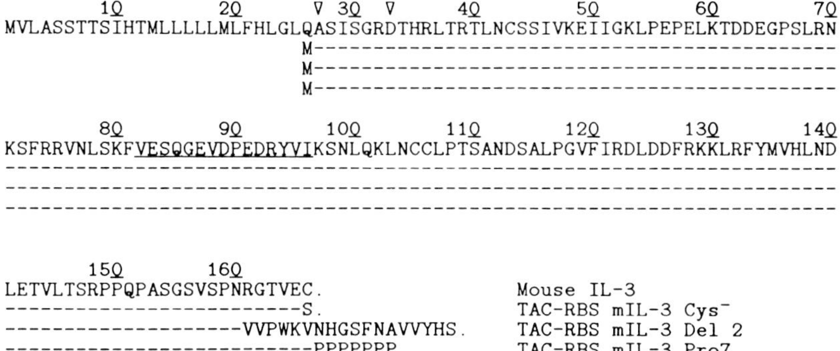

Figure 8 Amino acid sequences of IL-3 and *E. coli*-expressed mutants: The arrows indicate the two possible NH_2-termini of mature IL-3. The underlined sequence indicates the peptide used to immunize rats for the production of monoclonal antibodies.

Assays of both membrane and supernatant fractions for the ability to cause proliferation of an IL-3-dependent cell line revealed that most of the biological activity was in the membrane fraction and required extraction with 1% SDS before assay. In contrast to the lability of IL-3 during bacterial growth, the activity of the expressed IL-3 was relatively stable in cell extracts containing 1% SDS.

The effect of COOH-terminal mutations on bioactivity was measured by comparing the biological activity of the mutant proteins with the amount of antigen detected by the anti-IL-3 monoclonal antibody on Western blots. Because the monoclonal antibody was produced by immunizing with the IL-3 peptide from residue 82–96 (numbered from the initiator methionine), alterations at the COOH-terminus (amino acid 167) should not affect the ability of the antibody to recognize denatured mutant proteins. Table 1 shows that mIL-3 protein with the COOH-terminal cysteinyl residue replaced with serine is active, although the mutant protein appears to have a threefold decrease in relative bioactivity. The activity of the mIL-3 protein was tolerant to the addition of residues at the COOH-terminus (pTAC-RBS mIL-3 Pro7), although certain replacements at this terminus (pTAC-RBS mIL-3 de12) resulted in a 20-fold reduction in relative activity (see Table 1). These results are interesting because of the weak biological activity of a synthetic polypeptide representing residues 1–79 of IL-3 (34). This polypeptide was 10^4-fold less active than the

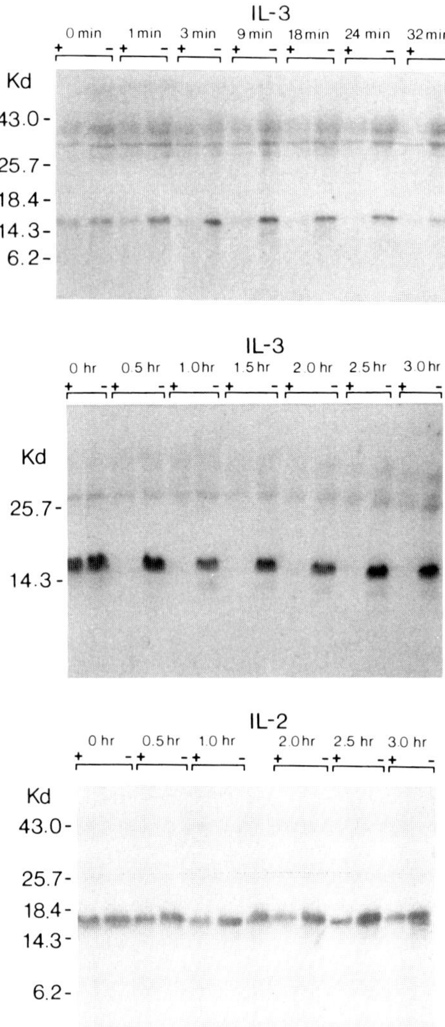

Figure 9 Stability of IL-3 and IL-2 in *E. coli* after inhibition of protein synthesis: Cultures of *E. coli* containing the expression plasmids (pTAC-RBS-IL-2) and (pTAC-RBS-IL-3) were induced with IPTG, and after an additional two generations of growth, half of each culture was treated with 100 μg/ml chloramphenicol. At the indicated times, aliquots were harvested and frozen. Proteins were extracted and analyzed by SDS-PAGE and Western blotting using the 10F4 anti-IL-3 and S4B6 anti-IL-2 monoclonal antibodies.

Table 1 Relative Activities of Normal and Mutant IL-3 Expressed in *E. coli*

Expressed protein	Activity (U/ml × 10^{-4})	Relative activity[a]
TAC-RBS mIL-3	22	1.00
TAC-RBS mIL-3 Cys$^-$	14	0.35
TAC-RBS mIL-3 del2	1	0.05
TAC-RBS mIL-3 Pro7	52	0.87

[a]The biological/antigenic activity ratio (measured by Western blotting, see Fig. 7) normalized to the value of mIL-3.

complete molecule, but even this weak activity indicates that a substantial part of the binding site must be present in the first 79 amino acids. The sensitivity of IL-3 bioactivity to some changes at the extreme COOH-terminal suggests that this region may also contribute to the binding site or that changes in this region may indirectly affect the binding site.

PURIFICATION OF RECOMBINANT INTERLEUKIN-3

Initially, we purified IL-3 from lysates or supernatants of yeast cells expressing the (pMFα1-IL3) secretion vector (discussed earlier). The material was purified by AcA54 gel permeation, followed by adsorption to sulfopropyl cation exchange resin. The eluted IL-3 was further purified by C8 reverse-phase HPLC, and two peaks of activity were obtained. These peak fractions, each contained a single species as visualized by silver-staining of SDS gels, with molecular weights of 20,000 and 25,000. The 20,000 components from both lysate and supernatant samples were subjected to microsequencing, and the expected NH_2-terminal sequence of mature IL-3 was obtained.

The amount of IL-3 synthesized by yeast cells was not as high as that obtained from mammalian expression systems; thus we undertook a more extensive purification of recombinant IL-3 from two long-term mammalian cell line sources. These were a C127 fibroblast line (S15D11) transformed with an IL-3 genomic clone in the BPV vector described earlier (pBPT72) and an L-cell line (B7) stably transfected with an IL-3 cDNA clone in the (pcD) vector (10). Supernatants from these two cell lines contained high levels of IL-3 (1–10 × 10^4 U/ml) as measured by the MTT colorimetric proliferation assay (36) using either the MC/9 or FDC-P1 cell lines (18,37).

One unit is defined as the amount of IL-3 that induced a half-maximal signal in the 3-(4,5-dimethyl-2 thiazolyl)-2,5-diphenyl-2H-tetrazolium bromide (MTT) assay, using 5×10^3 MC/9 cells in 0.1 ml. The levels of IL-3 bioactivity produced by the S15D11 and B7 cell lines are approximately one- to tenfold higher than the amount produced by Con A-induced antigen-specific T-cell lines, and 100 to 1000-fold higher than levels in WEHI-3 supernatants (T. Mosmann, unpublished observations), which have until recently served as the primary source of IL-3 (150 L provided approximately 2–10 μg IL-3; Ref. 11).

The method that we used for the purification of recombinant IL-3 (Table 2) is a modification of the procedure published by Ihle et al. (11). Briefly, cells were grown on Cytodex-3 microcarriers in medium containing 1–2% fetal bovine serum, and supernatants were concentrated tenfold using a Pellicon cassette system with a 10,000 molecular-weight-limit ultrafilter. The concentrated supernatants were applied to a DEAE-Sephacel column; the run-through and wash fractions contained 90% of the activity, purified 40- to 100-fold. A further fourfold purification of IL-3 was provided by hydroxyapatite batch chromatography, with 50% recovery. Reverse-phase chromatography was used to purify IL-3 to homogeneity. The columns were eluted with a shallow 30–45% acetonitrile, 0.1% TFA gradient. A single peak of IL-3 activity at 35.5% acetonitrile coeluted with a single, well-resolved protein peak, as detected by absorbance at 280 nm (J. Schreurs, unpublished results).

Overall, approximately 2400-fold purification was required to produce homogeneous IL-3 protein. From 2.5 L of starting material we recovered 480 μg of IL-3 with a 40% yield of bioactivity; thus the starting concentration of IL-3 in cell culture supernatants was estimated as 0.5 mg/L. The potency of this purified IL-3 was determined in an MC/9 proliferation assay alongside a sample of IL-3 purified from WEHI-3 supernatant (kindly provided by J. Ihle). The concentrations of IL-3 required for half-maximal responses were 4×10^{-12} and 3.3×10^{-12} M, respectively. These molarities were calculated from protein values determined by amino acid analysis. By Western blotting with a monoclonal anti-IL-3 antibody (see next section), IL-3 in the unpurified culture supernatants appeared as a distinct band at M_r 23,000 with additional higher–molecular-weight bands presumably representing additional glycosylation. The purified recombinant IL-3 migrated as a single M_r 23,000 silver-stained band on reducing SDS-PAGE (Fig. 10). Analysis by Aca 54 Ultrogel filtration showed that purified IL-3 eluted at M_r 38,000–43,000, presumably as a dimer.

Table 2 Purification of IL-3 from Mammalian Expression Systems

	Total activity (U)	% Yield (activity)	Total protein (mg)[a]	Specific activity (U/mg)	Fold purification
Crude	4.0×10^7	100	2574	1.5×10^4	1
DEAE-Sephacel	3.6×10^7	90	54	6.7×10^5	45
Hydroxylapatite	1.7×10^7	42	6.6	2.6×10^6	173
FPLC	1.7×10^7	40	0.48	3.5×10^7	2361

[a]Protein determinations were made assuming an OD_{280} value of 1.0 for a 1 mg/ml solution. The protein content of FPLC-purified IL-3 was determined by amino acid composition analysis.

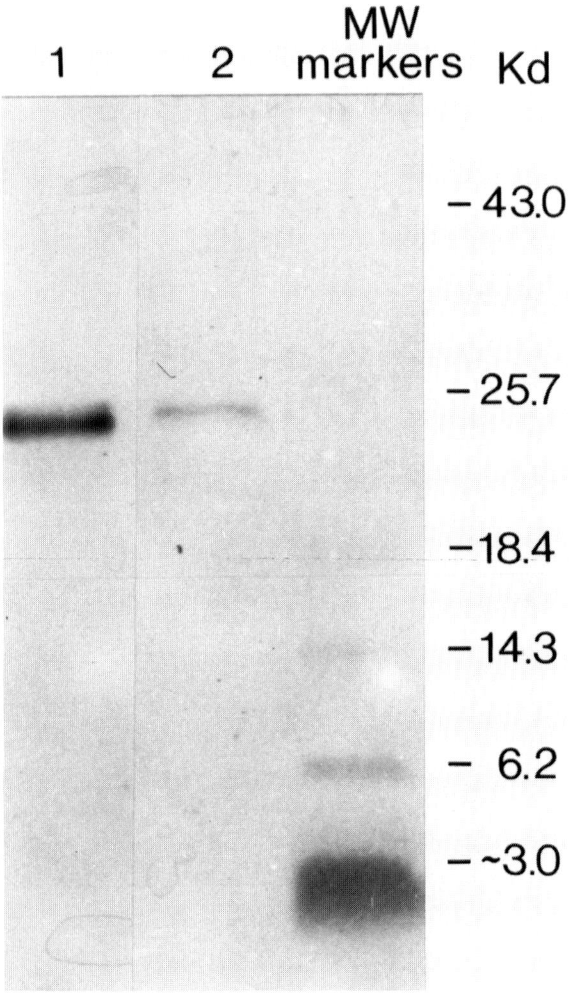

Figure 10 Homogeneity of purified recombinant IL-3: Purified IL-3 was analyzed by SDS-PAGE and silver staining. Lanes 1 and 2 contain approximately 600 and 60 ng IL-3, respectively.

MONOCLONAL ANTI-INTERLEUKIN-3 ANTIBODIES

When the cDNA clone for IL-3 was isolated, two methods for the production of anti-IL-3 antibodies were available. On the one hand, purified protein was immunogenic in rabbits (38), and whole T-cell supernatants injected into rats resulted in anti-IL-3 antisera (T. Mosmann, unpublished results). On the other hand, the known amino acid sequence of IL-3 could be used to synthesize peptides corresponding to IL-3 fragments, and these could be used to immunize rats. Using the latter approach, we immunized rats against two peptides representing amino acids 82–96 and 60–76 of IL-3 (numbering from the initiator methionine of IL-3).

Hybridomas were generated from the spleen cells of a rat immunized with the 82–96 peptide, and several hybridomas were selected that produced binding activity against both the immunizing peptide and native IL-3. The 10F4 IgG_{2a} monoclonal antibody has been characterized and used extensively in the detection and characterization of recombinant-expressed IL-3 by Western blotting (see Figs. 5, 7, and 9). This antibody recognizes mouse IL-3 synthesized in various cell types, including monkey, yeast, and bacterial expression systems (J. Abrams, unpublished results). In addition, another anti-IL-3 monoclonal antibody resulting from this fusion, 4B10, an IgM, has been used to develop a novel competitive enzyme immunoassay using an IL-3-β-galactosidase fusion protein (expressed in *E. coli*) as enzyme-labeled antigen. This assay has been used to detect IL-3 produced from *E. coli*, yeast, and mammalian sources. Neither 4B10 nor 10F4 antibody directly inhibits the biological activity of IL-3, indicating that: they do not have sufficient affinity to compete with the receptor for binding; or their determinants are not within, or adjacent to, the receptor binding site; or they recognize a determinant present only on a subpopulation of native IL-3 molecules. Regardless of their inability to neutralize activity, these monoclonal antibodies have proved invaluable for assessing the expression of IL-3 in yeast and *E. coli* expression systems.

BIOLOGICAL ACTIVITIES OF RECOMBINANT INTERLEUKIN-3

During our initial isolation of a cDNA clone for mouse IL-3 we used the mast cell growth factor activity (MCGF) to assess the clones by either hybrid selection of mRNA and translation in oocytes or by direct expression in monkey cells. We have also used the MCGF activity to test for activity of recombinant IL-3 synthesized in other systems. Biologically active IL-3 was produced in frog oocytes (13), and monkey (13), yeast (30), and bacterial cells (see Table 1). Several COOH-terminal-modified forms of IL-3 were synthesized in *E. coli*, and differences were seen in the relative activities. The MCGF activity of IL-3 derived from *E. coli* indicates that the relatively large amount of carbohydrate on IL-3 (four NH_2-linked attachment sites exist; Ref. 13) is not required for biological activity, at least in the proliferation assays. It is still possible that *E. coli*-derived IL-3 has altered in vivo properties, but this result, at least, indicates that *E. coli* expression can be useful for production of IL-3 in a biologically active form. This is also true for mouse IL-2, GM-CSF, IFN-γ, and human IL-2 and GM-CSF.

When we isolated a cDNA clone coding for MCGF activity, the sequence of the cDNA clone matched the limited NH_2-terminal sequence obtained for WEHI-3-derived IL-3 (12), and so it became important to determine the other reported bioactivities of IL-3 for two reasons—first, to confirm that the cDNA clone was in fact IL-3 by showing other activities in common and second, to provide final confirmation that the varied activities attributed to IL-3 could in fact be mediated by the cloned and expressed molecule in the absence of any other mouse lymphokine.

In addition to its MCGF activity, COS-IL-3 also stimulated proliferation of several IL-3-dependent cell lines, including FDC-P1 (37), DA-1, and NFS60 (unpublished observations). Although IL-3 alone stimulated proliferation of mast cell lines, the full proliferation of at least the MC/9 and MM3 (39) mast cell lines was obtained only in the presence of both IL-3 and BSF-1 (20,39–41). These two cell lines respond weakly to either IL-3 or BSF-1 alone, and strongly to the combination of both, whereas other cell lines such as DA-1 or FDC-P1 are apparently fully stimulated by IL-3 alone. The 20αSDH-inducing activity reported for IL-3 (1) was also present in COS-IL-3 preparations (15), as was the Thy1 antigen-inducing activity (15).

Interleukin-3 derived from monkey and yeast cells was also tested in two hemopoietic cell assays. The COS-IL-3 was found to sustain in vitro the cells responsible for spleen colony formation, and both COS- and yeast-IL-3 induced the growth of mixed colonies in methylcellulose bone marrow cell cultures (15). This latter activity, described as multi-CSF or hemopoietic cell growth factor (7) indicates the ability to support the growth of progenitor cells producing granulocytes, macrophages, mast cells, eosinophils, megakaryocytes, and erythroid cells (Table 3). In agreement with the results obtained with purified natural IL-3 (12), rIL-3 was able to stimulate growth of all of these cell types (see Table 3).

Table 3 Biological Activities of COS-IL-3 and Yeast-IL-3

				Multi-CSF					
	SDH	MCGF	THY-1	G	M	MC	EO	MEG	ER
COS-IL-3	+	+	+	+	+	+	+	+	+
Yeast-IL-3		+	+	+	+	+	+	+	+

The abbreviations G, M, MC, EO, MEG, and ER refer to the presence in hemopoietic colonies of granulocytes, macrophages, mast cells, eosinophils, megakaryocytes, and erythroid cells, respectively.

REFERENCES

1. Ihle, J. N., Pepersack, L., and Rebar, L. (1981). Regulation of T cell differentiation: In vitro induction of 20-α-hydroxysteroid dehydrogenase in splenic lymphocytes is mediated by a unique lymphokine. *J. Immunol. 126*:2184–2189.
2. Yung, Y. P., Eger, R., Tertian, G., and Moore, M. A. S. (1981). Long-term in vitro culture of murine mast cells. II. Purification of a mast cell growth factor and its dissociation from TCGF. *J. Immunol. 127*:794–799.
3. Razin, E., Cordon-Cardo, C., and Good, R. A. (1981). Growth of a pure population of mouse mast cells in vitro with conditioned medium derived from concanavalin A-stimulated splenocytes. *Proc. Natl. Acad. Sci. USA 78*:2559–2561.
4. Nabel, G., Galli, S. J., Dvorak, A. M., Dvorak, H. R., and Cantor, H. (1981). Inducer T lymphocytes synthesize a factor that stimulates proliferation of cloned mast cells. *Nature 291*:332–334.
5. Schrader, J. W., Lewis, S. J., Clark-Lewis, I., and Culvenor, J. G. (1981). The persisting (P) cell: Histamine content, regulation by a T cell-derived factor, origin from a bone marrow precursor, and relationship to mast cells. *Proc. Natl. Acad. Sci. USA 78*:323–327.
6. Dy, M., Lebel, B., Kamoun, P., and Hamburger, J. (1981). Histamine production during the anti-allograft response. *J. Exp. Med. 153*:293–309.
7. Bazill, G. W., Haynes, M., Garland, J., and Dexter, D. M. (1983). Characterization and partial purification of a haemopoietic cell growth factor in WEHI-3 cell conditioned medium. *Biochem. J. 210*:747–759.
8. Ihle, J. N., Lee, J. C., and Rebar, L. (1981). T cell recognition of Moloney leukemia virus proteins. III. T cell proliferative responses

against gp70 are associated with the production of a lymphokine inducing 20-alpha-hydroxysteroid dehydrogenase in splenic lymphocytes. *J. Immunol. 127*:2565–2570.

9. Lee, J. C., Hapel, A. J., and Ihle, J. N. (1982). Constitutive production of a unique lymphokine (IL-3) by the WEHI-3 cell line. *J. Immunol. 128*:2393–2398.
10. Miyatake, S., Yokota, T., Lee, F., and Arai, K. (1985). Structure of the chromosomal gene for murine interleukin-3. *Proc. Natl. Acad. Sci. USA 82*:316–320.
11. Ihle, J. N., Keller, J., Henderson, L., Frederick, K., and Palaszynski, E. (1982). Procedures for the purification of interleukin-3 to homogeneity. *J. Immunol. 129*:2431–2436.
12. Ihle, J. N., Keller, J., Oroszlan, S., Henderson, L. E., Copeland, T. D., Fitch, F., Prystowsky, M. B., Goldwasser, E., Schrader, J. W., Palaszynski, E., Dy, M., and Lebel, B. (1983). Biologic properties of homogeneous interleukin 3. I. Demonstration of WEHI-3 growth factor activity, mast cell growth factor activity, P cell-stimulating factor activity, colony-stimulating factor activity, and histamine-producing cell-stimulating factor activity. *J. Immunol. 131*:282–287.
13. Yokota, T., Lee, F., Rennick, D., Hall, C., Arai, N., Mosmann, T., Nabel, G., Cantor, H., and Arai, K. (1984). Isolation and characterization of a mouse cDNA clone that expresses mast-cell growth-factor activity in monkey cells. *Proc. Natl. Acad. Sci. USA 81*:1070–1074.
14. Fung, M., Hapel, A. J., Ymer, S., Cohen, D. R., Johnson, R. M., Campbell, H. D., and Young, I. G. (1984). Molecular cloning of cDNA for murine interleukin-3. *Nature 307*:233–237.
15. Rennick, D. M., Lee, F. D., Yokota, T., Arai, K., Cantor, H., and Nabel, G. J. (1985). A cloned MCGF cDNA encodes a multilineage hematopoietic growth factor: Multiple activities of interleukin 3. *J. Immunol. 134*:910–914.
16. Okayama, H. and Berg, P. (1983). A cDNA cloning vector that permits expression of cDNA inserts in mammalian cells. *Mol. Cell. Biol. 3*:280–289.
17. Nabel, G., Greenberger, J. S., Sakakeeny, M. A., and Cantor, H. (1981). Multiple biological activities of a cloned inducer T-cell population. *Proc. Natl. Acad. Sci. USA 78*:1157–1161.
18. Yokota, T., Arai, N., Lee, F., Rennick, D., Mosmann, T., and Arai, K. (1985). Use of a cDNA expression vector for isolation of mouse interleukin 2 cDNA clones: Expression of T-cell growth-factor activity after transfection of monkey cells. *Proc. Natl. Acad. Sci. USA 82*:68–72.
19. Lee, F., Yokota, T., Otsuka, T., Gemmell, L., Larson, N., Luh, J., Arai, K., and Rennick, D. (1985). Isolation of cDNA for a human granulocyte-macrophage colony-stimulating factor by functional expression in mammalian cells. *Proc. Natl. Acad. Sci. USA 82*:4360–4364.

20. Lee, F., Yokota, T., Otsuka, T., Meyerson, P., Villaret, D., Coffman, R., Mosmann, T., Rennick, D., Roehm, N., Smith, C., Zlotnik, A., and Arai, K. (1986). Isolation and characterization of a mouse interleukin cDNA clone that expresses BSF-1 activities and T cell and mast cell stimulating activities. *Proc. Natl. Acad. Sci. USA 83*:2061–2065.
21. Southern, P. J. and Berg, P. (1982). Transformation of mammalian cells to antibiotic resistance with a bacterial gene under control of the SV40 early region promoter. *J. Mol. Appl. Genet. 1*:327–341.
22. Law, M. F., Lowy, D. R., Dvoretzky, I., and Howley, P. M. (1981). Mouse cells transformed by bovine papilloma virus contain only extrachromosomal viral DNA sequences. *Proc. Natl. Acad. Sci. USA 78*: 2727–2731.
23. Fukunaga, R., Sokawa, Y., and Nagata, S. (1984). Constitutive production of human interferons by mouse cells with bovine papillomavirus as a vector. *Proc. Natl. Acad. Sci. USA 81*:5086–5090.
24. Pavlakis, G. N. and Hamer, D. H. (1983). Regulation of a metallothionein-growth hormone hybrid gene in bovine papilloma virus. *Proc. Natl. Acad. Sci. USA 80*:397–401.
25. Sambrook, J., Rodgers, L., White, J., and Gething, M. (1985). Lines of BPV-transformed murine cells that constitutively express influenza virus hemagglutinin. *EMBO J. 4*:91–103.
26. Law, M., Byrne, J. C., and Howley, P. M. (1983). A stable bovine papillomavirus hybrid plasmid that expresses a dominant selective trait. *Mol. Cell. Biol. 3*:2110–2115.
27. Lusky, M. and Botchan, M. (1981). Inhibition of SV40 replication in simian cells by specific pBR322 DNA sequences. *Nature 293*:79–81.
28. Frost, E. and Williams, J. (1978). Mapping temperature-sensitive and host range mutations of adenovirus type 5 by marker rescue. *Virology 91*:39–50.
29. Hitzeman, R. A., Leung, D. W., Perry, L. J., Kohr, W. J., Levine, H. L., and Goeddel, D. V. (1983). Secretion of human interferons by yeast. *Science 219*:620–625.
30. Miyajima, A., Otsu, K., Smith, C., Bond, M., Rennick, D., Arai, N., and Arai, K. (1985). Secretion of mature mouse interleukin-2 and interleukin-3 using the α-factor secretory system. *J. Cell. Biochem. Suppl. 9C*:156.
31. Julius, D., Brake, A., Blair, L., Kunisawa, R., and Thoner, J. (1984). Isolation of the putative structural gene for the lysine-arginine-cleaving endopeptidase required for processing of yeast prepro-alpha-factor. *Cell 37*:1075–1089.
32. Miyajima, A., Bond, M. W., Otsu, K., Arai, K., and Arai, N. (1985). Secretion of mature mouse interleukin-2 by *Saccharomyces cerevisiae*: Use of a general secretion vector containing promoter and leader sequences of the mating pheromone alpha-factor. *Gene 37*:155–161.

33. Clark-Lewis, I., Kent, S. B. H., and Schrader, J. W. (1984). Purification to apparent homogeneity of a factor stimulating the growth of multiple lineages of hemopoietic cells. *J. Biol. Chem. 259*:7488–7494.
34. Clark-Lewis, I., Aebersold, R., Ziltener, H., Schrader, J. W., Hood, L. E., and Kent, S. B. H. (1986). Automated chemical synthesis of a protein growth factor for hemopoietic cells, interleukin-3. *Science 231*: 134–139.
35. De Boer, H. A., Comstock, L. J., and Vasser, M. (1983). The *tac* promoter: A functional hybrid derived from the *trp* and *lac* promoters. *Proc. Natl. Acad. Sci. USA 80*:21–25.
36. Mosmann, T. (1983). Rapid colorimetric assay for cellular growth and survival: Application to proliferation and cytotoxicity assays. *J. Immunol. Methods 65*:55–63.
37. Ihle, J. N., Keller, J., Greenberger, J. S., Henderson, L., Yetter, R. A., and Morse, H. C. (1982). Phenotypic characteristics of cell lines requiring interleukin 3 for growth. *J. Immunol. 129*:1377–1383.
38. Palaszynski, E. W. and Ihle, J. N. (1984). Evidence for specific receptors for interleukin 3 on lymphokine-dependent cell lines established from long-term bone marrow cultures. *J. Immunol. 132*:1872–1876.
39. Mosmann, T. R., Cherwinski, H., Bond, M. W., Giedlin, M. A., and Coffman, R. L. (1986). Two types of murine helper T cell clone: 1. Definition according to profiles of lymphokine activities and secreted proteins. *J. Immunol. 136*:2348–2357.
40. Smith, C. A. and Rennick, D. M. (1986). Characterization of a murine lymphokine distinct from IL-2 and IL-3 possessing a TCGF activity and an MCGF activity that synergizes with IL-3. *Proc. Natl. Acad. Sci. USA 83*:1857.
41. Mosmann, T. R., Bond, M. W., Coffman, R. L., Ohara, J., and Paul, W. E. (1986). T cell and mast cell lines respond to B cell stimulatory factor-1. *Proc. Natl. Acad. Sci. USA 83*:5654–5658.

12

Molecular Cloning of Rodent IgE-Binding Factor Genes by Expression in Mammalian Cells

CHRISTINE L. MARTENS and KEVIN W. MOORE
DNAX Research Institute of Molecular and Cellular Biology, Palo Alto, California

KIMISHIGE ISHIZAKA
Johns Hopkins University School of Medicine, Baltimore, Maryland

Synthesis of immunoglobulin by B lymphocytes is regulated at several levels by T lymphocytes and their products. The known modes of this regulation include antigen-specific help and suppression, antigen-nonspecific help and suppression, idiotype-specific suppression, and heavy chain- or isotype-specific help and suppression. Studies of isotype-specific regulation of the synthesis of IgG (1-3), IgA (4,5), and IgE (6-10) have shown that the synthesis of a particular heavy-chain isotype by B cells can be regulated (augmented or suppressed) by T-cell factors that bind specifically to the Fc region of the immunoglobulin isotype that they regulate. These soluble factors apparently bear some structural relationship to the lymphocyte Fc receptor (1,11) and have been designated "immunoglobulin-binding factors," or Ig-BF.

Previous studies from the Ishizaka laboratory have characterized IgE-binding factors (IgE-BF) from rodent T lymphocytes that specifically regulate the IgE response. One of these factors selectively potentiates an in vitro IgE response (IgE-potentiating factor; Ref. 7), while another selectively suppresses the IgE response (IgE-suppressive factor; Ref. 6). Some evidence suggests that the IgE-potentiating factor and IgE-suppressive factor are closely related. Both factors are glycoproteins that have an affinity for IgE and can be fractionated by chromatography on IgE-Sepharose. The two factors have similar molecular sizes, 13–15 kDa, and share antigenic determinants (11). However, the two factors differ in their glycosylation patterns: IgE-potentiating factor exhibits affinity for lentil lectin and concanavalin A (Con A), while IgE-suppressive factor has an affinity for peanut agglutinin (PNA) but not Con A or lentil lectin (12). Several lines of evidence suggest that the same T cells have the capacity to produce both factors (13–15). These results have led to the proposal that IgE-potentiating factor and IgE-suppressive factor are polypeptides of similar primary structure, which differ in glycosylation and perhaps other features of their posttranslational processing (16).

Huff et al. (17) described a cloned rat-mouse T-hybridoma cell line that, upon incubation with IgE, forms at least three IgE-binding factors. One of these factors has a molecular mass (M_r) of about 13,000 and exhibits IgE-specific suppressive activity in vitro, while a second approximately 26,000 M_r IgE-binding factor has neither suppressive nor potentiating activity. Later, an approximately 60,000 M_r IgE-binding factor was identified in the hybridoma culture supernatant (18).

This hybridoma, 23B6, was used as a source of mRNA encoding IgE-binding factors in initial studies of the molecular biology of these immunoregulatory molecules. We identified and expressed cDNA clones that encode IgE-binding factor from this hybridoma cell line (19) and characterized the expressed gene products biochemically (18). These genes were identified as a subset of the endogenous, retroviruslike intracisternal A particle (IAP) gene family of the mouse, and immunochemical cross-reactivity of IgE-binding factor and IAP structural protein was demonstrated (36).

IDENTIFICATION OF IMMUNOGLOBULIN E-BINDING FACTOR COMPLEMENTARY DNA CLONES

When we began these studies, no structural information (amino acid sequence) for IgE-binding factor was available. A guinea pig antiserum that was known to recognize these factors was available (11) but proved to be unsuitable for use in molecular cloning experiments. We therefore relied upon the assays originally used to characterize IgE-binding factor: inhibition of IgE-specific rosette formation (20,21), affinity for IgE-coupled

Sepharose (22), and suppression or potentiation of an in vitro IgE response by antigen-primed rat lymphocytes (6,7,12).

Initial experiments demonstrated that IgE-binding factor activity could be detected in the supernatant of frog (*Xenopus*) oocytes that had been injected with RNA from the IgE-binding factor-producing hybridoma, 23B6 (19). Thus we constructed a cDNA library from poly(A)$^+$ RNA from IgE-induced 23B6 cells in the vector λgt10, and used the technique of hybrid selection and in vitro translation in *Xenopus* oocytes to identify IgE-binding factor cDNA clone fragments from this library. In this procedure, cDNA clones are denatured to make them single-stranded, bound to nitrocellulose filters, and incubated with a source of RNA, here RNA from the 23B6 hybridoma. The RNA that is homologous to the cDNA on the filter hybridizes, and nonhomologous messages may be washed away. The specific mRNA can then be eluted from the filter and assayed by incorporating it into an in vitro translation system that will translate the RNA into its protein product. *Xenopus* oocytes are very efficient at translating such messages, and may secrete the product into the supernatant fluid in which they are incubated. Using this procedure, several cDNA fragments were found that shared homology with mRNAs encoding IgE-binding factor. Products of the in vitro translation were active in inhibiting IgE-specific rosette formation and bound to IgE- but not to IgG-Sepharose. Thus the in vitro translation products shared functional characteristics with the IgE-binding factor from the 23B6 hybridoma (19).

COMPLEMENTARY DNA CLONES THAT DIRECT EXPRESSION OF RODENT IMMUNOGLOBULIN E-BINDING FACTORS IN COS7 MONKEY CELLS

To confirm results of hybrid selection and to obtain full-length cDNA clones, a cDNA library of poly(A)$^+$ RNA from IgE-induced 23B6 hybridoma cells was constructed in the mammalian cell expression vector, pcD (23). Expression of cDNA clones in this vector is driven by the SV40 early promoter; expression products can be generated by transient expression in COS7 cells (24,25). This library was screened using as a probe the longest of the cDNA fragments identified by hybrid selection (clone A18, approximately 1200 bp), and about 100 clones were picked. Plasmid DNA from each of these clones was introduced into COS7 monkey kidney cells for transient expression of the gene product.

Table 1 Expression of IgE-BF by Transfected COS7 Cells

DNA clone	Rosette inhibition[a] (%)	Rat IgE-Sepharose effluent/eluate	IgE cells[b]	IgG cells[b]
8.3	35	0/31	85	120
9.5	20	0/25	81	108
4.2	25	0/25	41	124
10.2	33	3/21	37	112
No IgE-BF	0	–	22	120
IgE-PF[c]	33	–	87	118

[a]Inhibition of IgE-specific rosettes.
[b]Antigen-primed rat mesenteric lymph node cells were incubated with IgE-BF samples as described (6,7,12). IgE- and IgG2-containing cells were enumerated by cytoplasmic immunofluorescence.
[c]IgE-BF produced by IgE induction of rat mesenteric lymph node cells in culture (27).

Assay of supernatants from transfection experiments with 70 of the cDNA clones yielded four cDNAs that direct synthesis in COS7 cells of secreted factors that inhibit IgE-specific rosette formation (19; Table 1). Supernatants from transient expression experiments with these four clones (4.2, 8.3, 9.5, and 10.2) were characterized further. Immunoglobulin E-binding factors in these supernatants all bound specifically to rat IgE-coupled Sepharose, and could be eluted at acid pH (see Table 1). Immunoglobulin E-binding factors in these supernatants did not bind to rat IgG_2-Sepharose, nor did they bind well to human IgE-Sepharose, as expected for a rodent IgE-binding factor (7,26).

TWO OF FOUR COMPLEMENTARY DNA CLONES DIRECT EXPRESSION OF IMMUNOGLOBULIN E-POTENTIATING FACTORS IN COS7 MONKEY CELLS

The IgE-Sepharose purified IgE-binding factors derived from clones 4.2, 8.3, 9.5, and 10.2 were tested for the selective ability to suppress or potentiate an IgE response by antigen-primed rat lymphocytes in vitro (6,7,12). The results of these experiments (19; see Table 1) showed that IgE-binding factor from transient expression of cDNA clones 8.3 and 9.5

enhanced the number of IgE-containing cells in these cultures approximately fourfold. Similar results were obtained with a preparation of IgE-potentiating factor derived from lymphocytes from a rat infected with the parasite *Nippostrongylus brasiliensis* (Nb) (7,27). In contrast, IgE-binding factor from transfections with cDNA clones 4.2 and 10.2 did not exhibit significant IgE-potentiating factor activity in vitro. Moreover, none of the IgE-binding factor preparations from the four cDNA clones suppressed the IgE response. In all experiments, the IgG_2 response remained unaffected, thus illustrating that the observed potentiating activity is specific for the IgE response.

Demonstration of potentiating activity of the expressed gene products was unexpected, as the 23B6 cell line from which these clones were isolated makes IgE-suppressive factor and no detectable IgE-potentiating factor under the conditions used to prepare cells for RNA isolation. Essentially all the IgE-binding factors made by the cells failed to bind to lentil lectin or Con A (17). Two possible explanations for the results were considered. First, IgE-potentiating factor mRNAs may be present in IgE-induced 23B6 cells, but the translation or secretion of these molecules is somehow inhibited. Alternatively, IgE-potentiating factor and IgE-suppressive factor may be encoded by the same mRNAs, but features of their posttranslational processing may differ depending upon conditions within the host cell.

Earlier studies suggested that a single T cell has the capacity to produce either IgE-potentiating factor or IgE-suppressive factor and that the two factors have common antigenic determinants. These results led Yodoi et al. (12) and Huff et al. (11) to propose that the biological activity of these factors is determined by the process of glycosylation of the same precursor molecules. Our results lend support to this hypothesis. Complementary DNA clones that express IgE-potentiating factor in COS7 monkey kidney cells were isolated from a rodent lymphoid cell line that produces an IgE-suppressive factor and no detectable IgE-potentiating factor. We tested whether or not expression of clone 8.3 in the presence of known inhibitors of glycosylation would result in IgE-binding factor with suppressive activity. We carried out the transfection in the presence of either glycosylation-inhibiting factor (28), a phospholipase inhibitory protein known to alter the biological activity of lymphocyte- and 23B6 hybridoma-produced IgE-binding factor, or tunicamycin. In both experiments, the IgE-binding factors produced by COS7 cells no longer had affinity for lentil lectin, and were active in suppressing an in vitro IgE response (29). These results strongly suggest that the polypeptides translated from mRNAs represented by the IgE-binding factor cDNA clones are processed differently by the host cells to give factors with suppressive and potentiating activities, respectively.

IN VITRO TRANSLATION OF IMMUNOGLOBULIN E-BINDING FACTOR MESSENGER RNA FROM YEAST CARRYING AN IMMUNOGLOBULIN E-BINDING FACTOR COMPLEMENTARY DNA CLONE

Because the primary structure of IgE-binding factors was unknown, it was necessary to demonstrate that the cDNA clones we identified encoded the structural genes for the factors. An alternative possibility was that the transfected cDNA clones induced expression of IgE-binding factor genes in the host cell. We established that these genes do encode IgE-binding factors by cloning a restriction fragment containing the entire coding sequence of IgE-binding factor clone 8.3 into the yeast expression vector (pAAR6) (30). This vector contains the alcohol dehydrogenase promoter and the *TRP1* gene as an auxotrophic selectable marker. The DNA was transformed into a tryptophan auxotroph, 20B-12, derived from a protease-deficient yeast strain (31). The poly(A)$^+$ RNA isolated from yeast cells carrying these plasmids was translated in *Xenopus* oocytes. Supernatants from oocytes were subjected to affinity chromatography on IgE-Sepharose, and the effluent and eluate fractions were tested for IgE-binding factor activity. Poly(A)$^+$ RNA from yeast carrying the cDNA clone in the correct 5′-3′ orientation was translated by *Xenopus* oocytes to give IgE-binding factor activity, while no activity was detected after injection of RNA derived from the corresponding clone in the opposite orientation. The results demonstrated that clone 8.3 is a structural gene that encodes a rodent IgE-binding factor (19).

The procedure of expressing a foreign gene in yeast after identification of an activity expressed in mammalian cells is generally applicable to the problems associated with cloning genes for which no structural data exist. Many biological assays for factors are subject to occasional inconsistencies in the population of target cells or to effects of unrelated molecules that may be unique to the expression system. Sometimes, the activity of a cloned gene product may not be identical with that of the originally defined factor because the original system contains a population of molecules with related, but not identical, properties or activities. An example of this was the discovery of two mast cell growth factor activities in the helper T-cell clone CL.Ly1^{+}2^{-}/9 (32). The gene encoding one of these activities was cloned and was found to be interleukin-3 (25); but the properties of IL-3 did not account for all of the mast cell growth factor activities found in the T-cell supernatant, thus suggesting the existence of a second similar factor. When this occurs it is imperative to demonstrate directly that the cloned gene actually encodes a structural gene for the factor being sought.

IMMUNOGLOBULIN E-BINDING FACTORS EXPRESSED IN COS7 CELLS ARE GLYCOPROTEINS OF 60,000 AND 11,000 MOLECULAR MASS

Gel filtration on Sephadex G-75 was used to determine the molecular size of recombinant IgE-binding factors. Transfection of cDNA clone 8.3 produced two peaks of IgE-binding factor activity that eluted at approximately 60,000 and 11,000 M_r. Expression of clone 10.2 in COS7 cells yielded IgE-binding factor activity that eluted near the void volume with an estimated molecular size of about 60,000.

The lectin-binding properties of these IgE-binding factors were determined following chromatography on IgE-Sepharose and Sephadex G-75. Immunoglobulin E-binding factors produced by transient expression of cDNA clones 8.3 and 10.2 all have affinity for lentil lectin. Lentil lectin eluates of the 60,000 and 11,000-M_r IgE-binding factors from clone 8.3

Table 2 Properties of Cloned, Expressed IgE-BF

IgE-BF	Mol. wt. (X 10^3)	Lentil lectin effluent/eluate	IgE cells[a]	IgG_2 cells[a]
None	–	0	38	124
Nb-rats[b]	13	0/25	114	109
8.3	11	0/31	112	107
8.3	60	6/32	105	121
10.2	60	0/40	57	107

[a]Biological activity assay as in Table 1.
[b]IgE-BF from rat mesenteric lymph node cells as in Table 1.

both selectively potentiated the in vitro IgE response without affecting the IgG_2 response (Table 2), while the 60,000-M_r binding factor from clone 10.2 had only marginal effect on the IgE response (see Table 2).

IMMUNOGLOBULIN E-BINDING FACTOR COMPLEMENTARY DNA CLONE 8.3 ENCODES A 62,000-M_r POLYPEPTIDE

The complete nucleotide sequence of IgE-binding factor cDNA clone 8.3 was determined (19). The sequence of this 3400 bp cDNA clone specifies a 556 amino acid (62,000 M_r) open-reading frame and a 3′ untranslated region of nearly 1400 nucleotides. There are two potential sites for N-linked glycosylation (Asn-X-[Ser/Thr]) and several sites where posttranslational proteolytic processing at tandem basic residues could occur. Because the expression of clone 8.3 in COS7 cells yields two molecular species of IgE-binding factor, the 11,000-M_r IgE-binding factor appears to be a product derived from the 60,000-M_r precursor by proteolytic cleavage. As both of these species have affinity for lentil lectin, the sites of the cleavages that generate the 11,000-M_r polypeptide must encompass one or both of the two potential sites for N-linked glycosylation. These data suggested that two IgE-binding factors produced by rodent T lymphocytes (60,000 and 13,000 M_r) might also share a precursor/product relationship.

IMMUNOGLOBULIN E-BINDING FACTOR COMPLEMENTARY DNA CLONES ARE HOMOLOGOUS TO MOUSE INTRACISTERNAL A PARTICLE GENES

In a comparison of the translated amino acid sequence of clone 8.3 with the amino acid sequence database (performed by Dr. R. Doolittle), a striking homology was found between amino acids 438–488 of the 8.3 sequence and the polymerases of several retroviruses. Chiu et al. (33) have identified a highly conserved sequence of 16 amino acids in the same region of retroviral polymerases; the 8.3 sequence (amino acids 438–450) shares 69% homology with the corresponding sequence of HTLV-I polymerase. The NH_2-terminal 437 amino acids encoded by clone 8.3 shared no significant homology with any other sequence in the data base.

This suggested homology between retroviral sequences and IgE-binding factor clone 8.3 was tested by blot hybridization. A nitrocellulose blot filter with restriction fragments of cloned retrovirus genes (provided by Drs. S. Aaronson and I.-M. Chiu) was probed with clone 8.3. The cDNA hybridized with a cloned mouse intracisternal A particle (IAP) gene (*IAP*81; Ref. 34) but not with DNA from several other cloned retroviral genes.

Heteroduplex analysis of the IgE-binding factor cDNA clone 8.3 with a cloned genomic IAP gene, *MIA*14 (35), demonstrated that clone 8.3 hybridized throughout its entire length to this IAP gene (36; Figs. 1,2). The heteroduplex also revealed that clone 8.3 has an internal deletion of approximately 3.4 kb relative to the genomic IAP gene. Thus although homology of the NH_2-terminal portion of clone 8.3 to sequences in the amino acid sequence database was not found, this clone appears to be completely homologous to a genomic IAP gene at the DNA level.

A comparison of the nucleotide sequence of clone 8.3 and two cloned IAP genes, *MIA*14 (35) and *IAP*62 (37), showed a very high degree of homology. The IgE-binding factor cDNA showed extensive homology at its 3′ end to a region of both IAP sequences that encode a long terminal repeat (LTR). Thus hybridization experiments and DNA sequence comparisons indicate that IgE-binding factor clone 8.3 is homologous to IAP genes.

The IAP genes are a family of closely related genes that are structurally similar to retrovirus proviral genomes. These genes are reiterated approximately 1000-fold in the genome of the laboratory mouse, *Mus musculus*, but IAP particles or gene products have not previously been associated with any known biological activity. The IAP genes are expressed in preimplantation embryos of the mouse (38) and in many neoplastic cells, including plasmacytomas (39). A recent report has demonstrated IAP transcripts and antigenic determinants in thymus and spleen of adult mice (40). The IAP particles resemble retrovirus particles morphologically but are not found outside the cell or transmitted horizontally (41). The IAP genes have been analyzed by Southern blot hybridization to genomic DNA, RNA blot hybridization, and restriction map analysis. Several cloned IAP genes give characteristic results in these analyses (35–44). We found that the restriction maps of four IgE-binding factor cDNA clones (Fig. 3) were virtually indistinguishable from those of cloned IAP genes, with shorter cDNAs apparently a result of internal deletions. Similarly, IAP genes that are less than full-length lack sequences found in the middle of the full-length clones. Further, RNA transcript sizes assessed by RNA blot hybridization, and mouse and rat genomic DNA blots probed with clone 8.3, gave results identical with those observed with mouse IAP genes as probe. When rat genomic DNA was probed with clone 8.3, a relatively

a.

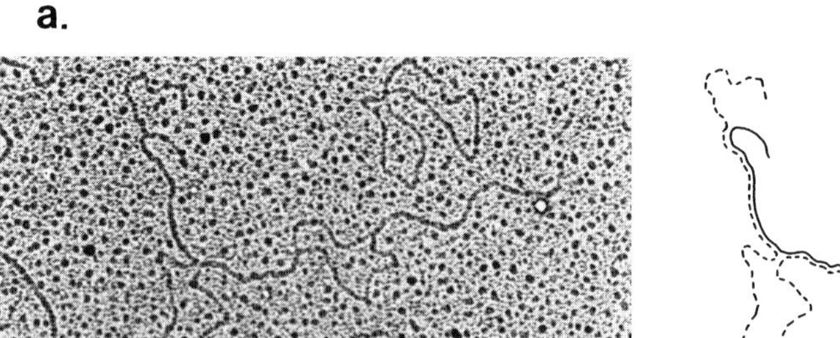

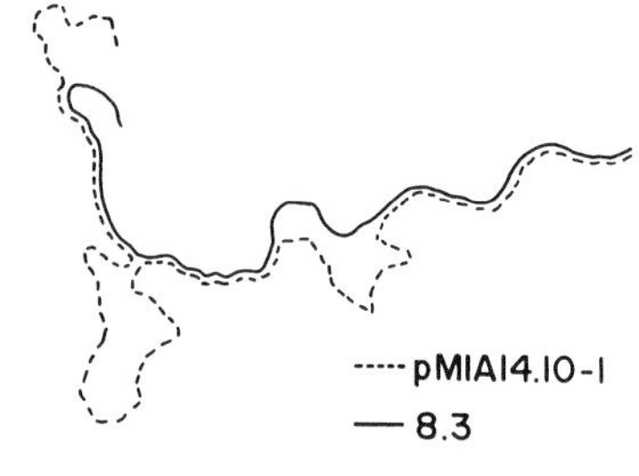

b.

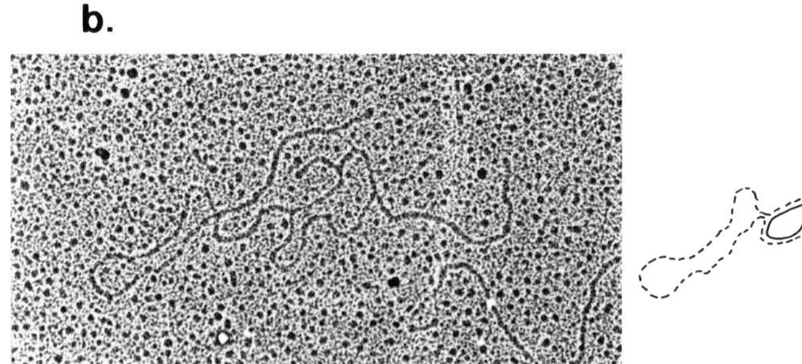

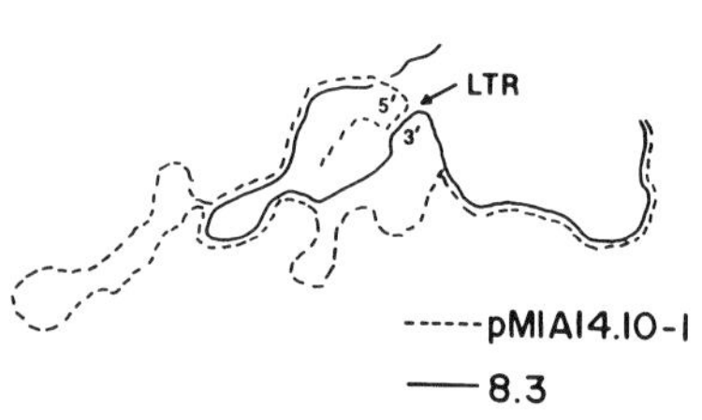

Figure 1 Heteroduplex analysis of genomic IAP clone (pMIA14.10) (35,43) with IgE-binding factor clone 8.3 (36). (a) Electron micrograph showing a heteroduplex of the IgE-binding factor clone 8.3 with the plasmid subclone (pMIA14.10-1) of the IAP gene. (b) Heteroduplex between the same two clones, showing hybridization of the 3′-LTR of clone 8.3 with the 5′-LTR of pMIA14.10-1. (*Source*: Ref. 36.)

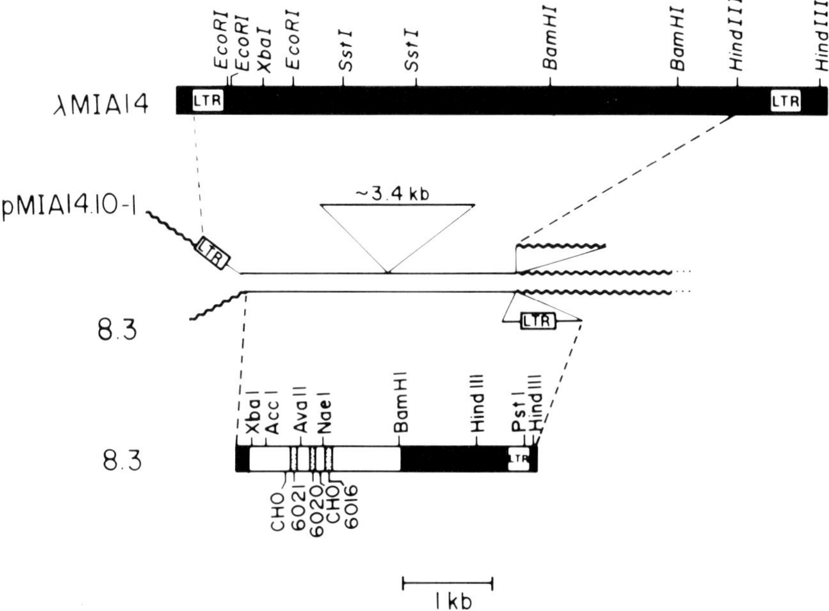

Figure 2 Line-drawn interpretation of heteroduplex shown in Fig. 1. Restriction sites, open-reading frame, and sites of N-linked glycosylation are indicated. The origins of synthetic peptides used in immunoabsorption experiments are indicated by hatched regions. Wavy lines indicate plasmid vector sequences.

weak pattern of several bands was observed; when mouse genomic DNA was probed, the pattern was one of very strong hybridization to many bands.

Thus IgE-binding factor cDNA clones and mouse IAP genes are similar in their restriction maps, patterns of transcripts detected in cells expressing IAPs, and reiteration frequencies in the mouse and rat genomes. Further, they share extensive homology as shown by DNA sequence comparisons and heteroduplex analysis. All these data indicated that the IgE-binding factor clone is a mouse IAP gene (36). No evidence was found for the existence of any segment of the IgE-binding factor gene that does not share homology with mouse IAP genes. We were unable to detect by genomic blot analysis any segment of rat DNA in IgE-binding factor clone

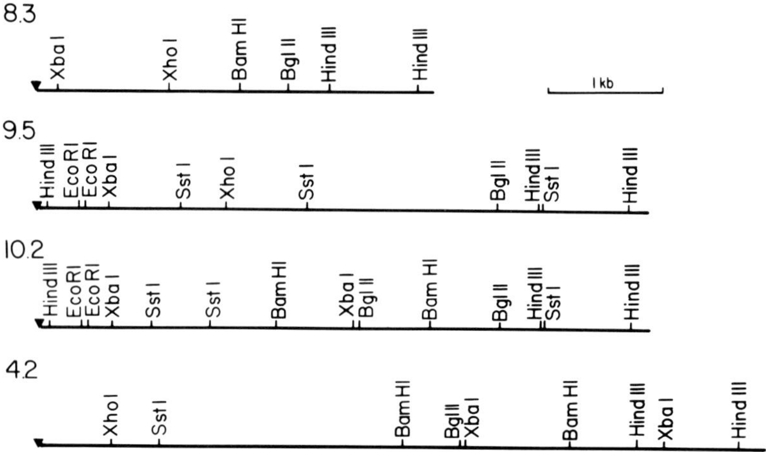

Figure 3 Restriction maps of four cDNA clones that encode rodent IgE-binding factor. The cDNA clone plasmid DNAs were cleaved with restriction endonucleases; single and double digests were electrophoresed on 1% agarose gels with appropriate-sized standards.

8.3 large enough to encode the 11,000-M_r IgE-binding factor. While we cannot rule out the presence of some small amount of non-IAP DNA in clone 8.3, the results give no indication that clone 8.3 is a recombinant gene containing both mouse IAP genetic material and rat sequences that might encode IgE-binding factor. These observations indicate that IgE-binding factor cDNA clone 8.3 is a member of the mouse IAP gene family.

It appears that only a small subset of IAP transcripts actually encodes IgE-binding factor. Many cells transcribe IAP genes abundantly but do not express detectable IgE-binding factor or Fc_ϵ receptors, such as NIH3T3 and mouse L cells. Also, only a small number of cross-hybridizing cDNA clones from the 23B6 library that were tested for IgE-binding factor activity were found to be positive (19).

IMMUNOGLOBULIN E-BINDING FACTOR SHARES ANTIGENIC DETERMINANTS WITH INTRACISTERNAL A PARTICLE PROTEINS

To demonstrate the relationship between IAPs and IgE-binding factors at the protein level, we tested IgE-binding factor from several soutces for reactivity with rabbit antisera against IAP particles (from P. Calarco, Ref. 45) and against purified IAP structural protein p73 (46). Samples of IgE-binding factor were absorbed with these antisera or with normal rabbit serum, immune complexes were removed by passage over goat anti-rabbit IgG-coupled Sepharose, and the absorbed samples were assessed for the presence of IgE-binding factor by inhibition of IgE-specific rosette formation. Two different anti-IAP antisera absorbed IgE-binding factor activity produced by expression of clone 8.3 in COS7 cells (Table 3), and both of these antisera also recognized IgE-binding factor produced by the 23B6 hybridoma.

To produce antisera with more limited specificities, we obtained synthetic peptides corresponding to portions of the predicted amino acid sequence of the IgE-binding factor encoded by clone 8.3 (36). Because the 11,000-M_r IgE-binding factor has affinity for lentil lectin, it must contain one or both of the carbohydrate attachment sites found in the sequence of clone 8.3; thus the synthetic peptides were chosen from sequences near these two sites. One of these peptides, 6021, was able to block most of the reactivity of one anti-IAP antiserum (PC) with 11,000-M_r IgE-binding factor expressed from clone 8.3 (see Table 3). The DNA sequence that encodes this peptide shares exact homology with the corresponding sequence in the IAP clone MIA14; this peptide apparently contains the major antigenic determinant on the 11,000-M_r IgE-binding factor which is recognized by the anti-IAP antiserum. Sepharose-coupled peptide 6021 was also used to purify antibodies from a second anti-IAP antiserum (A1.3). These specific antibodies recognized IgE-binding factor produced by expression of clone 8.3 and by the 23B6 hybridoma. Finally, this peptide as well as a second peptide (6020) was used as an immunogen in rabbits; the resulting antibodies reacted both with purified IAP protein p73 and with IgE-binding factor from the 23B6 hybridoma (see Table 3). Thus the relationship between IAPs and IgE-binding factor was demonstrated at both the protein and DNA levels.

Evidence has been presented that antigenic determinant(s) are shared between rat IgE-binding factor and the lymphocyte Fc_ϵ receptor (11). Immunoglobulin-binding factors that regulate other isotypes have been described, and a relationship between these factors and lymphocyte Fc receptors has been suggested (1–5,47,48). In light of the finding that rodent IgE-binding factors are encoded by a subset of the IAP gene family, it is tempting to speculate that related IAP genes might encode Fc receptors and Ig-binding factors specific for the other immunoglobulin isotypes.

Table 3 IgE-BF and IAP Proteins are Immunochemically Related

Source of IgE-BF	Absorbed with	RI (%)[a]
8.3–60 kDa	anti-IAP A1.3[b]	8
8.3–60 kDa	NRS[c]	20
8.3–11 kDa	anti-IAP A1.3[b]	3
8.3–11 kDa	anti-IAP PC[d]	4
8.3–11 kDa	anti-IAP PC + 6020[e]	0
8.3–11 kDa	anti-IAP PC + 6021[e]	20
8.3–11 kDa	NRS	37
23B6	anti-IAP A1.3	0
23B6	anti-IAP PC	9
23B6	anti-6020[f]	0
23B6	anti-6021[f]	13
23B6	NRS	36

[a]Inhibition of IgE-specific rosettes, as described (20,21).
[b]Antiserum against electrophoretically purified IAP protein p73 (46).
[c]Normal rabbit serum.
[d]Antiserum against deoxycholate-treated IAP particles (45).
[e]Synthetic peptides were used in the antibody reaction at a final concentration of 10 μg/ml (36).
[f]Rabbit antisera raised against ovalbumin conjugates of synthetic peptides (36).

ADVANTAGES OF CLONING BY DIRECT EXPRESSION

The experiments described here would have been impossible without the powerful tool of direct expression of cDNA clones in mammalian cells. There are several aspects of our findings that may be noted. First, these rodent IgE-binding factor genes are members of a large multigene family; only a few members of that family actually encode IgE-binding factor. Indirect techniques such as hybrid selection were inadequate to identify the small subset of active genes. Also, without direct expression of the cDNA clones we could not have ruled out the possibility in hybrid selection experiments that nonspecifically trapped RNA unrelated to the cDNA was translating into the activity we assayed.

Second, direct expression provides a straightforward approach to cloning genes for molecules for which little or no structural data exist. An important reservation is that the gene, once cloned, must be related back to the "activity" being assayed to prevent being misled by artifactual problems. In this work we described two approaches that we used to relate the IgE-binding factor cDNA clone 8.3 to the original IgE-binding factor produced by normal cells. The coding sequence of clone 8.3 was recloned into a yeast expression vector; RNA from these yeast cells translated into IgE-binding factor activity. In addition, antisera raised against synthetic peptides derived from the translated nucleotide sequence of the cloned IgE-binding factor gene were shown to react with cloned and expressed IgE-binding factor as well as with IgE-binding factor from the hybridoma. These two approaches, although time-consuming, unequivocally identified clone 8.3 as a structural gene encoding IgE-binding factor.

Third, direct expression allowed us to study the biochemical characteristics of the expressed molecules. These studies revealed, for example, the precursor/product relationship between the 60,000- and 11,000-M_r IgE-binding factor produced by expression of clone 8.3.

Fourth, as glycosylation appears to play an important role in the function of IgE-binding factor (11–16), expression of the cloned genes in mammalian cells will allow a full investigation of the involvement of carbohydrate side chains in the activity of these molecules. Expression in prokaryotic systems produces nonglycosylated molecules only; yeast cells do add carbohydrate, but the extent and pattern of glycosylation may differ from the products expressed in mammalian cells.

Finally, identification of the IgE-binding factor cDNA clones as IAP genes has opened an extremely interesting field of research. No biological activity had previously been associated with these abundantly expressed genes. Expression of IAP gene products in COS7 cells should allow a systematic study of the biochemistry and perhaps other functions of IAP gene products in the future.

ACKNOWLEDGMENTS

We are grateful to Dr. Paula Jardieu, Dr. Thomas Huff, Dr. Judy Mietz, Dr. Edward Kuff, and Dr. Mary Trounstine for contributing to the results discussed here. This work was supported in part by USPHS research grant AI-11202 to K. I.

REFERENCES

1. Lowy, I., Brezin, C., Neauport-Sautes, C., Theze, J., and Fridman, W. H. (1983). Isotype regulation of antibody production: T-cell hybrids can be selectively induced to produce IgG_1 and IgG_2 subclass-specific suppressive immunoglobulin-binding factors. *Proc. Nat. Acad. Sci. USA 80*:2323–2327.
2. Bich-Thuy, L. T. and Revillard, J. P. (1982). Selective suppression of human B-lymphocyte differentiation into IgE-producing cells by soluble Fcγ receptors. *J. Immunol. 129*:150–152.
3. Bich-Thuy, L. T., Samarut, C., Brochier, J., Fridman, W. H., and Revillard, J. P. (1980). Suppression of mitogen-induced peripheral B-cell differentiation by soluble Fcγ receptors released from lymphocytes. *Eur. J. Immunol. 10*:894–898.
4. Hoover, R. G., Gebel, H. M., Dieckgraefe, B. K., Hickman, S., Rebbe, N. F., Hirayama, N., Ovary, Z., and Lynch, R. G. (1981). Occurrence and potential significance of increased numbers of T-cells with Fc receptors in meyloma. *Immunol. Rev. 56*:115–139.
5. Yodoi, J., Adachi, M., Teshigawara, K., Miyamainaba, M., Masuda, T., and Fridman, W. H. (1983). T cell hybridomas coexpressing Fc receptors (FcR) for different isotypes. II. IgA-induced formation of suppressive IgA binding factor(s) by a murine T hybridoma bearing FcγR and FcαR. *J. Immunol. 131*:303–310.
6. Hirashima, M., Yodoi, J., and Ishizaka, K. (1980). Regulatory role of IgE-binding factors from rat T lymphocytes. III. IgE-specific suppressive factor with IgE-binding activity. *J. Immunol. 125*:1442–1448.
7. Suemura, M., Yodoi, J., Hirashima, M., and Ishizaka, K. (1980). Regulatory role of IgE-binding factors from rat T-lymphocytes. I. Mechanisms of enhancement of IgE responses by IgE-potentiating factor. *J. Immunol. 125*:148–154.
8. Suemura, M., Shiho, O., Deguchi, H., Yamamura, Y., Bottcher, I., and Kishimoto, T. (1981). Characterization and isolation of IgE class-specific suppressor factor (IgE-TsF). I. The presence of binding site(s) for IgE and of H-2 gene products in IgE-TsF. *J. Immunol. 127*:465–471.
9. Suemura, M., Ishizaka, A., Kobatake, S., Sugimura, K., Maeda, K., Nakanishi, K., Kishimoto, S., Yamamura, Y., and Kishimoto, T. (1983). Inhibition of IgE production in B-hybridomas by IgE class-specific suppressor factor from T-hybridomas. *J. Immunol. 130*:1056–1060.
10. Saryan, J. A., Leung, D. Y. M., and Geha, R. S. (1983). Induction of human IgE synthesis by a factor derived from T cells of patients with hyper-IgE states. *J. Immunol. 130*:242–247.
11. Huff, T. F., Yodoi, J., Uede, T., and Ishizaka, K. (1984). Presence of an antigenic determinant common to rat IgE-potentiating factor, IgE-suppressive factor, and Fcϵ receptors on T- and B-lymphocytes. *J. Immunol. 132*:406–412.

12. Yodoi, J., Hirashima, M., and Ishizaka, K. (1982). Regulatory role of IgE-binding factors from rat T-lymphocytes. V. The carbohydrate moieties in IgE-potentiating factors and IgE-suppressive factors. *J. Immunol. 128*:289–295.
13. Yodoi, J., Hirashima, M., and Ishizaka, K. (1981). Lymphocytes bearing Fc receptors for IgE. V. Effect of tunicamycin on the formation of IgE-potentiating factor and IgE-suppressive factor by Con A-activated lymphocytes. *J. Immunol. 126*:877–882.
14. Yodoi, J., Hirashima, M., and Ishizaka, K. (1981). Lymphocytes bearing Fc receptors for IgE. VI. Suppressive effect of glucocorticoids on the expression of Fc_{ϵ} receptors and glycosylation of IgE-binding factors. *J. Immunol. 127*:471–476.
15. Yodoi, J., Hirashima, M., Hirata, F., DeBlas, A. L., and Ishizaka, K. (1981). Lymphocytes bearing Fc receptors for IgE. VII. Possible participation of phospholipase A_2 in the glycosylation of IgE-binding factors. *J. Immunol. 127*:476–482.
16. Huff, T. F., Uede, T., Iwata, M., and Ishizaka, K. (1983). Modulation of the biologic activities of IgE-binding factors. III. Switching of a T-cell hybrid clone from the formation of IgE-suppressive factor to the formation of IgE-potentiating factor. *J. Immunol. 131*:1090–1095.
17. Huff, T. F., Uede, T., and Ishizaka, K. (1982). Formation of rat IgE-binding factor by rat-mouse T cell hybridomas. *J. Immunol. 129*: 509–514.
18. Jardieu, P., Moore, K., Martens, C., and Ishizaka, K. (1985). Relationship among IgE-binding factors with various molecular weights. *J. Immunol. 135*:2727–2735.
19. Martens, C. L., Huff, T. F., Jardieu, P., Trounstine, M. L., Coffman, R. L., Ishizaka, K., and Moore, K. W. (1985). cDNA clones encoding IgE-binding factors from a rat-mouse T-cell hybridoma. *Proc. Natl. Acad. Sci. USA 82*:2460–2464.
20. Yodoi, J. and Ishizaka, K. (1979). Lymphocytes bearing receptors for IgE. I. Presence of human and rat T lymphocytes with Fc_{ϵ} receptors. *J. Immunol. 122*:2577–2583.
21. Yodoi, J. and Ishizaka, K. (1980). Lymphocytes bearing Fc receptors for IgE. IV. Formation of IgE-binding factors by rat T-lymphocytes. *J. Immunol. 124*:1322–1329.
22. Yodoi, J., Hirashima, M., and Ishizaka, K. (1980). Regulatory role of IgE-binding factors from rat T-lymphocytes. II. Glycoprotein nature and source of IgE-potentiating factor. *J. Immunol. 125*:1435–1441.
23. Okayama, H. and Berg, P. (1983). A cDNA cloning vector that permits expression of cDNA inserts in mammalian cells. *Mol. Cell. Biol. 3*: 280–289.
24. Gluzman, Y. (1981). SV40-transformed simian cells support the replication of early SV40 mutants. *Cell 23*:175–182.

25. Yokota, T., Lee, F., Rennick, D., Hall, C., Arai, N., Mosmann, T., Nabel, G., Cantor, H., and Arai, K. (1984). Isolation and characterization of a mouse cDNA clone that expresses mast cell growth factor activity in monkey cells. *Proc. Natl. Acad. Sci. USA 81*:1070–1074.
26. Huff, T. F. and Ishizaka, K. (1984). Formation of IgE-binding factors by human T-cell hybridomas. *Proc. Natl. Acad. Sci. USA 81*:1514–1518.
27. Suemura, M. and Ishizaka, K. (1979). Potentiation of IgE response in vitro by T-cells from rats infected with *Nippostrongylus brasiliensis. J. Immunol. 123*:918–924.
28. Uede, T., Hirata, F., Hirashima, M., and Ishizaka, K. (1983). Modulation of the biologic activities of IgE-binding factors. I. Identification of glycosylation-inhibiting factor as a fragment of lipomodulin. *J. Immunol. 130*:878–884.
29. Martens, C. L., Jardieu, P., Trounstine, M. L., Stuart, S. G., Ishizaka, K., and Moore, K. W. (1987). Potentiating and suppressive IgE-binding factors are expressed by a single cloned gene. *Proc. Natl. Acad. Sci. USA* (in press).
30. Ammerer, G. (1983). Expression of genes in yeast using the ADCI promoter. *Methods Enzymol. 101*:192–201.
31. Jones, E. W. (1976). Proteinase mutants of *Saccharomyces cerevisiae. Genetics 85*:23–33.
32. Smith, C. A. and Rennick, D. M. (1986). Characterization of a murine lymphokine distinct from IL-2 and IL-3 possessing a TCGF activity and an MCGF activity that synergizes with IL-3. *Proc. Natl. Acad. Sci. USA 83*:1857–1861.
33. Chiu, I. M., Callahan, R., Tronick, S. R., Schlom, J., and Aaronson, S. A. (1984). Major *pol* gene progenitors in the evolution of oncoviruses. *Science 223*:364–370.
34. Ono, M., Cole, M. D., White, A. T., and Huang, R. C. (1980). Sequence organization of cloned intracisternal A-particle genes. *Cell 21*:465–473.
35. Lueders, K. K. and Kuff, E. L. (1980). Intracisternal A-particle genes: Identification in the genome of *Mus musculus* and comparison of multiple isolates from a mouse gene library. *Proc. Natl. Acad. Sci. USA 77*:3571–3575.
36. Moore, K. W., Jardieu, P., Mietz, J. A., Trounstine, M. L., Kuff, E. L., Ishizaka, K., and Martens, C. L. (1986). Rodent IgE-binding factor genes are members of an endogenous retrovirus-like gene family. *J. Immunol. 136*:4283–4290.
37. Christy, R. J., Brown, A. R., Gourlie, B. B., and Huang, R. C. (1985). Nucleotide sequences of murine intracisternal A-particle gene LTRs have extensive variability within the R region. *Nucl. Acids Res. 13*:289–302.
38. Biczysko, W., Pienkowski, M., Solter, D., and Koprowski, H. (1973). Virus particles in early mouse embryos. *J. Natl. Canc. Inst. 51*:1041–1050.

39. Wivel, N. A. and Smith, G. H. (1971). Distribution of intracisternal A-particles in a variety of normal and neoplastic mouse tissues. *Int. J. Cancer* *7*:167–175.
40. Kuff, E. L. and Fewell, J. W. (1985). Intracisternal A-particle gene expression in normal mouse thymus tissue: Gene products and strain-related variability. *Mol. Cell. Biol.* *5*:474–483.
41. Minna, J. D., Lueders, K. K., and Kuff, E. L. (1974). Expression of genes for intracisternal A-particle antigen in somatic cell hybrids. *J. Natl. Canc. Inst.* *52*:1211–1217.
42. Kuff, E. L., Feenstra, A., Lueders, K., Smith, L., Hawley, R., Hozumi, N., and Shulman, M. (1983). Intracisternal A-particle genes as moveable elements in the mouse genome. *Proc. Natl. Acad. Sci. USA* *80*:1922–1996.
43. Kuff, E. L., Smith, L. A., and Lueders, K. K. (1981). Intracisternal A-particle genes in *Mus musculus*: A conserved family of retrovirus-like elements. *Mol. Cell. Biol.* *1*:216–227.
44. Wujcik, K. M., Morgan, R. A., and Huang, R. C. (1984). Transcription of intracisternal A-particle genes in mouse myeloma and Ltk$^-$ cells. *J. Virol.* *52*:29–36.
45. Huang, T. T. and Calarco, P. (1981). Immunoprecipitation of intracisternal A-particle-associated antigens from preimplantation mouse embryos. *J. Natl. Canc. Inst.* *67*:1129–1133.
46. Kuff, E. L., Callahan, R., and Howk, R. S. (1980). Immunological relationship between the structural proteins of intracisternal A-particles of *Mus musculus* and the M432 retrovirus of *Mus cervicolor*. *J. Virol.* *33*:1211–1214.
47. Fridman, W. H., Neauport-Sautes, C., Daeron, M., Yodoi, J., Lowy, I., Brezin, C., Vaquero, C., Gelabert, M. J., and Theze, J. (1984). Induction of Fc receptors and immunoglobulin-binding factors in T-cell clones. *Mol. Immunol.* *21*:1243–1251.
48. Kiyono, H., Mosteller-Barnum, L. M., Pitts, A. M., Williamson, S. I., Michalek, S. M., and McGhee, J. R. (1985). Isotype-specific immunoregulation. IgA-binding factors produced by Fcα receptor-positive T cell hybridomas regulate IgA responses. *J. Exp. Med.* *161*:731–747.

13

Interferon: From Rarity to Plenty, Simplicity to Complexity

SIDNEY PESTKA*
Roche Institute of Molecular Biology, Roche Research Center, Nutley, New Jersey

The natural interferons (IFN), usually as crude preparations, provided all of the materials for fundamental and clinical studies until 1980 when several groups succeeded in introducing genes coding for individual human interferons into bacteria, making it possible to express the corresponding interferon proteins. Thus it then became feasible to prepare individual subtypes of human leukocyte (α) interferon as well as human fibroblast (β) interferon through bacterial fermentation. Just as it has been necessary to develop purification schemes for the isolation of the natural interferons to remove other potentially active interferons and lymphokines, as well as other proteins, so purification techniques for the preparation of homogeneous recombinant interferons had to be designed that would remove the contaminating bacterial proteins from the interferon (IFN). This chapter summarizes procedures involved in the preparation and construction of recombinant interferons. In addition, as an example, the purification of recombinant human IFN-αA by monoclonal antibodies is described. The last section of this chapter summarizes its biological activities.

**Present affiliation*: UMDNJ–Robert Wood Johnson Medical School, Piscataway, New Jersey.

ISOLATION OF RECOMBINANTS

The advent of recombinant DNA technology permitted the cloning of genes from one organism into another. Genes, formerly difficult to obtain, were now available to study their structure, function, transcription, and expression. Because a vast base of knowledge had already been developed providing a solid understanding of the regulation of the expression of many genes in *Escherichia coli*, the ground was prepared to use these regulatory elements for expression of foreign genes in bacteria. Interferon was among the first human proteins expressed in *E. coli* (1,2).

Because recombinant DNA technology offered an opportunity to produce large amounts of human interferons economically, many scientific teams set out to clone them in bacteria. Several groups achieved the isolation of recombinants for a few human α-interferon subtypes (3,4) and for β-interferon (4-8) achieving their goals by somewhat different but analogous approaches. I describe the cloning of a recombinant human α-interferon as an illustration of these procedures.

Isolating human interferon DNA sequences was a formidable task because it meant preparing DNA recombinants from cellular mRNA that was present at a low level. This task had never been accomplished previously for a protein whose structure was unknown. In addition, to reconstruct properly DNA recombinants that would express natural interferon, it was useful to know the partial amino acid sequence of the proteins, particularly at the NH_2- and COOH-terminal ends. Without this information synthesis of natural human interferon in bacteria would not have been possible. Thus purification of the human interferons and determination of their structure (9-17) assisted us and others in these efforts.

To isolate recombinants containing the human DNA corresponding to the sequence of an α-interferon, our approach involved a number of procedures. First, it was necessary to isolate and measure the interferon mRNA. This was accomplished several years earlier when interferon mRNA was translated in cell-free extracts (Fig. 1) (18,19) and in frog oocytes (20-23). The next step was to prepare sufficient mRNA from cells synthesizing interferon, and this was accomplished with both fibroblasts and leukocytes (24,25).

A library of complementary DNA (cDNA) was prepared from a template of partially purified mRNA isolated from human leukocytes synthesizing interferon (details of this and the other steps in the procedure are shown schematically in Fig. 2 and are described in the figure caption). The dC-tailed double-stranded DNA obtained was hybridized to dG-tailed DNA

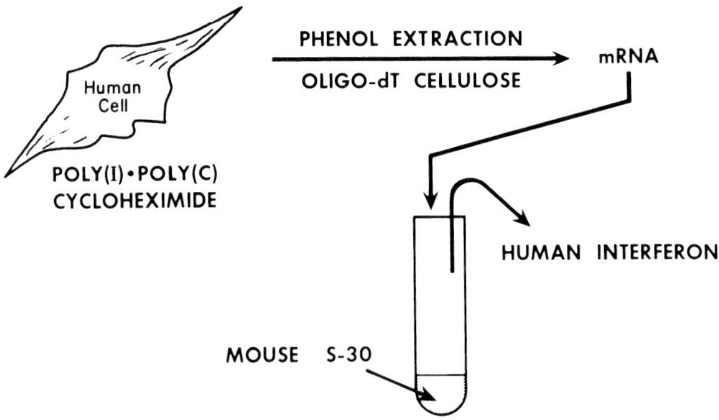

Figure 1 Interferon synthesis in a cell-free system. Human fibroblasts were stimulated to produce interferon by treatment with the inducer, poly (I)•poly (C). Four hours later, the total RNA present was extracted from the cells with phenol, and the fraction enriched in mRNA was selected on an oligo(dT)-cellulose column. An S-30 supernatant translation fraction was prepared from mouse cells. This was able to translate the various mRNA species, including that for IFN-β, into the corresponding proteins. The interferon formed was detected in a standard antiviral assay. In this way, biologically active human interferon was synthesized in the test tube for the first time. By injecting the mRNA into intact frog oocytes, the mRNA could be measured at 0.01–0.001 the levels that could be detected in the cell-free extracts (*Source*: from Ref. 1).

from plasmid (pBR322) that had been cleaved at the *Pst*I restriction nuclease site and introduced into *E. coli* by transformation. About 14,000 tetracycline-resistant and ampicillin-sensitive transformants were obtained. This provided a large group of cDNA recombinants with DNA copies of all the mRNAs extracted from the leukocytes. The next and the hardest part of the procedure was to find in this large library of recombinant plasmids those that contained DNA that encoded interferon. If we had been able to begin with pure interferon mRNA, it would have been a simple task. However we did not have pure interferon mRNA. We began with a mixture of mRNA molecules, only a few of which were interferon-specific. We could show their presence by translating the RNA and assaying the products for interferon activity (as in Fig. 1). In this situation, we had to devise an indirect two-stage procedure. In the first stage, we screened all the bacterial colonies to find those with cDNA made from the RNA of induced cells;

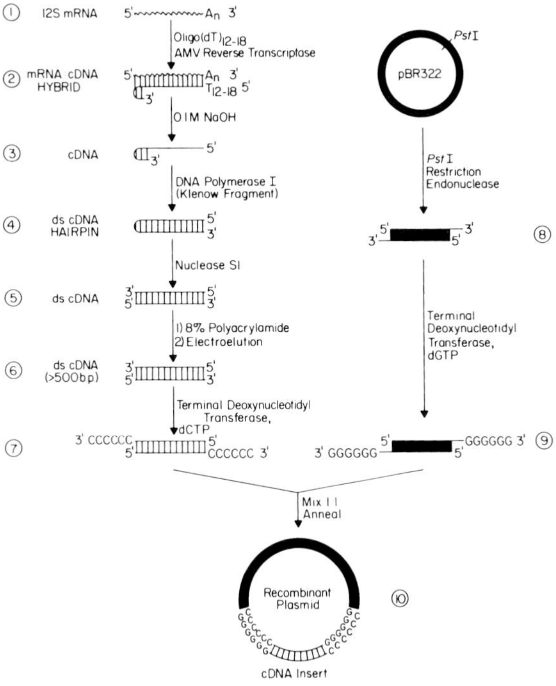

Figure 2 Preparation of interferon DNA recombinants from mRNA. *Step 1.* A human leukocyte suspension was induced to form interferon by stimulation with Sendai virus. Six hours later, an extract was made, from which mRNA was prepared that was enriched in 12S mRNA by differential centrifugation. *Step 2.* The mRNA fraction was used as a template with AMV reverse transcriptase in the presence of all four deoxynucleotide triphosphates and oligo$(dT)_{12\text{-}18}$ as a primer to generate a DNA strand complementary to the mRNA (cDNA) forming mRNA:cDNA hybrids. *Step 3.* Treatment with 0.1 M NaOH digested away the RNA, leaving a cDNA fragment with a self-annealed 3′ end. *Step 4.* Extension of the chain with DNA polymerase I (Klenow fragment) produced a double-stranded (ds) cDNA containing a hairpin loop. *Step 5.* Treatment with nuclease S1 opened the hairpin loop. *Step 6.* The ds-cDNA was sized on an 8% polyacrylamide gel followed by electroelution to give a fraction containing at least 500 bp. *Step 7.* Treatment with terminal deoxynucleotidyl transferase in the presence of dCTP added cytosine homopolymer tails at the 3′ ends of each strand. *Step 8.* The plasmid pBR322 was cleaved (linearized) at the *Pst*I site with *Pst*I restriction endonuclease. *Step 9.* Homopolymer tails of oligodeoxyguanylate (oligo-dG) were added to the 3′ ends of the linearized plasmid DNA with terminal deoxynucleotidyl transferase in the

among these there might have been some carrying interferon cDNA. We therefore screened all of the recombinants for their ability to bind to mRNA from cells synthesizing interferon (induced cells) but not to mRNA from uninduced cells (those not producing interferon) (Fig. 3). To do this, individual transformant colonies were screened by colony hybridization for the presence of induced-specific sequences with ^{32}P-labeled interferon mRNA (mRNA from induced cells) as a probe. In the presence of excess mRNA from uninduced cells (see Fig. 3), recombinants that were representative of mRNA sequences existing only in induced cells should be evident on hybridization. This screening procedure allowed us to discard about 90% of the colonies: because their plasmids carried no induced cDNA, these could not encode interferon (4,26).

In the second stage, we had to identify among the remaining 10% those recombinants containing the interferon DNA sequences (i.e., about 1400). To do this, we pooled the recombinant plasmids in groups of 10 and examined these for the presence of interferon-specific sequences by an assay that depends upon hybridization of interferon mRNA to plasmid DNA (4,27). Plasmid DNA from 10 recombinants was isolated and covalently bound to diazobenzyloxymethyl (DBM) paper (Fig. 4). Messenger RNA from induced cells was hybridized to each filter. Unhybridized mRNA was removed by washing. After the specifically hybridized mRNA was eluted, both fractions were translated in *Xenopus laevis* oocytes. Once a positive group had been found (one in which the specifically hybridized mRNA yielded interferon after microinjection into frog oocytes), it was necessary to identify the specific clone or clones containing interferon cDNA. The 10 individual colonies were grown, the plasmid DNAs were prepared, and each individual DNA was examined by mRNA hybridization as described earlier (see Fig. 4). By these procedures a recombinant, plasmid 104 (p104), containing most of the coding sequence for a human α-interferon, was identified (4). The DNA sequence was determined and corresponded to what was then known of the amino acid sequence of purified human leukocyte interferon (14,15). The cDNA insert in (p104)

---

presence of dGTP. *Step 10.* The two fragments with complementary sticky ends were mixed in equal proportions and annealed to yield a recombinant plasmid. A larger number of similar plasmids not containing interferon genetic information were also formed during this procedure. This cDNA library contained copies of all the mRNA in these cells including interferon-specific mRNA (*Source*: from Ref. 1).

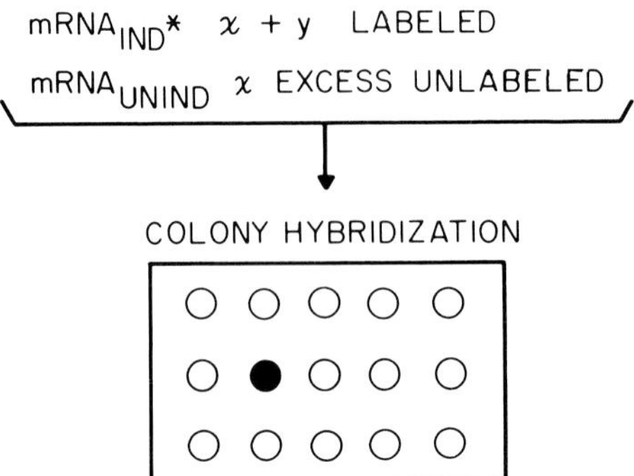

Figure 3 Schematic outline of hybridization procedure. *Escherichia coli* cells were transformed with the recombinant plasmids generated as described in Fig. 2. Colonies derived from individual transformed bacterial cells were transferred to filter paper, fixed, and probed with a ^{32}P-labeled mRNA preparation from cells producing interferon and therefore enriched in interferon mRNA (x + y). The hybridization was performed in the presence of excess unlabeled mRNA from uninduced cells (x). This procedure identified bacterial colonies containing DNA coding for the protein specifically formed in induced leukocytes, including interferon. The induced-specific sequences (y) include interferon sequences as well as others that are induced concomitantly with interferon (*Source*: from Ref. 1).

contains the sequence corresponding to more than 80% of the amino acids in leukocyte interferon but not for those at its amino-terminal end. It was therefore used as a probe for finding a full-length copy of the interferon cDNA sequence that could be used for expression of human leukocyte interferon in *E. coli.* In addition, (p104) DNA was used to isolated DNA sequences corresponding to α-interferons directly from a human gene bank.

Examination of the coding regions of the leukocyte interferon genes that have been isolated in our laboratory, and in others, have shown that these correspond to a family of homologous proteins, the α-interferon subtypes (for reviews and additional citations see Refs. 1,2,28) which are closely related to each other and yet each unique in amino acid sequence (Fig. 5). Thus the previously discovered heterogeneity in human leukocyte interferon was shown to be, at least in part, the result of distinct genes

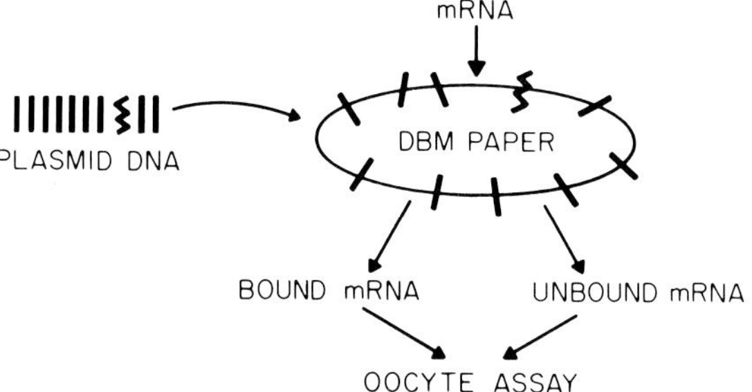

Figure 4 Schematic illustration of screening of recombinants with DBM paper. Plasmid DNA was isolated from a pool of colonies, e.g., 10 colonies as shown in the figure, and bound covalently to diazobenzyloxymethyl (DBM) paper. To detect a recombinant containing an interferon sequence (shown as a zig-zag in the illustration), mRNA prepared from cells synthesizing interferon was hybridized to the bound DNA. After unhybridized mRNA had been removed by washing, the specifically hybridized mRNA was eluted and translated in *X. laevis* oocytes. By this procedure, those pools of clones in which at least one recombinant contained an interferon sequence were identified. Thereafter, individual clones in each pool were separately screened by the same procedure. Unbound mRNA was microinjected into oocytes as well as a control to ascertain that the mRNA was not destroyed by the manipulations.

representing each expressed human leukocyte interferon sequence. The cloned human IFN-αA, which was the first we isolated, corresponds to the natural interferons that we purified from the mixture present in leukocyte interferon by high-performance liquid chromatography (HPLC) and termed α_2 and β_1. [The natural interferons that we isolated from the mixture present in leukocyte interferon by HPLC (9–11) were then designated α_1, α_2, β_1, β_2, β_3, γ_1, γ_2, γ_3, γ_4, γ_5, and δ. Unfortunately, the same terminology was later applied to designate leukocyte, fibroblast, and immune interferons, respectively as α, β, and γ. The α_2 and β_1 indicated here refer to two different leukocyte interferon fractions.]

By procedures similar to those described for (p104), (p101) was shown to contain the sequence for human fibroblast interferon (4). Thus the nucleotide sequences coding for human leukocyte and fibroblast interferons were identified.

	S1 S10	S20	S23	1 10	20	30	40	50	60	70
IFN-α consensus	MALSFSLLMA	VLVLSYKSIC	SLG	CDLPQTHSLG	NRRALILLAQ	MGRISPFSCL	KDRHDFGFPQ	EEFDGNQFQK	AQAISVLHEM	IQQTFNLFST
IFN-αK (α6)	...P.A....	LV...C..S.	..D	....	H..TMM....	.R...L....	......R...	....	.E.......V	....
IFN-α5 (αG)	...P.V....	LV..NC....	...	.........S	...T.MIM..	....	....	....	....	....
IFN-αA (α2)	...T.A..V.	L....C..S.	.V.	....	S..T.M....	.RK..L....	....	...-......	.ET.P.....	...I......
IFN-αD (α1)	..SP.A...V	LV...C..S.	...	....E....D	...T.M....	.S....S...	M.........	....	.P.......L	...I....T.
IFN-αH1 (αH2)	...P...M..	LV...C..S.	...	.N.S.....N	...T.M.M..	.R........	......E...	....	....	M.........
IFN-αB2 (α8)	...T.Y..V.	LV......FS	...	....	....	.R........	......E...	....DK....	....	....
IFN-αB	...T.Y.MV.	LV......FS	...	....	....	.R........	......E...	....DK....	....	....
IFN-α4b	....	....	...	....	....	.....H....	.........E	.....H....	T.........	....
IFN-αC	....	....	...	....	........G.	....	......RI..	....	....	....
IFN-αL (▼α10)	....	.........*	...	.......T.R	........G.	....	......RI..	....	....	....
IFN-αJ1 (α7)	..R......V	....	...	.........R	....	....	....E.R..E	.....H....	T.........	....
IFN-αJ2	..R......V	....	...	.........R	....	....	....E.R..E	.....H....	T.........	....
IFN-αI	....	....	...	....	....	....	...P...L..	....	T.........	....
IFN-αF	....	....	...	....	....	....	....	....	....	....
IFN-αWA	....	....	...	....	....	.....H....	...Y......	.V........	.....AF...	....
IFN-αGx-1	...P...M..	LV...C..S.	...	.N.S.....N	...T.MIM..	....	....	....	....	....
IFN-α76	....	....	...	....	....	.....H....	.........E	.....H....	....	....
IFN-α88		....	...	....	....	....	.......L..	....	T.........	....

	80	90	100	110	120	130	140	150	160	166
IFN-α consensus	KDSSAAWDES	LLEKFSTELY	QQLNDLEACV	IQEVGVEETP	LMNEDSILAV	RKYFQRITLY	LTEKKYSPCA	WEVVRAEIMR	SFSFSTNLQK	RLRRKD
IFN-αK (α6)	....V....R	..D.LY....	....	M...W.GG..	....	....	....	....	...S.R...E	.....E
IFN-αG (α5)	.....T...T	..D..Y....	.........M	M......D..	...V....T.	....	....	....	...L.A...E	.....E
IFN-αA (α2)	.........T	..D..Y....	....	..G...T...	..K.......	....	.K........	....	...L.....E	S..S.E
IFN-αD (α1)	.........D	..D..C....	....	M..ER.G...	...V......	K...R.....	....	....	.L.L.....E	.....E
IFN-αH1 (αH2)	.N.......T	.....YI..F	..M.......	....	....	K.........	.M........	....	....	......
IFN-αB2 (α8)	......L..T	..DE.YI..D	.......S..	M.....I.S.	..Y.......	....	.......S..	....	...L.I....	..KS.E
IFN-αB	......L..T	..DE.YI..D	VLC	D.....I.S.	..Y.......	....	.......S..	....	...L.I....	..KS.E
IFN-α4b	E......EQ.	....	....	....	...V......	....	....	....	.L........	......
IFN-αC	E......EQ.	....	....	....	....	....	.I.R......	....	.L........	......
IFN-αL (▼α10)	E......EQ.	........I.	....	....	....	....	.I.R......	....	.L........	......
IFN-αJ1 (α7)	E......EQ.	....	....	....	.....F....	....	.M........	....	........K.	G.....
IFN-αJ2	E......EQ.	....	....	....	.....F....	....	.M........	....	....	......
IFN-αI	E......EQ.	....	....N.....	.....M....	....	....	....	....	.L........	I.....
IFN-αF	.....T.EQ.	.........N	.....M....	....	...V......	K.........	....	....	...L.KIF.E	.....E
IFN-αWA	.........T	..D..YI..F	....	T.......IA	....	....	.MG.......	....	....	G.....
IFN-αGx-1	.....T...T	..D..Y....	.........M	M......D..	...V....T.	....	....	....	...L.A...E	.....E
IFN-α76	E......EQ.	....	....	....	....	....	....	....	.L........	......
IFN-α88	E......EQ	....	....N.....	.....M....	....	....	....	....	.L........	......

Figure 5 The amino acid sequences of human leukocyte interferon (IFN-α) species derived from cDNA or genomic DNA sequences. Sequences, including the signal peptide (S1–S23), are presented in comparison with a consensus sequence (see Ref. 28 for a detailed list of citations). Corresponding residues are presented only when they differ from the consensus sequence. Residues that are common to all listed sequences are underlined in the consensus sequence. Sequences A–L are from the laboratories of Pestka, Goeddel, and colleagues, whereas sequences with numeric designations are from the laboratory of Weissmann and colleagues. Closely related sequences are listed together. The cloned αL(Ψα10) sequence has a termination codon within the signal sequence (indicated by an asterisk) and may therefore represent a pseudogene; however the coding region for the mature protein is otherwise normal. The following interferons are of identical amino acid sequence: αK = α6; αJ = α7; αB2 = α8; αL = Ψα10. The following interferons are identical except for the residues shown in parentheses: IFN-αA (Lys-23), IFN-α2 (Arg-23); IFN-αD (Val-114), IFN-α1 (Ala-114); IFN-αJ1 (Lys-159, Gly-161), IFN-αJ2 (Gln-159, Arg-161), IFN-α7 (Lys-159, Gly-161); IFN-αH1 (Phe-152), IFN-αH2 (Leu-152). A gap was introduced at position 44 in IFN-αA to provide for maximum alignment with the other species. Gaps are indicated by dashes. In several positions, alternative amino acids could be chosen for the consensus sequence: S11, V or L; 78, D or E; 79, E or Q; 80, S or T; 83, D or E; 86, S or Y; 154, F or L; 166, D or E.

CONSTRUCTION OF EXPRESSION VECTORS

Expression of Human Leukocyte Interferon in *Escherichia coli*

As noted before, (p104) contained most of the sequence for a human α-interferon but did not contain the sequence coding for the amino-terminus of the protein. Accordingly, (p104) was used to screen additional cDNA recombinants, and several that hybridized to its unique interferon-coding sequence were identified (29). Most contained interferon DNA sequences of sufficient size to code for an entire α-interferon protein.

Our first full-length recombinant isolate corresponded to IFN-αA (4,29), and its entire *Pst*I insert was sequenced. Existing knowledge about interferon protein sequences permitted us to determine the correct translational reading frame and hence to predict the entire amino acid sequence for the interferon encoded by this recombinant. The mature IFN-αA was expressed directly by reconstruction of the recombinant (29). The leader sequence of the protein was removed and an ATG translation-initiation codon was placed immediately preceding the codon for the first amino acid of mature leukocyte interferon. Next, a 300-bp *Eco*RI fragment of *E. coli* DNA was constructed, containing the tryptophan (*trp*) promoter-operator and the *trp* leader ribosome-binding site, but stopping short of the ATG sequence needed to initiate translation of the leader peptide of the *trp* regulatory region. This DNA fragment was attached to the reconstructed human leukocyte interferon preceding the ATG codon (Fig. 6). Inserted into *E. coli*, the recombinant yielded high levels of activity, about 2×10^8 units (about 1 mg) of interferon per liter of culture. The interferon protein produced in *E. coli* behaves similarly to interferon formed directly by human leukocytes: it is stable to acid treatment, is neutralized by antiserum to human leukocyte interferon, and it binds to monoclonal antibodies specific for human leukocyte interferon. It can be purified to homogeneity with the use of monoclonal antibodies (30,31). With improvements in fermentation and in the bacterial strains, high levels of human α-interferons (1×10^{10} U/L; 50 mg/L) can be reached in large-scale cultures. Similar high levels have been produced with other interferons and other eukaryotic proteins.

Expression of Human Fibroblast Interferon in *Escherichia coli*

A bacterial clone containing β (fibroblast) interferon DNA was identified (4,8). In contrast to the multiple species of α-interferon, experiments have

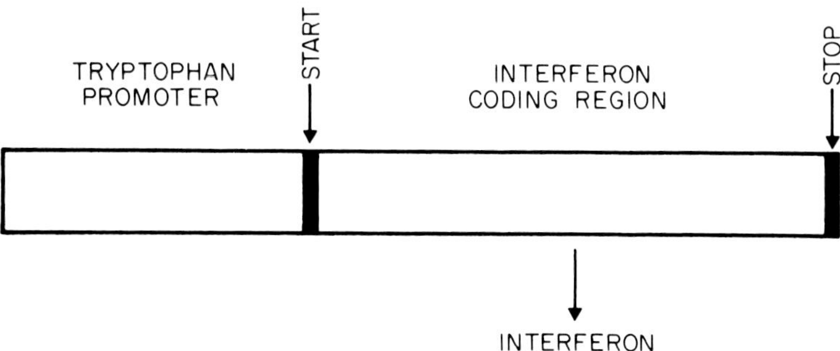

Figure 6 Regulation of interferon expression in *E. coli.* A 300-bp fragment of *E. coli* DNA was prepared with the restriction endonuclease *Eco*RI. This contained the tryptophan (*trp*) promoter-operator and ribosome-binding site. The complete DNA sequence coding for IFN-αA was prepared and an ATG codon (which is the signal for the initiation of translation of the mRNA into a protein) was placed immediately in front of the codon for the first amino acid of the mature protein. The *Eco*RI *trp* promoter-operator fragment was ligated distal to this ATG codon and inserted into plasmids. Bacteria transformed with a plasmid containing this control region and the interferon-coding sequence formed interferon in large amounts in the absence of tryptophan. Leukocyte IFN-αA expression was thus regulated by the *trp* promoter-operator (*Source*: from Ref. 1).

indicated that there is only a single human β-interferon gene that corresponds to this recombinant. To express mature human IFN-β directly in *E. coli*, a series of plasmids that placed the synthesis of the 166-amino acid polypeptide under *trp* promoter control (see Fig. 6) were constructed (8). The IFN-β produced in bacteria is similar to that formed by human fibroblasts by several criteria. It contains the same amino acid sequences; has the same relative antiviral activity on human and bovine cells; and is neutralized by rabbit antibodies to fibroblast-derived interferon but not by antibodies to human leukocyte interferon. However IFN-β made in bacteria is not glycosylated, whereas that made by human cells contains carbohydrate (32,33).

There are three cysteines in human IFN-β, one free cysteine (Cys-17) and two (Cys-31 and Cys-141) involved in a single disulfide bridge. Because the free cysteine permits aggregates of Hu-IFN-β to form (33,33a), Lin et al. (33b) have synthesized a modified interferon where Cys-17 is replaced by Ser-17: [Ser-17] Hu-IFN-β. This new IFN-β is biologically as active as the natural or recombinant IFN-β made in animal cells or in *E. coli.* They report that it is more stable than the natural interferon with Cys-17.

Other Expression Vectors

Although *E. coli* has been the preponderant host used for the production of recombinant proteins, other host-vector systems have been studied and may be used more in the future. For example, the human interferons have been expressed in yeast vectors (34,35). In addition, the regulatory regions of eukaryotic viruses have been utilized to obtain expression of interferons in animal cells (36–40). Furthermore, by direct transformation of cells with the human IFN-β gene together with the gene for dihydrofolate reductase resistance, the human interferon gene has been amplified in Chinese hamster cells (41). With the use of such eukaryotic vectors, glycosylated human β-interferon has been produced at high levels. Human IFN-α has also been expressed in silkworm with the use of a baculovirus vector (41a).

CONSTRUCTION OF SYNTHETIC INTERFERONS

With the isolation of multiple α-interferon cDNA and genomic recombinants, it was possible to construct hybrid molecules. Those recombinants that have restriction endonuclease sites in common can simply be cut and religated to the respective complementary segments. For example, human IFN-αA and IFN-αD were cut at their common *Bgl*II and *Pvu*II restriction endonuclease sites and religated, giving rise to hybrid molecules (42–44) (Fig. 7).

Because IFN-αD exhibits greater antiviral activity on bovine cells than on human cells, whereas IFN-αA has approximately similar activity on both, it was of interest to examine the activity of the hybrid molecules. Their antiviral activity seems to correlate with the amino-terminal half of the molecule, the antiviral activity of the A/D hybrids resembling that of IFN-αA, and the antiviral activity of the D/A hybrids resembling that of IFN-αD. Interestingly, some hybrid molecules have activities that are not exhibited by either of the parent molecules. For example, the hybrid IFN-αA/D (*Bgl*II) is quite active on mouse cells, whereas neither parent molecule is. It seems that a change in a single amino acid of IFN-αA is able to alter the activity of the molecule. An astronomical number of novel interferon molecules can be generated by making hybrids, by amino acid substitutions,

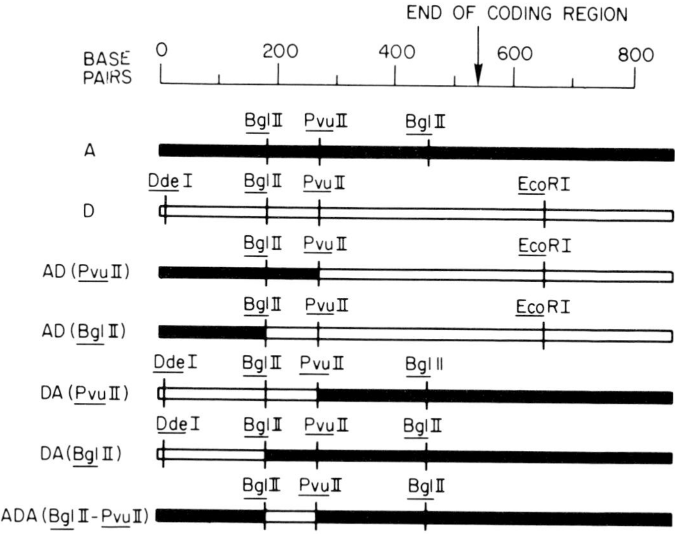

Figure 7 Schematic restriction maps of the plasmid DNA regions coding for the mature proteins of IFN-αA and IFN-αD, showing the sites for cleavage by the restriction enzymes *Bgl*II and *Pvu*II. Hybrids A/D, D/A, and A/D/A were formed by ligating the appropriate segments generated with *Bgl*II and *Pst*I.

and by other alterations. Thus it may be possible to find molecules with specific properties, e.g., with potent antiviral activity but without antiproliferative activity or certain side effects; or to tailor the molecules to exhibit the properties desired, such as high antitumor activity. One such site-specific mutation has replaced the cysteine at position 17 in IFN-β with a serine to provide a molecule with greater stability and activity (33b,45). Many site-specific mutations and various modifications of the interferons have been prepared (45a,45b).

PURIFICATION OF RECOMBINANT INTERFERONS

To purify interferons expressed in bacteria the procedures for purification of any protein from bacteria can, in general, be followed. The bacteria need to be broken to prepare a crude extract. Following this, various ion-exchange or sizing chromatographic steps can be utilized to purify the

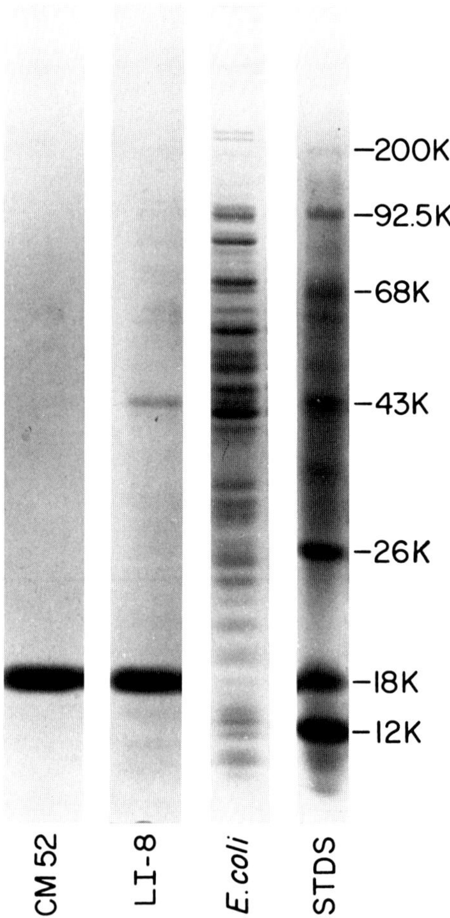

Figure 8 Sodium dodecyl sulfate-polyacrylamide gel electrophoresis of human interferon produced from *E. coli.* Lane LI-8: material eluted from a specific monoclonal antibody column; lane CM-52: the same material after final purification; *E. coli*: total proteins from an S30 extract of bacterial cells producing IFN-αA; STDS: standard molecular weight markers, as indicated. Approximately 20 μg of each fraction was used for electrophoresis. The gel was stained with 2.5% Coomassie brilliant blue (30,31).

molecules. If a specific monoclonal antibody is available that binds the interferon, its use in an affinity column can greatly simplify the purification. As an example, the purification of recombinant human IFN-αA is described.

Purification of Recombinant Human Interferon-αA

Monoclonal antibodies to the human leukocyte interferons can be used to purify recombinant human IFN-αA produced in bacteria (30,31). After *E. coli* containing this interferon are disrupted, unbroken cells and cellular debris are removed by centrifugation. The interferon and soluble bacterial proteins remain in the cell lysate. Nucleic acids (DNA and RNA) that make the lysate viscous, and thus difficult to handle easily, are precipitated by polymin P. The soluble proteins remaining in the lysate are concentrated, if necessary, and passed directly through an immunoabsorbent column containing a monoclonal antibody to human leukocyte interferon. The antibodies bind only the interferon; all of the other components and proteins pass through the column. After the column has been washed, the IFN-αA bound to the column is eluted with an acidic solution (30,31) yielding a virtually pure interferon solution (Fig. 8). The column is washed and neutralized so that it can be used again. The interferon solution is concentrated by passage over a column of carboxymethylcellulose (30,31). The specific activity of the purified IFN-αA made in bacteria is very similar to that of the same human α-interferon subtype synthesized by human leukocytes.

BIOLOGICAL ACTIONS

The recombinant IFN-αA exhibits antiviral activity and antiproliferative activity comparable with those of crude and purified natural leukocyte interferons (44,46). It stimulates natural killer cell activity (47) and cellular differentiation of muscle (48), and it inhibits cloning efficiency of human myeloid cells (49). In studies of human melanoma cells, it was found that interferon is a potent stimulator of differentiation (50). We have analyzed the effects of various human interferons produced in bacteria and the antileukemic compound mezerein (MEZ) on growth and melanogenesis in human melanoma cells. In four human melanoma cell lines, recombinant human fibroblast interferon (IFN-β) was more active than recombinant human leukocyte interferons [IFN-αA, IFN-αD, or IFN-αA/D (*Bgl*)] in inhibiting cellular proliferation. Mezerein, an analogue of the tumor promoter 12-*O*-tetradecanoyl-phorbol-13-acetate (TPA), can itself inhibit growth of cells as well as stimulate differentiation of melanoma cells. The combination of interferon and mezerein resulted in a very potent synergistic inhibition of cellular proliferation in all four melanoma cell lines examined. The results indicated that the antiproliferative effect of interferon toward melanoma cells can be enhanced by treatment with mezerein and that this synergistic effect is associated with an enhancement of terminal differentiation. Because a major problem limiting the utility of interferon as an antitumor agent in vivo may be the development of resistant cell populations, the combination of interferon with agents capable of inducing tumor cell differentiation may help to circumvent this problem and thereby increase the clinical efficacy of interferon as an antitumor agent.

Monoclonal antibodies reactive with the surface of human breast carcinoma cells have been generated and characterized (51). The immunogens used were membrane-enriched fractions of metastatic carcinoma lesions. Recombinant interferon has been employed to enhance the expression of specific tumor-associated antigens on the surface of tumor cells already expressing the antigen and to induce their specific expression on the surface of carcinoma cells not previously expressing the antigen. Such enhancement of tumor antigens can improve gamma scanning for the detection of tumor masses and may serve to improve tumor immunotherapy with monoclonal antibodies.

Currently, IFN-αA is being used in clinical trials in humans (52) as an antitumor agent as well as an antiviral agent (see other chapters in this volume).

The differentiation of human leukemic HL-60 cells from their preponderantly promyelocyte form to a neutrophil-like state can be induced by the addition of dimethylsulfoxide (DMSO) or retinoic acid (RA) to the growth medium (53–57). Within 2 days after the addition of DMSO or retinoic acid to growing HL-60 cells, the binding of IFN-αA to treated cells increases significantly relative to its binding to untreated cells (58–60). The difference in binding of IFN-αA between the treated and untreated cells continues to increase for at least 3 days. These results are in qualitative agreement with those of Yonehara et al. (61). Analysis of binding curves of IFN-αA to neutrophil-like and promyelocytic HL-60 cells leads to the conclusion that the increased binding of ^{125}I-labeled IFN-αA to neutrophil-like cells is primarily the result of an increase in the number of binding sites on these cells.

The increased binding of ^{125}I-labeled IFN-αA to differentiating HL-60 cells precedes terminal differentiation to banded or segmented neutrophils and more likely correlates approximately with the transition to myelocytes. The increased binding is significant by 24 hr after exposure to DMSO and thus is a reasonably early change in the macromolecules defining cellular phenotype. It seems reasonable to suggest that the increased binding of interferon may be tightly linked to the differentiation of these cells.

It is interesting that, of the tissue culture cells we have examined, including Daudi, U937, KG-1, and HL-60 cells, the promyelocytic HL-60 line has the lowest binding of IFN-αA, whereas the differentiated neutrophil-like HL-60 cells show binding closer to that of the other cultured lines (58). The changes noted in IFN-αA binding to HL-60 cells during myeloid differentiation and during monocytoid differentiation (58,61) may ultimately be useful in examining the expression and control of the IFN-α receptor.

INTERACTIONS OF INTERFERONS WITH CELLS

Shortly after pure interferons were available, they were labeled to study their binding to cells (62). The interferon receptors appear to consist of two types: one that binds IFN-α and IFN-β, but not IFN-γ; the second recognizes IFN-γ, but not IFN-α or IFN-β. The synergy of IFN-α and IFN-β on the one hand with IFN-γ on the other is a result of their respective binding to different receptors and resultant distinct mechanistic pathways. Although synergy or additivity is usually the case with IFN-α/IFN-β and IFN-γ, it is possible that their individual pathways may conflict so that they may antagonize their respective actions. Synergy has been demonstrated for their antiviral and antiproliferative activity, antagonism for some macrophage functions.

The Interferon Receptors and Their Chromosomal Locations

The initial event in IFN action is its binding to specific cell surface receptors (62–65). Considerable evidence from the binding and competition of various IFNs to cells has led to the conclusion that there are separate receptors for the leukocyte (IFN-α) and immune (IFN-γ) interferons (66–72). Fibroblast interferon (IFN-β) clearly binds to the IFN-α receptor (68,69,73, 74). There remains disagreement over whether or not IFN-β can also bind to the IFN-γ receptor, although the weight of the evidence suggests that it does not (66,68,71,74–78). The human IFN-α receptor (or its binding subunit) has been identified as a covalent complex with ^{125}I-labeled IFN-α of a relative molecular mass (M_r) of about 150,000 by SDS-polyacrylamide gel electrophoresis (SDS-PAGE) following covalent coupling with bifunctional reagents (67). It appears to be a glycoprotein and is not linked by disulfide bonds to other membrane proteins (67). The IFN-α receptor (or its binding subunit) has been solubilized from cell membranes with detergents as a complex with bound IFN-α (79) or in a form capable of binding IFN-α (80,81). Analysis of the IFN-α and IFN-β sensitivity of various mutant human cells and rodent-human somatic cell hybrids led to the conclusion that the gene encoding the Hu-IFN-α and IFN-β receptor is located on human chromosome 21 (70,82-86). Further evidence comes from the pattern of binding ^{125}I-labeled IFN-α to mutant human cells and to somatic cell hybrids (70,87). Finally, antibodies directed against a membrane protein encoded by chromosome 21 can block IFN-α/β action and binding (70,72,83,84) and can specifically immunoprecipitate a covalent ^{125}I-labeled IFN-α_2 receptor complex (70).

A covalent complex of IFN-γ and its binding site (receptor) of M_r 105,000-125,000 on SDS-PAGE has been demonstrated with ^{125}I-labeled IFN-γ (68-75) or, more recently, with ^{32}P-labeled Hu-IFN-γ (88). By photoaffinity labeling of cultured fibroblasts, a covalent complex of M_r about 230,000 was identified with a photoactivatable ^{125}I-labeled IFN-γ derivative (89). Evidence linking sensitivity to Hu-IFN-γ to chromosome 21 has been presented (90; reviewed in 91). However sensitivity to IFN-γ does not clearly segregate with human chromosome 21 (85,86) and ^{125}I-labeled IFN-γ does not bind to mouse-human somatic cell hybrids carrying human chromosome 21 (70).

We have recently reported the labeling of human IFN-γ with ^{32}P to high specific radioactivity (78,92). The high radioactive specific activity of this reagent permits great sensitivity in probing for the presence of the IFN-γ receptor by binding and covalent cross-linking (88). By cross-linking of ^{32}P-labeled Hu-IFN-γ to various human-hamster, and human-mouse somatic cell hybrid lines, the human chromosome encoding the IFN-γ receptor-binding subunit was located to the long arm of human chromosome 6 (93). However although the Hu-IFN-γ receptor is expressed in the human-rodent hybrids, the protein does not confer on several hybrids the ability to be protected by Hu-IFN-γ from killing by vesicular stomatitis virus.

CONCLUDING COMMENTS

Of the interferons, leukocyte interferon-αA was the first interferon produced in bacteria to be tested in man, but other leukocyte interferons as well as fibroblast and immune interferon are now being tested. Some types, individual species, and combinations of interferon may be more effective than others against particular diseases and under particular conditions. Moreover, it may be possible as more is learned about the mechanisms involved to tailor interferon molecules to optimize particular effects.

Finally, it should be noted that the introduction of a recombinant interferon into clinical trials in humans was achieved in record time by the rapid transfer of technology from laboratory-level basic science to appropriate pharmaceutical areas. This required the enthusiasm, dedication, and cooperation of many individuals as well as guidance from the staff of the Division of Biologics of the Food and Drug Administration. Clinical trials are progressing on schedule and results will be forthcoming continually in the months and years ahead.

ACKNOWLEDGMENTS

I thank my many colleagues and coworkers whose contributions are cited for making all of these achievements possible; Louise Brenner and Kathy Cairoli for expert assistance in the preparation of this manuscript.

REFERENCES

1. Pestka, S. (1983). The human interferons–from protein purification and sequence to cloning and expression in bacteria: Before, between, and beyond. *Arch. Biochem. Biophys. 221*:1–37.
2. Pestka, S. (1983). The purification and manufacture of human interferons. *Sci. Am. 249*:36–43.
3. Nagata, S., Taira, H., Hall, A., Johnsrud, H., Streuli, M., Escodi, J., Boll, W., Cantell, K., and Weissmann, C. (1980). Synthesis in *E. coli* of a polypeptide with human leukocyte interferon activity. *Nature 284*: 316–320.
4. Maeda, S., McCandliss, R., Gross, M., Sloma, A., Familletti, P. C., Tabor, J. M., Evinger, M., Levy, W. P., and Pestka, S. (1980; 1981). Construction and identification of bacterial plasmids containing nucleotide sequence for human leukocyte interferon. *Proc. Natl. Acad. Sci. USA 77*:7010–7013; *78*:4648.
5. Taniguchi, T., Ohno, S., Fujii-Kuriyama, Y., and Muratmatsu, M. (1980). The nucleotide sequence of human fibroblast interferon cDNA. *Gene 10*:11–15.
6. Derynck, R., Content, J. E., De Clercq, E. G., Volckaert, G., Tavernier, J., Devos, R., and Fiers, W. (1980). Isolation and structure of a human fibroblast interferon gene. *Nature 285*:542–547.

7. Houghton, M., Steward, A. G., Doel, S. M., Emtage, J. S., Eaton, M. A. W., Smith, M. E., Patel, P. T., Lewis, H. M., Porter, A. G., Birch, J. R., Cartwright, T., and Carey, N. H. (1980). The amino-terminal sequence of human fibroblast interferon as deduced from reverse transcripts obtained using synthetic oligonucleotide primers. *Nucl. Acids Res. 8*: 1913–1931.
8. Goeddel, D. V., Sheppard, H. M., Yelverton, E., Leung, D., Crea, R., Sloma, A., and Pestka, S. (1980). Synthesis of human fibroblast interferon by *E. coli. Nucl. Acids Res. 8*:4057–4074.
9. Rubinstein, M., Rubinstein, S., Familletti, P. C., Miller, R. S., Waldman, A. A., and Pestka, S. (1978). Human leukocyte interferon purified to homogeneity. *Science 202*:1289–1290.
10. Rubinstein, M., Rubinstein, S., Familletti, P. C., Miller, R. S., Waldman, A. A., and Pestka, S. (1979). Human leukocyte interferon: Production, purification to homogeneity, and initial characterization. *Proc. Natl. Acad. Sci. USA 76*:640–644.
11. Rubinstein, M., Levy, W. P., Moschera, J. A., Lai, C.-Y., Hershberg, R. D., Bartlett, R. T., and Pestka, S. (1979). Human leukocyte interferon: Isolation and characterization of several molecular forms. *Arch. Biochem. Biophys. 210*:307–318.
12. Zoon, K. C., Smith, M. E., Bridgen, P. J., Zur, N. D., and Anfinsen, C. B. (1979). Purification and partial characterization of human lymphoblastoid interferon. *Proc. Natl. Acad. Sci. USA 76*:5601–5605.
13. Allen, G. and Fantes, K. H. (1980). A family of structural genes for human lymphoblastoid (leukocyte-type) interferon. *Nature 287*: 408–411.
14. Levy, W. P., Shively, J., Rubinstein, M., Del Valle, U., and Pestka, S. (1980). Amino-terminal amino acid sequence of human leukocyte interferon. *Proc. Natl. Acad. Sci. USA 77*:5102–5104.
15. Levy, W. P., Rubinstein, M., Shively, J., Del Valle, U., Lai, C.-Y., Moschera, J., Brink, L., Gerber, L., Stein, S., and Pestka, S. (1981). Amino acid sequence of a human leukocyte interferon. *Proc. Natl. Acad. Sci. USA 78*:6186–6190.
16. Shively, J. E., Del Valle, U., Blacher, R., Hawke, D., Levy, W. P., Rubinstein, M., Stein, S., McGregor, W. C., Tarnowski, J., Bartlett, R., Lee, D., and Pestka, S. (1982). Microsequence analysis of peptides and proteins. IV. Structural studies on human leukocyte interferons. *Anal. Biochem. 126*:318–326.
17. Hobbs, D. and Pestka, S. (1982). Purification and characterization of interferons from a continuous myeloblastic cell line. *J. Biol. Chem. 257*:4071–4076.
18. Pestka, S., McInnes, J., Havell, E. A., and Vilcek, J. (1975). Cell-free synthesis of human interferon. *Proc. Natl. Acad. Sci. USA 72*:3898–3901.

19. Thang, N. N., Thang, D. C., De Maeyers, E., and Montagnier, L. (1975). Biosynthesis of mouse interferon by translation of its messenger RNA in a cell-free system. *Proc. Natl. Acad. Sci. USA 72*:3975–3977.
20. Reynolds, F. H. Jr., Premkumar, E., and Pitha, P. M. (1975). Interferon activity produced by translation of human interferon messenger RNA in cell-free ribosomal systems and in *Xenopus* oocytes. *Proc. Natl. Acad. Sci. USA 72*:4881–4885.
21. Cavalieri, R. L., Havell, E. A., Vilcek, J., and Pestka, S. (1977). Synthesis of human interferon by *Xenopus laevis* oocytes: Two structural genes for interferons in human cells. *Proc. Natl. Acad. Sci. USA 74*: 3287–3291.
22. Cavalieri, R. L., Havell, E. A., Vilcek, J., and Pestka, S. (1977). Induction and decay of human fibroblast interferon mRNA. *Proc. Natl. Acad. Sci. USA 74*:4415–4419.
23. Cavalieri, R. L. and Pestka, S. (1977). Synthesis of interferon in heterologous cells, cell-free extracts, and *Xenopus laevis* oocytes. *Tex. Rep. Biol. Med. 35*:117–123.
24. McCandliss, R., Sloma, A., and Pestka, S. (1981). Isolation and cell-free translation of human interferon mRNA from fibroblasts and leukocytes. *Methods Enzymol. 79*:51–59.
25. Familletti, P. C., McCandliss, R., and Pestka, S. (1981). Production of high levels of human leukocyte interferon from a continuous human myeloblast cell culture. *Antimicrob. Agents Chemother. 20*:5–9.
26. Maeda, S., Gross, M., and Pestka, S. (1981). Screening of colonies by RNA-DNA hybridization with mRNA from induced and uninduced cells. *Methods Enzymol. 79*:613–618.
27. McCandliss, R., Sloma, A., and Pestka, S. (1981). Use of DNA bound to filters for selection of interferon-specific nucleoc acid sequences. *Methods Enzymol. 79*:618–622.
28. Pestka, S. (1986). Interferon from 1981 to 1986. *Methods Enzymol. 119*:3–14.
29. Goeddel, D. V., Yelverton, E., Ullrich, A., Heyneker, H. L., Miozzari, G., Holmes, W., Seeburg, P. H., Dull, T., May, L., Stebbing, N., Crea, R., Maeda, S., McCandliss, R., Sloma, A., Tabor, J., Gross, M., Familletti, P. C., and Pestka, S. (1980). Human leukocyte interferon produced by *E. coli* is biologically active. *Nature 287*:411–416.
30. Staehelin, T., Hobbs, D. S., Kung, H.-F., Lai, C.-Y., and Pestka, S. (1981). Characterization of recombinant human leukocyte interferon (IFLrA) with monoclonal antibodies. *J. Biol. Chem. 256*:9750–9754.
31. Staehelin, T., Hobbs, D. S., Kung, H.-F., and Pestka, S. (1981). Purification of recombinant human leukocyte interferon (IFLrA) with monoclonal antibodies. *Methods Enzymol. 78*:505–512.
32. Knight, E. Jr. (1976). Purification and initial characterization from human diploid cells. *Proc. Natl. Acad. Sci. USA 73*:520–523.

33. Friesen, H.-J., Stein, S., Evinger, M., Familletti, P. C., Moschera, J., Meienhoffer, J., Shively, J., and Pestka, S. (1981). Purification and molecular characterization of human fibroblast interferon. *Arch. Biochem. Biophys. 206*:432–450.
33a. Knight, E., Jr. and Fahey, D. (1982). Human interferon-β: Effects of deglycosylation. *J. Interferon Res. 2*:421–429.
33b. Mark, D., Lu, S., Creasey, A., Yamamoto, R., and Lin, L. (1984). Site-specific mutagenesis of the human fibroblast interferon gene. *Proc. Natl. Acad. Sci. USA 81*:5662–5666.
34. Hitzeman, R. A., Leung, D. W., Perry, L. J., Kohr, W. J., Levine, H. L., and Goeddel, D. V. (1973). Secretion of human interferons by yeast. *Science 219*:620–625.
35. Schaber, M. D., DeChiara, T. M., and Kramer, R. A. (1986). Yeast vectors for production of interferon. *Methods Enzymol. 119*:416–423.
36. Zinn, K., Mellon, P., Ptashne, M., and Maniatis, T. (1982). Regulated expression of an extrachromosomal human β-interferon gene in mouse cells. *Proc. Natl. Acad. Sci. USA 79*:4897–4901.
37. Canaani, D. and Berg, P. (1982). Regulated expression of human interferon β_1 gene after transduction into cultured mouse and rabbit cells. *Proc. Natl. Acad. Sci. USA 79*:5166–5170.
38. Devos, R., Cheroutre, Y., Taya, W., Degrave, W., Van Heuverswyn, H., and Fiers, W. (1982). Molecular cloning of human immune interferon cDNA and its expression in eukaryotic cells. *Nucl. Acids Res. 10*: 2487–2501.
39. Derynck, R., Gray, P. W., Yelverton, E., Leung, D. W., Shepard, H. M., Lawn, R. M., Ullrich, A., Najarian, R., Pennica, D., Hagie, F. E., Hitzeman, R. A., Sherwood, P. J., Levinson, A. D., and Goeddel, D. V. (1982). Synthesis of human interferons and analogs in heterologous cells. In *From Genes to Protein*: *Translation into Biotechnology.* Edited by F. Ahmad, J. Schultz, E. E. Smith, and W. J. Whelan. Academic Press, New York, pp. 249–259.
40. Mulcahy, L., Kann, M., Kelder, B., Rehberg, E., Pestka, S., and Stacey, D. W. (1986). Use of rous sarcoma viral genome to express human fibroblast interferon. *Methods Enzymol. 119*:383–396.
41. Innis, M. I. and McCormick, F. (1986). Procedures for expression, modification, and analysis of human fibroblast interferon (IFN-β) genes in heterologous cells. *Methods Enzymol. 119*:397–403.
41a. Maeda, S., Kawai, T., Obinata, M., Fujiwara, H., Horiuchi, T., Saeki, Y., and Furusawa, M. (1985). Production of human alpha-interferon in silkworm using a baculovirus vector. *Nature 315*:592–594.
42. Streuli, M., Hall, A., Boll, W., Stewart, W. E. II, Nagata, M., and Weissmann, C. (1981). Target cell specificity of two species of human interferon-α produced in *Escherichia coli* and of hybrid molecules derived from them. *Proc. Natl. Acad. Sci. USA 78*:2848–2852.

43. Seck, P. K., Apperson, S., Stebbing, N., Gray, P. W., Leung, D., Shepard, H. M., and Goeddel, D. V. (1981). Antiviral activities of hybrids of two major human leukocyte interferons. *Nucl. Acids Res. 9*:6153–6166.
44. Rehberg, E., Kelder, B., Hoal, E. G., and Pestka, S. (1982). Specific molecular activities of recombinant and hybrid leukocyte interferons. *J. Biol. Chem. 257*:11497–11502.
45. Lin, L. S., Yamamoto, R., and Drummond, R. J. (1986). Purification of recombinant human interferon β expressed in *Escherichia coli. Methods Enzymol. 119*:183–192.
45a. Chang, N. T., Kung, H-F., and Pestka, S. (1982). Synthesis of a human leukocyte interferon with a modified carboxy terminus in *Escherichia coli. Arch. Biochem. Biophys. 221*:585–589.
45b. DeChiara, T. M., Erlitz, F., and Tarnowski, S. J. (1986). Procedures for in vitro DNA mutagenesis of human leukocyte interferon sequences. *Meth. Enzymol. 119*:403–415.
46. Evinger, M., Maeda, S., and Pestka, S. (1981). Recombinant human leukocyte interferon produced in bacteria has antiproliferative activity. *J. Biol. Chem. 256*:2113–2114.
47. Herberman, R. B., Ortaldo, J. R., Mantovani, A., Hobbs, D. S., Kung, H. F., and Pestka, S. (1982). Effect of human recombinant interferon on cytotoxic activity of natural killer (NK) cells and monocytes. *Cell. Immunol. 67*:160–167.
48. Fisher, P., Miranda, A., Babiss, L. E., Pestka, S., and Weinstein, I. B. (1983). Opposing effects of interferon produced in bacteria and of tumor promoters on myogenesis in human myoblast cultures. *Proc. Natl. Acad. Sci. USA 80*:2961–2965.
49. Grant, S., Bhalla, K., Weinstein, I. B., Pestka, S., and Fisher, P. B. (1982). Differential effect of recombinant human leukocyte interferon on human leukemic and normal myeloid progenitor cells. *Biochem. Biophys. Res. Commun. 108*:1048–1055.
50. Fisher, P. B., Prignoli, D. R., Hermo, H. Jr., Weinstein, I. B., and Pestka, S. (1985). Effects of combined treatment with interferon and mezerein on melanogenesis and growth in human melanoma cells. *J. Interferon Res. 5*:11–22.
51. Schlom, J., Greiner, J., and Horan, H. P. (1984). Monoclonal antibodies to breast cancer-associated antigens as potential reagents in the management of breast cancer. *Cancer 54*:2777–2794.
52. Gutterman, J. V., Fine, S., Quesada, J., Horning, S. J., Levine, J. F., Alexanian, R., Bernhardt, R., Kramer, M., Spiegel, H., Colburn, W., Trown, P., Merigan, T., and Dziewanowska, Z. (1982). Recombinant leukocyte A interferon: Pharmacokinetics, single-dose tolerance, and biologic effects in cancer patients. *Ann. Intern. Med. 96*:549–556.
53. Collins, S. J., Ruscetti, F. W., Gallagher, R. E., and Gallo, R. C. (1978). Terminal differentiation of human promyelocytic leukemia cells induced

by dimethyl sulfoxide and other polar compounds. *Proc. Natl. Acad. Sci. USA 75*:2458-2462.
54. Gallagher, R., Collins, S., Trujillo, J., McCredie, K., Ahearn, M., Tsai, M. S., Metzgar, R., Aulakh, G., Ting, R., Ruscetti, F., and Gallo, R. (1979). Characterization of the continuous differentiating myeloid cell line (HL-60) from a patient with acute promyelocytic leukemia. *Blood 54*:713–733.
55. Collins, S. J., Ruscetti, F. W., Gallagher, R. E., and Gallo, R. C. (1979). Normal functional characteristics of cultured human promyelocytic leukemia cells (HL-60) after induction of differentiation by dimethylsulfoxide. *J. Exp. Med. 149*:969-974.
56. Honma, Y., Takenaga, K., Kasukabe, T., and Hozumi, M. (1980). Induction of differentiation of cultured human promyelocytic leukemia cells by retinoids. *Biochem. Biophys. Res. Commun. 95*:507–512.
57. Breitman, T. R., Selonick, S. E., and Collins, S. J. (1980). Induction of differentiation of the human promyelocytic leukemia cell line (HL-60) by retinoic acid. *Proc. Natl. Acad. Sci. USA 77*:2936-2940.
58. Langer, J. A. and Pestka, S. (1985). Changes in binding of alpha interferon IFN-αA to HL60 cells during myeloid differentiation. *J. Interferon Res. 5*:637-649.
59. Langer, J. A. and Pestka, S. (1985). Procedures for studying binding of interferon to human cells in suspension cultures. *Methods Enzymol. 119*:305–312.
60. Pestka, S., Langer, J. A., Fisher, P. B., Weinstein, I. B., Ortaldo, R., and Herberman, R. B. (1985). The human interferons: From the past and into the future. In *Mediators in Cell Growth and Differentiation.* Edited by R. J. Ford and A. L. Maizel. Raven Press, New York, pp. 261–281.
61. Yonehara, S., Yonehara, M., Yamaguchi, T., and Nagata, S. (1984). Relationship between interferon system and differentiation of human promyelocytic leukemia cell HL60. (Abstr 1) *Antiviral Res. 3*:49.
62. Zoon, K. C. and Arnheiter, H. (1984). Studies of the interferon receptors. *Pharmacol. Ther. 24*:259-278.
63. Friedman, R. M. (1967). Interferon binding: The first step in establishment of antiviral activity. *Science 156*:1760-1761.
64. Chany, C. (1976). Membrane-bound interferon specific cell receptor system: Role in the establishment and amplification of the antiviral state. *Biomedicine 24*:148-157.
65. Aguet, M. and Mogensen, K. E. (1983). Interferon receptors. In *Interferon 5.* Edited by I. Gresser. Academic Press, New York, pp. 1–22.
66. Branca, A. A. and Baglioni, C. (1981). Evidence that types I and II interferons have different receptors. *Nature 294*:768-770.
67. Joshi, A. R., Sarkar, F. H., and Gupta, S. L. (1982). Crosslinking of human leukocyte interferon α-2 to its receptor on human cells. *J. Biol. Chem. 257*:13884-13887.

68. Sarkar, F. H. and Gupta, S. L. (1984). Receptors for human γ interferon: Binding and crosslinking of ^{125}I-labeled recombinant γ interferon to receptors on WISH cells. *Proc. Natl. Acad. Sci. USA 81*:5160–5164.
69. Sarkar, F. H. and Gupta, S. L. (1984). Interferon receptor interaction. Internalization of interferon α_2 and modulation of its receptor on human cells. *Eur. J. Biochem. 140*:461–467.
70. Raziuddin, A., Sarkar, F. H., Dutkowski, R., Shulman, L., Ruddle, F. H., and Gupta, S. L. (1984). Receptors for human α and β interferon but not for γ interferon are specified by human chromosome 21. *Proc. Natl. Acad. Sci. USA 81*:5504–5508.
71. Orchansky, P., Novick, D., Fisher, D. G., and Rubinstein, M. (1984). Type I and type II interferon receptors. *J. Interferon Res. 4*:275–282.
72. Shulman, L. M., Kamarck, M. E., Slate, D. L., Ruddle, F. H., Branca, A. W., Baglioni, C., Maxwell, B. L., Gutterman, J., Anderson, P., Nagler, C., and Vilcek, J. (1984). Antibodies to chromosome 21 coded cell surface components block binding of human α interferon but not γ interferon to human cells. *Virology 137*:422–427.
73. Branca, A. A. and Baglioni, C. (1982). Down-regulation of the interferon receptor. *J. Biol. Chem. 257*:13197–13200.
74. O'Rourke, E. C., Drummond, R. J., and Creasey, A. A. (1984). Binding of ^{125}I-labeled recombinant β interferon (ISN-β Ser_{17}) to human cells. *Mol. Cell. Biol. 4*:2745–2749.
75. Littman, S. J., Faltynek, C. R., and Baglioni, C. (1985). Binding of human recombinant ^{125}I-interferon γ to receptors on human cells. *J. Biol. Chem. 260*:1191–1195.
76. Anderson, P., Yip, Y. K., and Vilcek, J. (1982). Specific binding of ^{125}I-human interferon-γ to high affinity receptors on human fibroblasts. *J. Biol. Chem. 257*:11301–11304.
77. Thompson, M. R., Zhang, Z.-Q., Fournier, A., and Tan, Y. H. (1985). Characterization of human β-interferon-binding sites on human cells. *J. Biol. Chem. 260*:563–567.
78. Rashidbaigi, A., Kung, H.-F., and Pestka, S. (1985). Characterization of receptors for immune interferon in U937 cells with ^{32}P-labeled human recombinant immune interferon. *J. Biol. Chem. 260*:8514–8519.
79. Eid, P. and Mogensen, K. E. (1983). Isolated interferon α-receptor complexes stabilized in vitro. *FEBS Lett. 156*:157–160.
80. Faltynek, C. R., Branca, A. A., McCandless, S., and Baglioni, C. (1983). Characterization of an interferon receptor on human lymphoblastoid cells. *Proc. Natl. Acad. Sci. USA 80*:3269–3273.
81. Traub, A., Feinstein, S., Gez, M., Lazar, A., and Mizrahi, A. (1985). Purification of properties of the α-interferon receptor of human lymphoblastoid (Namalva) cells. *J. Biol. Chem. 259*:13872–13877.
82. Tan, Y. H., Tischfield, J., and Ruddle, F. (1973). The linkage of genes of the human interferon-induced antiviral protein and indophenol oxidase-B traits to chromosome G-21. *J. Exp. Med. 137*:317–330.

83. Revel, M., Bash, D., and Ruddle, F. H. (1976). Antibodies to a cell-surface component coded by human chromosome 21 inhibit action of interferon. *Nature 260*:139–141.
84. Tan, Y. H. (1976). Chromosome 21 and the cell growth inhibitory effect of human interferon preparations. *Nature 260*:141–143.
85. Zhang, Z.-X., de Clercq, E., Heremans, H., Verhaegen-Lewalle, M., and Content, J. (1982). Antiviral and anticellular activities of human and murine type I and type II interferons in human cells monosomic, disomic and trisomic for chromosome 21 (41405). *Proc. Soc. Exp. Biol. Med. 170*:103–111.
86. De Ley, M. and Billiau, A. (1982). Responsiveness of human cells trisomic for chromosome 21 to the antiviral action of human immune interferon. *Antiviral Res. 2*:97–102.
87. Epstein, C. J., McManus, N. H., and Epstein, L. B. (1982). Direct evidence that the gene product of the human chromosome 21 locus, IFRC, is the interferon α receptor. *Biochem. Biophys. Res. Commun. 107*: 1060–1066.
88. Rashidbaigi, A., Kung, H.-F., and Pestka, S. (1985). Study of the receptor for immune interferon in human histiocytic lymphoma U937 cells with a ^{32}P-labeled human recombinant immune interferon. *Fed. Proc. 44*:1435.
89. Anderson, P. and Nagler, C. (1984). Photoaffinity labeling of an interferon-γ receptor on the surface of cultured fibroblasts. *Biochem. Biophys. Res. Commun. 120*:828–833.
90. Weil, J., Epstein, C. J., Epstein, L. B., Sedmak, J. J., Sabran, J. L., and Grossberg, S. E. (1983). A unique set of polypeptides is induced by γ interferon in addition to those induced in common with α and β interferons. *Nature 301*:437–439.
91. Epstein, C. J. and Epstein, L. B. (1983). Genetic control of the response to interferon in man and mouse. In *Lymphokines*. Vol. 8. Edited by E. Pick. Academic Press, New York, pp. 277–301.
92. Kung, H.-F. and Bekesi, E. (1986). Phosphorylation of human immune interferon (IFN-γ). *Methods Enzymol. 119*:296–301.
93. Rashidbaigi, A., Langer, J. A., Jung, V., Jones, C., Morse, H. G., Tischfield, J. A., Trill, J. J., Kung, H.-F., and Pestka, S. (1986). The gene for the human interferon receptor is located on chromosome 6. *Proc. Natl. Acad. Sci. USA 83*:384–388.

14
Molecular Biology of Human Lymphotoxin

PATRICK W. GRAY
Genentech, Inc., South San Francisco, California

Lymphotoxin (LT) is secreted from mitogen-activated lymphocytes and was initially identified by its anticellular effect on several tumor cell lines (1-3). Lymphotoxin exhibits a spectrum of activities on cell lines, including cytolysis and cytostasis to no growth inhibition. Some primary cell cultures are growth stimulated by LT (4). This anticellular specificity for tumor cells led to in vivo studies that suggest that crude preparations containing LT have an antitumor effect (5-8).

The purification of LT proved difficult because of the small amount and apparent heterogeneity of material secreted from activated lymphocyte cultures. The reported sizes of LT ranged from a relative molecular mass (M_r) of 10,000 to greater than 200,000 M_r (9). Aggarwal et al. (10) reported the purification of LT to homogeneity and demonstrated that a 20,000-M_r band observed by sodium dodecyl sulfate polyacrylamide gel electrophoresis (SDS-PAGE) retained biological activity. This form of LT was purified from the human lymphoblastoid cell line RPMI-1788 and had an apparent M_r of 60,000-70,000 when measured by molecular sieve chromatography. The 20,000-M_r form appears to be derived from a 25,000-M_r form of LT, which was subsequently characterized by Aggarwal et al. (11). Natural LT is thus susceptible to aggregation and degradation phenomena, which may account for the previously described heterogeneity. Additional complexity was caused by the presence of other cytotoxic factors, such as tumor necrosis factor (TNF). Although the 1788-derived LT appeared to be less heterogeneous than that reported previously, antibodies raised against it neutralized all of the cytolytic activity produced by nonadherent lymphocytes (12,13). These results suggest that LT is the preponderant cytotoxic lymphokine produced by the nonadherent fraction of peripheral blood mononuclear cells.

CLONING OF LYMPHOTOXIN COMPLEMENTARY DNA

Lymphotoxin activity is quantitated by observation of cytolysis of a susceptible tumor cell line. The murine fibroblast line L-929 (14) is particularly sensitive to lysis by LT in a rapid assay: Cells are treated with actinomycin D (which increases assay sensitivity by about tenfold) and then exposed to LT for 18 hr. Cells are next stained with crystal violet, and only viable cells absorb the dye. Much of the assay is amenable to automation.

Lymphotoxin was isolated from stimulated RPMI-1788 cultures by chromatography on controlled pore glass, DEAE-cellulose, and lentil lectin Sepharose, followed by preparative native polyacrylamide gel electrophoresis (10,11). The resulting homogeneous LT and proteolytic LT fragments were subjected to microsequence analysis and 155 residues of LT were determined. A small number of COOH-terminal residues were not determined because of the limited availability of material and the hydrophobic nature of this region.

A synthetic LT gene was constructed that encoded the 155 residues determined by sequencing, preceded by an ATG translational initiation codon (15). The design of this synthetic gene presumed that the unknown COOH-terminal residues would not be necessary for biological activity; this has been observed for some other proteins such as interferon-α (IFN-α) (16) and interferon-gamma (IFN-γ) (17). The LT synthetic gene was constructed in three segments from synthetic oligonucleotides 16–20 bases in length (15,18). The three segments were individually cloned, sequenced, and then ligated together with an expression plasmid containing a trp promoter. *Escherichia coli* cultures containing this expression plasmid were grown, but extracts were inactive when assayed on murine L-929 cells. This suggested that the COOH-terminal residues, which were not identified by protein sequencing (and consequently left out of the synthetic gene), were necessary for LT activity.

The three segments of the synthetic LT gene were utilized as probes for the identification of a natural LT cDNA sequence (15). Human peripheral blood mononuclear cells were stimulated with mitogens and utilized for the isolation of mRNA. Complementary DNA was prepared from the mRNA

```
   1                                                               AGGGGCTCCGCACAGCAG
  19 GTGAGGCTCTCCTGCCCCATCTCCTTGGGCTGCCCGTGCTTCGTGCTTTGGACTACCGCCCAGCAGTGTCCTGCCC
  95 TCTGCCTGGCCTCGGTCCTCCTGCACCTGCTGCCTGGATCCCCGGCCTGCCTGGGCCTGGGCCTTGGTTCTCCCC

     -34             -30                                     -20
     met thr pro pro glu arg leu phe leu pro arg val cys gly thr thr leu his leu
 171 ATG ACA CCA CCT GAA CGT CTC TTC CTC CCA AGG GTG TGT GGC ACC ACC CTA CAC CTC

                         -10                                 -1  1
     leu leu leu gly leu leu leu val leu leu pro gly ala gln gly Leu Pro Gly Val
 228 CTC CTT CTG GGG CTG CTG CTG GTT CTG CTG CCT GGG GCC CAG GGG CTC CCT GGT GTT

                         10                                      20
     Gly Leu Thr Pro Ser Ala Ala Gln Thr Ala Arg Gln His Pro Lys Met His Leu Ala
 285 GGC CTC ACA CCT TCA GCT GCC CAG ACT GCC CGT CAG CAC CCC AAG ATG CAT CTT GCC

                             30                                      40
     His Ser Thr Leu Lys Pro Ala Ala His Leu Ile Gly Asp Pro Ser Lys Gln Asn Ser
 342 CAC AGC ACC CTC AAA CCT GCT GCT CAC CTC ATT GGA GAC CCC AGC AAG CAG AAC TCA

                                 50                                      60
     Leu Leu Trp Arg Ala Asn Thr Asp Arg Ala Phe Leu Gln Asp Gly Phe Ser Leu Ser
 399 CTG CTC TGG AGA GCA AAC ACG GAC CGT GCC TTC CTC CAG GAT GGT TTC TCC TTG AGC

                                     70                                      80
     Asn Asn Ser Leu Leu Val Pro Thr Ser Gly Ile Tyr Phe Val Tyr Ser Gln Val Val
 456 AAC AAT TCT CTC CTG GTC CCC ACC AGT GGC ATC TAC TTC GTC TAC TCC CAG GTG GTC

                                         90
     Phe Ser Gly Lys Ala Tyr Ser Pro Lys Ala Thr Ser Ser Pro Leu Tyr Leu Ala His
 513 TTC TCT GGG AAA GCC TAC TCT CCC AAG GCC ACC TCC TCC CCA CTC TAC CTG GCC CAT

     100                                     110
     Glu Val Gln Leu Phe Ser Ser Gln Tyr Pro Phe His Val Pro Leu Leu Ser Ser Gln
 570 GAG GTC CAG CTC TTC TCC TCC CAG TAC CCC TTC CAT GTG CCT CTC CTC AGC TCC CAG

         120                                     130
     Lys Met Val Tyr Pro Gly Leu Gln Glu Pro Trp Leu His Ser Met Tyr His Gly Ala
 627 AAG ATG GTG TAT CCA GGG CTG CAG GAA CCC TGG CTG CAC TCG ATG TAC CAC GGG GCT

             140                                     150
     Ala Phe Gln Leu Thr Gln Gly Asp Gln Leu Ser Thr His Thr Asp Gly Ile Pro His
 684 GCG TTC CAG CTC ACC CAG GGA GAC CAG CTA TCC ACC CAC ACA GAT GGC ATC CCC CAC

                 160                                     170 171
     Leu Val Leu Ser Pro Ser Thr Val Phe Phe Gly Ala Phe Ala Leu
 741 CTA GTC CTC AGC CCT AGT ACT GTC TTC TTT GGA GCC TTC GCT CTG TAG AACTTGGAAAAA

 801 TCCAGAAAGAAAAAATAATTGATTTCAAGACCTTCTCCCCATTCTGCCTCCATTCTGACCATTTCAGGGGTCGTCA
 877 CCACCTCTCCTTTGGCCATTCCAACAGCTCAAGTCTTCCCTGATCAAGTCACCGGAGCTTTCAAAGAAGGAATTCT
 953 AGGCATCCCAGGGGACCCACACTCCCTGAACCATCCCTGATGTCTGTCTGGCTGAGGATTTCAAGCCTGCCTAGGA
1029 ATTCCCAGCCCAAAGCTGTTGGTCTTGTCCACCAGCTAGGTGGGGCCTAGATCCACACACAGAGGAAGAGCAGGCA
1105 CATGGAGGAGCTTGGGGGATGACTAGAGGCAGGGAGGGGACTATTTATGAAGGCAAAAAAATTAAATTATTTATTT
1181 ATGGAGGATGGAGAGAGGGAATAATAGAAGAACATCCAAGGAGAAACAGAGACAGGCCCAAGAGATGAAGAGTGAG
1257 AGGGCATGCGCACAAGGCTGACCAAGAGAGAAAGAAGTAGGCATGAGGGATCACAGGGCCCCAGAAGGCAGGGAAA
1333 GGCTCTGAAAGCCAGCTGCCGACCAGAGCCCCACACGGAGGCATCTGCACCCTCGATGAAGCCCAATAAACCTCTT
1409 TTCTCTGA-polyA tail
```

Figure 1 Sequence and translation of human LT cDNA. The sequence begins at the proposed start of the mRNA (20). Consequently, this sequence contains 100 extra residues at the 5′ end that were not identified by cDNA cloning (15). The signal sequence is presented in lower-case letters.

and cloned in the vector λgt10. This library of 10,000 phage was screened with the synthetic radiolabeled LT gene segments under conditions of low stringency (19). Several phage hybridized to all three segments, and the longest cDNA insert was sequenced.

The lymphotoxin cDNA sequence and encoded protein sequence are presented in Fig. 1. The LT cDNA structure is typical of other characterized cDNAs. The 5′-untranslated region is 170 bp long (20). The 3′-untranslated region is 626 bp in length and contains the consensus polyadenylation addition sequence AATAAA just upstream of the poly(A) tail. The longest open-reading frame predicts a sequence that is completely homologous with the determined LT protein sequence. This is preceded by a 34-residue sequence that has characteristics of a signal sequence (21). The encoded COOH-terminal region of the cDNA predicted an additional 16 residues that were not identified by protein sequencing. Using a PstI restriction endonuclease site common to both sequences, DNA encoding these 16 residues was spliced into the previously constructed expression plasmid. Cultures containing the resulting hybrid synthetic gene/natural cDNA plasmid produced cytolytic activity when assayed on L-929 cells. This activity could be inhibited by polyclonal and monoclonal sera prepared against natural LT, but preimmune serum did not affect the recombinant LT (15).

LYMPHOTOXIN PROTEIN STRUCTURE

The expression of LT in *E. coli* made possible the preparation and isolation of recombinant LT that would be useful for characterizing its biological activities and physicochemical properties. A murine monoclonal antibody derived to natural LT was isolated (C. V. Benton and T. S. Bringman, unpublished) and utilized for immunoaffinity purification (15). Essentially homogeneous recombinant LT can be isolated from *E. coli* cultures by ammonium sulfate precipitation followed by chromatography on the monoclonal antibody-conjugated column.

Recombinant LT derived from *E. coli* is not glycosylated and consequently exhibits a lower relative molecular weight (M_r) (18,600 compared with 25,000) than natural LT. Other biochemical characteristics of recombinant LT are very similar to natural LT. Both preparations tend to aggregate under nondenaturing conditions and to chromatograph on molecular sieving columns as multimers. Both natural and recombinant LT have similar thermolability profiles, with a $T^{1/2}$ of 75°C. Both preparations are insensitive to proteases such as trypsin, chymotrypsin, *Staphylococcus aureus* V8 protease, lysine C peptidase, and thermolysin (22).

The COOH-terminal region of LT is probably buried in the interior of the molecule because this region comprises mostly hydrophobic residues and because LT is resistant to carboxypeptidase treatment. The NH_2-terminus of natural LT is relatively more hydrophilic and susceptible to proteolysis. Two forms of LT have been isolated from RPMI-1788 cells that differ in their NH_2-termini (11); the smaller form (20,000 M_r) lacks 23 residues compared with the larger form (25,000 M_r). Both of these forms of LT have similar specific activities and both have been engineered for expression in *E. coli* (15,18).

The cytolysis of tumor cells by LT appears to be mediated by a specific cell surface receptor (23). Human LT from both natural and recombinant sources was radiolabeled with [^{3}H] propionyl succinimidate at lysine residues. This labeled LT was fully active in cell lysis and bound with high affinity (Kd = 6.7 × 10^{-11} M) to a single class of receptors on murine L-929 cells that contained an average of 3200 binding sites per cell. Binding was specific and could be competitively inhibited with unlabeled LT or with

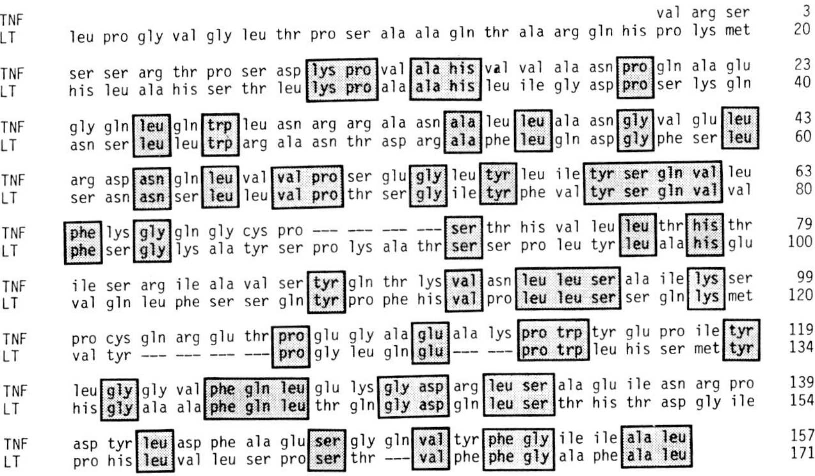

Figure 2 Homology of the primary sequences of mature LT (15) and TNF (24).

antibodies specific for LT. The amount of LT bound to cells was directly proportional to the amount of observed cell lysis.

The primary sequence of LT is unique and exhibits no significant homology with other toxins reported in the Dayhoff database. However significant homology is observed with tumor necrosis factor (TNF), which was cloned (24) and purified to homogeneity (25) by a group at Genentech about the same time as LT. The mature forms of LT and TNF share 35%

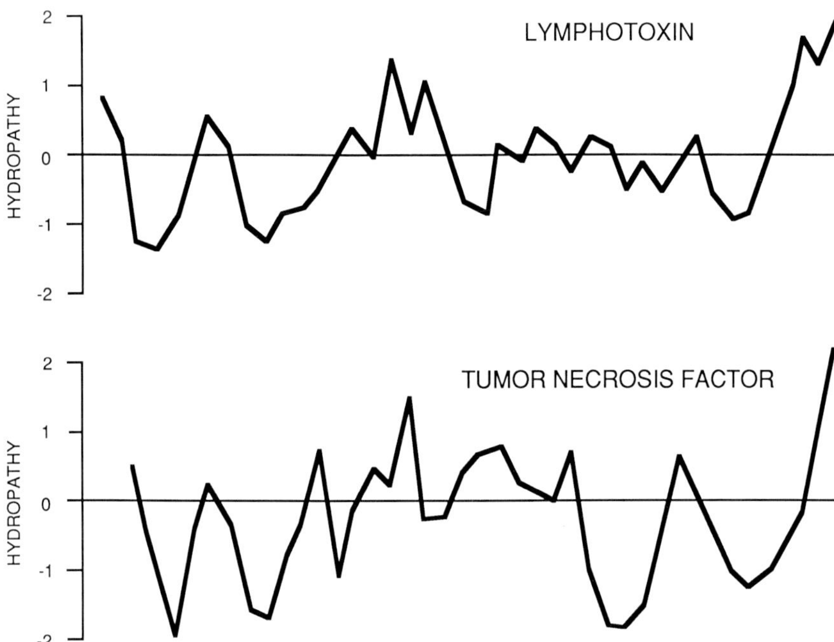

Figure 3 Comparison of hydropathy profiles of LT (top) and TNF (bottom) by the method of Kyte and Doolittle (37), using a width of 10 residues and a jump of four residues.

protein homology, as presented in Fig. 2. In addition, numerous conservative amino acid changes can be observed in this alignment. This homology suggests that LT and TNF have similar structures, which is supported by comparisons of hydrophobicity plots, presented in Fig. 3. Although the signal sequences are not homologous, the secreted forms of LT and TNF each have a relatively hydrophilic amino terminal region and a major hydrophobic COOH-terminus. This similarity is reflected in the biological activities of LT and TNF, described later. Notable distinctions of protein structure of LT and TNF include glycosylation (LT only) and a disulfide bond (TNF only).

LYMPHOTOXIN GENE STRUCTURE

The human LT gene was isolated from a human genomic-λ library using the synthetic LT gene as a probe (20). The gene contains three intervening sequences and is about 3-kb pairs in length, as shown in Fig. 4. The first intron (287 bp) interrupts the 5′-untranslated region, while the second (86 bp) and third (247 bp) introns interrupt the signal and mature sequences, respectively. As shown by Northern blot hybridization, the primary transcript is processed into a 16S mRNA (15). The LT transcript is preceded by a characteristic "TATA" box (TATAAA) 28 bp upstream from the putative cap site (20).

The LT gene structure is similar to that of the TNF gene (20), which also contains three introns. These genes are encoded by human chromosome 6 near the loci for the major histocompatibility complex. As shown by Pennica and Goeddel (26), only 1200 bp separate the 3′ end of the LT gene from the 5′ end of the TNF gene. Only the last exon of each gene is significantly homologous (56%) at the DNA level, as shown in Fig. 5. Because the last exon of each gene codes for more than 80% of each secreted protein, the resultant mature proteins are quite homologous, as shown in Fig. 2.

The transcription of the LT and TNF genes is quite distinct. The TNF is released from macrophages 2–24 hr after induction, while LT is secreted by lymphocytes 8–72 hr following stimulation (13). Consistent with their independent regulation, little homology is observed in the promoter regions of the LT and TNF genes (20).

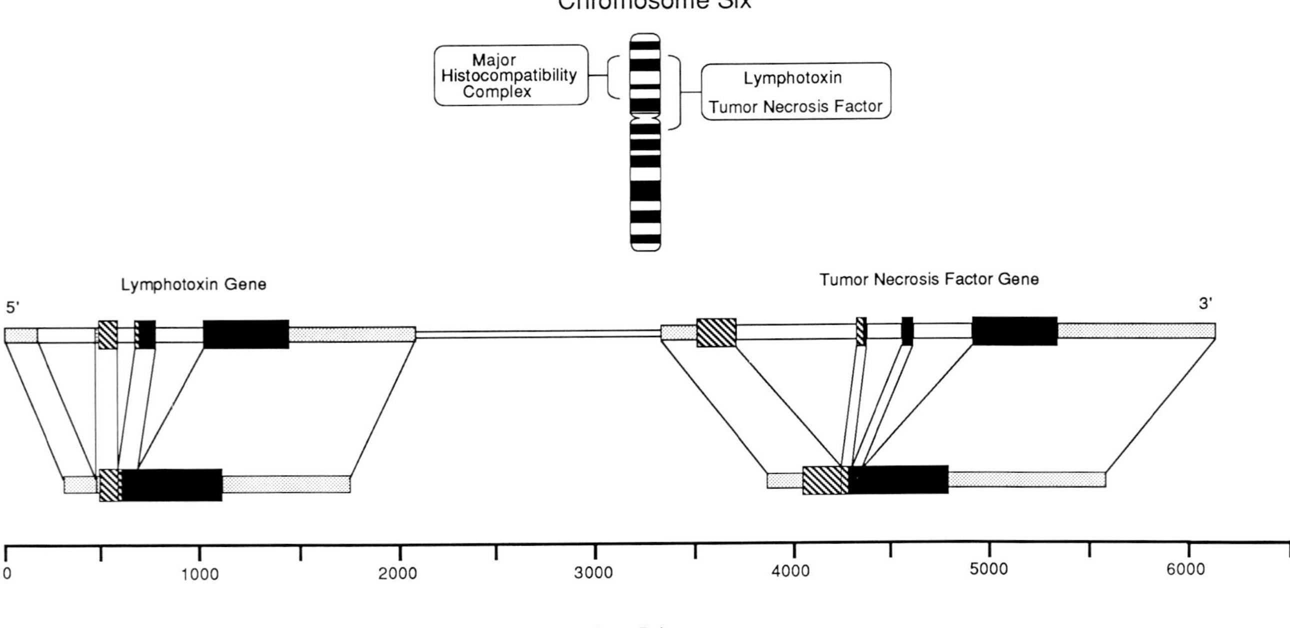

Figure 4 Map of the human LT and TNF genes. Chromosomal localization is presented on top. The primary transcript of each gene contains three introns (open boxes) which are excised to produce the mRNA (bottom). Mature coding sequences are presented as filled boxes, the signal sequence is a hatched box, and 5′- and 3′-untranslated regions are stippled.

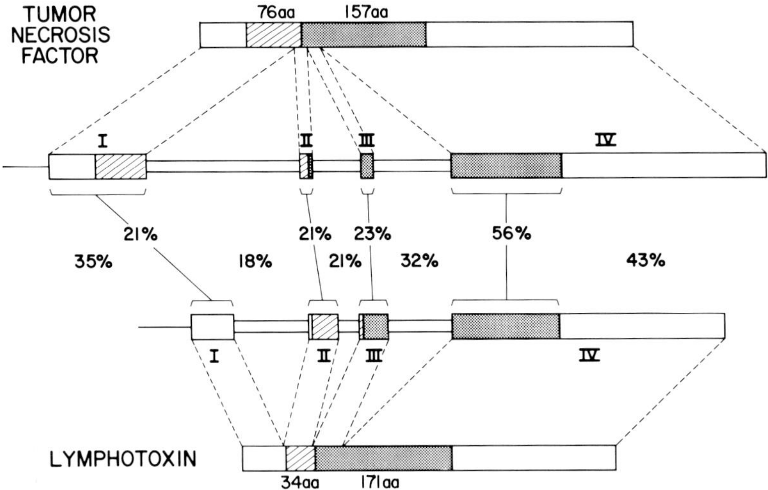

Figure 5 The DNA homology of regions of the human LT and TNF genes. Only the last exon of each gene is significantly homologous.

BIOLOGICAL ACTIVITY OF LYMPHOTOXIN

Lymphotoxin was initially characterized by its anticellular activity. It causes rapid lysis of some tumor lines, exhibits antiproliferative activity on others, and does not affect still others (15,27). It does not inhibit growth of normal cell lines and stimulates the growth of some primary cell cultures (4).

Lymphotoxin exhibits an antitumor effect in vivo. In the classic tumor necrosis assay (28), LT causes hemorrhagic necrosis of methylcholanthrene-induced sarcoma in susceptible mice (15). This is a rapid effect that occurs within 24 hr following intratumoral injection.

This factor also appears to be an important regulatory molecule of the immune system. It can stimulate granulocytes in an antibody-dependent cellular cytotoxicity assay (29,30) and stimulates osteoclasts to resorb bone tissue in vitro (31).

Lymphotoxin and IFN-γ exhibit a potent synergistic effect in antiproliferative assays in vitro (12,32,33). This synergy may be a result of an increase in LT receptor number induced by IFN-γ (34). The potent antitumor activity found in natural preparations of lymphokines may be a result of synergistic activity of small amounts of both LT and IFN-γ (12).

Tumor necrosis factor exhibits all of the biological activities that have so far been ascribed for LT. This is probably a result of their recognition by the same cell surface receptor (34). Lymphotoxin and TNF may work in concert with each other by having similar bioactivities but independent modes of regulation.

Other cytotoxic agents derived from hematopoietic cells have been described. Although antibodies to LT and TNF appear to neutralize all of the murine L-929 cell cytotoxicity of PBLs, other cytotoxic lymphokines may exist that are more species-specific. Natural killer cells produce an anticellular factor that has been partially purified (35,36). Cytotoxic T lymphocytes produce a granule-encapsulated protein (cytolysin) that causes lysis of both normal and neoplastic cells. Antibodies and DNA probes specific for LT and TNF will be useful in understanding the relationship of these cytotoxic factors to LT and TNF.

The cloning of LT cDNA was necessary for characterizing LT and understanding the heterogeneity of cytotoxic molecules. The availability of recombinant LT should aid the biological analysis of this lymphokine and help to define its role in the immune system and in controlling neoplasia.

REFERENCES

1. Granger, G. A. and Kolb, W. P. (1968). Lymphocyte in vitro cytotoxicity: Mechanisms of immune and non-immune small lymphocyte mediated target L-cell destruction. *J. Immunol. 101*:111–120.
2. Ruddle, N. H. and Waksman, B. H. (1968). Cytotoxicity mediated by soluble antigen and lymphocytes in delayed hypersensitivity. III. Analysis of mechanism. *J. Exp. Med. 128*:1267–1279.
3. Rosenau, W. (1968). Lymphotoxin, a review and analysis. *Fed. Proc. 27*:34–38.
4. Sugarman, B. J., Aggarwal, B. B., Hass, P. E., Figari, I. S., Palladino, M. A., and Shepard, H. M. (1985). Recombinant human tumor necrosis factor-α: Effects on proliferation of normal and transformed cells in vitro. *Science 230*:943–945.
5. Papermaster, B. W., Gilliland, C. D., McEntire, J. E., Smith, M. E., and Buchok, S. J. (1980). Lymphokine-mediated immunotherapy studies in mouse tumor systems. *Cancer 45*:1248–1253.
6. Evans, C. H. (1982). Lymphotoxin—an immunologic hormone with anticarcinogenic and antitumor activity. *Cancer Immunol. Immunother. 12*:181–190.
7. Khan, A., Hill, N. O., Ridgway, H., and Webb, K. (1982). In *Human Lymphokines.* Edited by A. Khan and N. O. Hill. Academic Press, New York, pp. 621–632.

8. Ransom, J. H., Evans, C. H., and DiPaolo, J. A. (1982). Lymphotoxin prevention of diethylnitrosamine carcinogenesis in vivo. *J. Natl. Cancer Inst. 69*:741–744.
9. Granger, G. A., Yamamoto, R. S., Fair, D. S., and Hiserodt, J. C. (1978). The human LT system. I. Physico-chemical heterogeneity of LT molecules released by mitogen-activated human lymphocytes in vitro. *Cell. Immunol. 38*:388–402.
10. Aggarwal, B. B., Moffat, B., and Harkins, R. N. (1984). Human lymphotoxin. Production by a lymphoblastoid cell line, purification and initial characterization. *J. Biol. Chem. 259*:686–691.
11. Aggarwal, B. B., Henzel, W. J., Moffat, B., Kohr, W. J., and Harkins, R. N. (1985). Primary structure of human lymphotoxin derived from 1788 lymphoblastoid cell line. *J. Biol. Chem. 260*:2334–2344.
12. Stone-Wolff, D. S., Yip, Y. K., Kelker, H. C., Le, J., Henriksen-De Stefano, D., Rubin, B. Y., Rinderknecht, E., Aggarwal, B. B., and Vilcek, J. (1984). Interrelationships of human interferon-gamma with lymphotoxin and monocyte cytotoxin. *J. Exp. Med. 159*:828–843.
13. Nedwin, G. E., Svedersky, L. P., Bringman, T. S., Palladino, M. A., and Goeddel, D. V. (1985). Effect of interleukin-2, interferon-γ, and mitogens on the production of tumor necrosis factors α and β. *J. Immunol. 135*:2492–2497.
14. Kramer, J. J. and Granger, G. A. (1972). The in vitro induction and release of a cell toxin by immune C57B1–6 mouse peritoneal macrophages. *Cell. Immunol. 3*:88–100.
15. Gray, P., Aggarwal, B. B., Benton, C. V., Bringman, T. S., Henzel, W. J., Jarrett, J. A., Leung, D. W., Moffat, B., Ng, P., Svedersky, L. P., Palladino, M. A., and Nedwin, G. E. (1984). Cloning and expression of cDNA for human lymphotoxin, a lymphokine with tumor necrosis activity. *Nature 312*:721–724.
16. Levy, W. P., Rubinstein, M., Shively, S., Del Valle, U., Lai, C.-Y., Moschera, J., Brink, L., Gerber, L., Stein, S., and Pestka, S. (1981). Amino acid sequence of a human leukocyte interferon. *Proc. Natl. Acad. Sci. USA 78*:6186–6190.
17. Burton, L. E., Gray, P. W., Goeddel, D. V., and Rinderknecht, E. (1985). Modifications of recombinant human and murine interferon-γ and their biochemical characteristics. In *The Biology of the Interferon System 1984.* Edited by H. Kirchner and H. Schellekens. Elsevier Science, Amsterdam, pp. 403–409.
18. Nedwin, G. E., Jarrett-Nedwin, J. A., Leung, D. W., and Gray, P. W. (1985). Cloning and expression of the cDNA for human lymphotoxin. In *Cellular and Molecular Biology of Lymphokines.* Edited by C. Sorg and A. Schimpl. Academic Press, New York, pp. 675–684.
19. Gray, P. W. and Goeddel, D. V. (1983). Cloning and expression of murine immune interferon cDNA. *Proc. Natl. Acad. Sci. USA 80*:5842–5846.

20. Nedwin, G. E., Naylor, S. L., Sakaguchi, A. Y., Smith, D., Jarrett-Nedwin, J., Pennica, D., Goeddel, D. V., and Gray, P. W. (1985). Human lymphotoxin and tumor necrosis factor genes: Structure, homology, and chromosomal localization. *Nucl. Acids Res. 13*:6361–6373.
21. Kreil, G. (1981). Transfer of proteins across membranes. *Ann. Rev. Biochem. 50*:317–348.
22. Aggarwal, B. B. (1985). Human lymphotoxin. *Methods Enzymol. 116*: 441–448.
23. Hass, P. E., Hotchkiss, A., Mohler, M., and Aggarwal, B. B. (1985). Characterization of specific high affinity receptors for human lymphotoxin on mouse fibroblasts. *J. Biol. Chem. 260*:12214–12218.
24. Pennica, D., Nedwin, G. E., Hayflick, J. S., Seeburg, P. H., Derynck, R., Palladino, M. A., Kohr, W. J., Aggarwal, B. B., and Goeddel, D. V. (1984). Human tumor necrosis factor: Precursor structure, expression, and homology to lymphotoxin. *Nature 312*:724–729.
25. Aggarwal, B. B., Kohr, W. J., Hass, P. E., Moffat, B., Spencer, S. A., Henzel, W. J., Bringman, T. S., Nedwin, G. E., Goeddel, D. V., and Harkins, R. N. (1985). Human tumor necrosis factor. Production, purification, and characterization. *J. Biol. Chem. 260*:2345–2354.
26. Pennica, D. and Goeddel, D. V. (1986). Cloning of human and murine tumor necrosis factor genes: Characterization and bioactivities. *Lymphokines* (in press).
27. Williamson, B. D., Carswell, E. A., Rubin, B. Y., Prendergast, J. S., and Old, L. J. (1983). Human tumor necrosis factor produced by human B cell lines: Synergistic cytotoxic interaction with human interferon. *Proc. Natl. Acad. Sci. USA 80*:5397–5401.
28. Carswell, E. A., Old, L. J., Kassel, R. L., Green, S., Fiore, N., and Williamson, B. (1975). An endotoxin-induced serum factor that causes necrosis of tumors. *Proc. Natl. Acad. Sci. USA 72*:3666–3670.
29. Kondo, L. L., Rosenau, W., and Wara, D. W. (1981). Role of lymphotoxin in antibody-dependent cell-mediated cytotoxicity. *J. Immunol. 126*:1131–1133.
30. Shalaby, M. R., Aggarwal, B. B., Rinderknecht, E., Svedersky, L. P., Finkle, B. S., and Palladino, M. A. (1985). Activation of human polymorphonuclear neutrophil functions by gamma interferon and tumor necrosis factors. *J. Immunol. 135*:2069–2073.
31. Bertolini, D. R., Nedwin, G. E., Bringman, T. S., Smith, D. D., and Mundy, G. R. (1986). Stimulation by bone resorption and inhibition of bone formation in vitro by human tumor necrosis factor. *Nature 319*:516–518.
32. Lee, S. H., Aggarwal, B. B., Rinderknecht, E., Assisi, F., and Chiu, H. (1984). The synergistic antiproliferative effect of γ-interferon and human lymphotoxin. *J. Immunol. 133*:1083–1086.

33. Williams, T. W. and Bellanti, J. A. (1983). In vitro synergism between human interferons and human lymphotoxins: Enhancement of lymphotoxin-induced target cell killing. *J. Immunol. 130*:518–520.
34. Aggarwal, B. B., Eessalu, T. E., and Hass, P. E. (1986). Characterization of receptors for human tumor necrosis factor and their regulation by γ-interferon. *Nature 318*:665–667.
35. Wright, S. C. and Bonavida, B. (1981). Selective lysis of NK-sensitive target cells by a soluble mediator released from murine spleen cells and human peripheral blood lymphocytes. *J. Immunol. 126*:1516–1521.
36. Farram, E. and Targen, S. R. (1983). Identification of human natural killer soluble cytotoxic factors (NKCF) derived from NK-enriched lymphocyte populations: Specificity of generation and killing. *J. Immunol. 130*:1252–1256.
37. Kyte, J. and Doolittle, R. F. (1982). A simple method for displaying the hydropathic character of a protein. *J. Mol. Biol. 157*:105–132.

15

Tumor Necrosis Factors Alpha and Beta

DIANE PENNICA, M. REFAAT SHALABY, and MICHAEL A. PALLADINO, JR.
Genentech, Inc., South San Francisco, California

Over the past 25 years there have been numerous reports describing potent immunoregulatory and antitumor activities present in the supernatants of activated lymphoid cell populations. These nonspecific soluble factors, later termed *lymphokines* or more generally *cytokines*, have been an area of intense interest as scientists attempt to dissect the complex and apparently paradoxical interrelationships of specific immune responses and the involvement of nonspecific lymphokine mediators. One major obstacle in the attempt to simplify this area of immunology was the constantly increasing list of newly described factors. Depending upon the bioassay developed to measure a specific activity and the method of lymphokine induction, it was unclear which of the lymphokines were, in fact, responsible for the observed activities.

A major breakthrough came in 1981 with the announcement of the molecular cloning of the complementary DNA (cDNA) for one of these lymphokines, human gamma interferon (HuIFN-γ) (1). The genes for other biologically active proteins such as interleukin-2 (IL-2) (2), and murine IFN-γ (3) have been also cloned.

At the Fourth International Lymphokine Workshop held in 1984 in Schloss Elmau, West Germany, the list of recombinant cytokines was extended to included interleukin-1 (4,5), B-lymphoblastoid cell line-derived tumor necrosis factor-beta (TNF-β) (also referred to as lymphotoxin) (6), and macrophage-derived tumor necrosis factor-alpha (TNF-α) (also referred to as cachectin) (7).

Possibly no other lymphokine has been more controversial than tumor necrosis factor, because the in vivo activities ascribed to TNF were considered to be mediated by lipopolysaccharide contaminants in the TNF preparations purified from serum.

It is the purpose of this chapter to (a) review the history of macrophage-derived TNF-α and the other closely related B-lymphoblastoid and lymphocyte derived factor, TNF-β (previously called lymphotoxin), (b) describe how the techniques of protein biochemistry and molecular biology were used to identify and synthesize human TNF-α (HuTNF-α), murine TNF-α (MuTNF-α), and human TNF-β (HuTNF-β), and (c) describe some antitumor activities as well as some recently discovered immunoregulatory activities of these proteins.

HISTORY OF THE TUMOR NECROSIS FACTORS

The first descriptions of TNF-like activities can possibly be traced to a play by George Bernard Shaw, *The Doctor's Dilemma*, and to scientific reports by Coley and Bruns (8,9) who described regression of certain tumors in patients either recovering from bacterial infections or in patients intentionally injected with bacterial toxins. Gratia and Linz in 1931 (10) and Shear and colleagues in 1943 (11) demonstrated that endotoxins can induce hemorrhagic necrosis of certain transplanted tumors in mice. Endotoxins however are not directly cytotoxic to tumor cells in vitro. It was not until 1952 that Algire (12) demonstrated that the hemorrhagic necrosis was possibly the result of endotoxin-induced hypotension leading to vascular collapse and the resulting tumor necrosis.

In 1975 Carswell and colleagues showed that serum from mice infected with Bacillus Calmette Guerin (BCG) and subsequently treated with endotoxin contained a substance capable of inducing tumor necrosis in certain transplantable tumors in mice (13). They called this substance tumor necrosis factor (TNF) and advanced the hypothesis that endotoxin-induced tumor necrosis was mediated by the release of TNF from activated macrophages. Tumor necrosis factor was also found to be cytotoxic to a number of transformed cell lines in vitro (13–18). Recently Williamson et al. and Rubin et al. have described a B-cell produced "TNF-like" factor that they have named TNF (LUK II) (19,20).

Prior to the Carswell studies, another agent had also been shown to exert antitumor activities. Govaerts in 1960 and Rosenau and Moon in 1961 demonstrated that lymphocytes from specifically sensitized animals could lyse allogeneic target cells in vitro (21,22). In 1968, three groups described a cytotoxic factor(s) produced by antigen- or mitogen-stimulated lymphocytes that also caused target cell lysis (23–25). This factor, initially referred to as *lymphocyte cytotoxic factor(s)*, was consequently renamed *lymphotoxin* by Granger (24–26) and others and more recently *tumor necrosis factor*-beta (TNF-β) (27). The specific reasons for this latest nomenclature change will be discussed in detail in this chapter. We will use the new nomenclature throughout this chapter.

HUMAN TUMOR NECROSIS FACTOR-α

Adherent cells isolated from human peripheral blood mononuclear cells stimulated with BCG and endotoxin produce a factor with tumor necrosis activity (7). This factor named HuTNF-α showed in vivo activities similar to those of murine TNF originally discovered in the sera of mice injected with BCG and subsequently treated with endotoxin (13,16,18,28–30). Antiserum raised against partially purified preparations of HuTNF-α completely neutralized its cytotoxic activity on L929 cells but not the activity of HuTNF-β preparations (31). Purification and characterization of the human factor proved difficult because of the limited quantities of protein that could be obtained from peripheral blood adherent cells.

Alternatively, a panel of human tumor cell lines of hematopoetic origin were screened for their ability to produce HuTNF-α. Two of these, HL-60 and U937, were found to secrete HuTNF-α following stimulation with 4-β-phorbol-1,2β-myristate-13α-acetate (PMA). Measurable levels of HuTNF-α were detectable as early as 2 hr after PMA stimulation of HL-60 cells. Therefore this cell line was used for both the protein purification and the cDNA isolation (7,31).

The HL-60-produced HuTNF-α was purified to homogeneity by controlled-pore glass, DEAE-cellulose chromatography, Mono Q fast-protein liquid chromatography, and reverse-phase high-performance chromatography (RP-HPC) (31). HL-60-produced HuTNF-α was determined to be a protein of approximately 17,000 relative molecular weight (M_r). Microsequencing was performed to determine the NH_2-terminal amino acid sequence of purified HuTNF-α and additional sequence information was obtained from peptides derived by proteolytic digestion of HuTNF-α with trypsin, *Staphylococcus aureus* V8 protease, and chymotrypsin.

Oligo(dT)-primed poly(A^+) RNA from PMA-induced HL-60 cells was used to prepare a cDNA library of approximately 200,000 clones in the

```
HUMAN TNF-β    NH2-Leu Pro Gly Val Gly Leu Thr Pro Ser Ala Ala Gln Thr Ala Arg Gln His Pro Lys Met His Leu Ala His Ser Thr Leu Lys Pro Ala
HUMAN TNF-α                                                                        NH2-Val Arg Ser Ser Ser Arg Thr Pro Ser Asp Lys Pro Val
MURINE TNF-α                                                                       NH2-Leu Arg Ser Ser Ser Gln Asn Ser Ser Asp Lys Pro Val

HUMAN TNF-β    Ala His Leu Ile Gly Asp Pro Ser Lys Gln Asn Ser Leu Leu Trp --- --- --- Arg Ala Asn Thr Asp Arg Ala Phe Leu Gln Asp Gly Phe
HUMAN TNF-α    Ala His Val Val Ala Asn Pro Gln Ala Glu Gly Gln Leu Gln Trp Leu Asn Arg Arg Ala Asn --- --- --- Ala Leu Leu Ala Asn Gly Val
MURINE TNF-α   Ala His Val Val Ala Asn His Gln Val Glu Glu Gln Leu Glu Trp Leu Ser Gln Arg Ala Asn --- --- --- Ala Leu Leu Ala Asn Gly Met

HUMAN TNF-β    Ser Leu Ser Asn Asn Ser Leu Leu Val Pro Thr Ser Gly Ile Tyr Phe Val Tyr Ser Gln Val Val Phe Ser Gly Lys Ala Tyr Ser Pro Lys
HUMAN TNF-α    Glu Leu Arg Asp Asn Gln Leu Val Val Pro Ser Glu Gly Leu Tyr Leu Ile Tyr Ser Gln Val Leu Phe Lys Gly Gln Gly Cys --- Pro ---
MURINE TNF-α   Asp Leu Lys Asp Asn Gln Leu Val Val Pro Ala Asp Gly Leu Tyr Leu Val Tyr Ser Gln Val Leu Phe Lys Gly Gln Gly Cys --- Pro ---

HUMAN TNF-β    Ala Thr Ser Ser Pro Leu Tyr Leu Ala His Glu Val Gln Leu Phe Ser Ser Gln Tyr Pro Phe His Val Pro Leu Leu Ser Ser Gln Lys Met
HUMAN TNF-α    --- Ser Thr --- His Val Leu Leu Thr His Thr Ile Ser Arg Ile Ala Val Ser Tyr Gln Thr Lys Val Asn Leu Leu Ser Ala Ile Lys Ser
MURINE TNF-α   --- Asp Tyr --- --- Val Leu Leu Thr His Thr Val Ser Arg Phe Ala Ile Ser Tyr Gln Glu Lys Val Asn Leu Leu Ser Ala Val Lys Ser

HUMAN TNF-β    Val Tyr --- --- --- --- Pro --- Gly Leu Gln Glu --- Pro Trp Leu His Ser Met Tyr His Gly Ala Ala Phe Gln Leu Thr Gln Gly Asp
HUMAN TNF-α    Pro Cys Gln Arg Glu Thr Pro Glu Gly Ala Glu Ala Lys Pro Trp Tyr Glu Pro Ile Tyr Leu Gly Gly Val Phe Gln Leu Glu Lys Gly Asp
MURINE TNF-α   Pro Cys Pro Lys Asp Thr Pro Glu Gly Ala Glu Leu Lys Pro Trp Tyr Glu Pro Ile Tyr Leu Gly Gly Val Phe Gln Leu Glu Lys Gly Asp

HUMAN TNF-β    Gln Leu Ser Thr His Thr Asp Gly Ile Pro His Leu Val Leu Ser Pro Ser Thr --- Val Phe Phe Gly Ala Phe Ala Leu - COOH
HUMAN TNF-α    Arg Leu Ser Ala Glu Ile Asn Arg Pro Asp Tyr Leu Asp Phe Ala Glu Ser Gly Gln Val Tyr Phe Gly Ile Ile Ala Leu - COOH
MURINE TNF-α   Gln Leu Ser Ala Glu Val Asn Leu Pro Lys Tyr Leu Asp Phe Ala Glu Ser Gly Gln Val Tyr Phe Gly Val Ile Ala Leu - COOH
```

Figure 1 Comparison of rHuTNF-α, rMuTNF-α, and rHuTNF-β sequences. Identical amino acids are boxed. The 79-amino-acid presequence regions of rHuTNF-α and rMuTNF-α are not included. Broken lines indicate amino acid deletions in the sequences.

vector λgt10. The library was screened using a ^{32}P-labeled synthetic 42-base-long oligonucleotide, synthesized using the amino acid sequence data obtained from one of the nine tryptic peptides analyzed. Of the nine hybridizing clones that were obtained, seven hybridized to a [^{32}P] cDNA probe prepared from mRNA obtained from HL-60 cells stimulated for 4 hr with PMA. Two overlapping cDNA clones were obtained that contained 1643 nucleotides and had an open-reading frame encoding 233 amino acids. Comparison of the NH_2-terminal amino acid sequence of natural HuTNF-α with the amino acid sequence obtained from the cDNA sequence showed that the mature polypeptide of 157 amino acids (Fig. 1) was preceded by a sequence of 76 residues which is probably involved in TNF secretion as it is not observed on mature HuTNF-α (7). From the cDNA sequence, a relative molecular weight of 17,356 was calculated for the mature protein, which agrees with the value obtained for the HL-60-produced HuTNF-α monomer on sodium dodecyl sulfate-polyacrylamide gels (SDS-PAGE). The cDNA sequence was engineered for direct expression in *Escherichia coli* under transcriptional control of the *E. coli trp* promoter. Extracts of *E. coli* containing the (pTNFtrp) plasmid contained a prominent polypeptide (recombinant HuTNF-α, rHuTNF-α) that migrated with HL-60-produced HuTNF-α on SDS-PAGE and contained significant cytotoxic activity in the L929 bioassay.

MURINE TUMOR NECROSIS FACTOR-α

The accessibility of a cDNA probe for rHuTNF-α permitted the isolation of the cDNA for MuTNF-α. Of the six macrophage cell lines tested, P388D1, J774A1, RAW 264.7, WR19M.1, WEH1-3, and PU5-1.8, the PU5-1.8 cell line consistently secreted the highest levels of MuTNF activity.

Northern blot analysis was performed to determine whether this activity was due to MuTNF-α, MuTNF-β, or a previously uncharacterized cytotoxic factor. Messenger RNA was isolated 5 hr after PMA induction of PU5-1.8 cells and probed with a ^{32}P-labeled fragment from either the HuTNF-α or HuTNF-β cDNA clones. A band migrating at approximately 18 S hybridized strongly to the rHuTNF-α probe, while no hybridization was seen with the HuTNF-β probe. Because high-stringency hybridization conditions were used, the cytotoxic factor was most likely murine TNF-α.

Oligo(dT)-primed poly(A^+) RNA from PMA-induced PU5-1.8 cells was used to prepare a cDNA library in λgt-10. A MuTNF-α cDNA clone was identified in the cDNA library prepared by using mRNA from the murine macrophagelike cell line PU5-1.8 that was induced for 5 hr with PMA. A

^{32}P-labeled HuTNF-α cDNA probe strongly hybridized to approximately 0.02% of the clones from a cDNA library. Comparison of the encoded amino acid sequence from one of the cDNA clones revealed a strong (approximately 79%) homology to the amino acid sequence of rHuTNF-α. The isolated MuTNF-α cDNA encoded a polypeptide consisting of a 79-amino-acid presequence region followed by the sequence for mature MuTNF-α of 156 amino acids (see Fig. 1). When engineered for direct expression in *E. coli*, the MuTNF-α cDNA directed the synthesis of biologically active recombinant MuTNF-α (rMuTNF-α) as determined by the L929 bioassay (32).

HUMAN TUMOR NECROSIS FACTOR-β

The HuTNF-β was first characterized as a factor in supernatants of mitogen-stimulated mononuclear cells that had cytolytic/cytostatic activities on neoplastic cell lines but which showed little or no anticellular activities on primary cell cultures and normal cell lines (23–25). Purification and subsequent characterization of HuTNF-β proved difficult because of the limited quantity of active protein secreted by primary lymphocyte cultures. Recently, HuTNF-β was successfully purified from supernatants of PMA-stimulated RPMI-1788 B-lymphoblastoid cells grown in serum-free RPMI-1640 medium (33). Purification was accomplished by DEAE-cellulose chromatography, preparative isoelectric focusing, lentil lectin-Sepharose chromatography, and preparative polyacrylamide gel electrophoresis. The HuTNF-β migrated on SDS-PAGE as two bands of M_r 25,000 and 20,000. The M_r 25,000 species represented 95% of the material and the remaining 5% consisted of the M_r 20,000 form. A sequence of 155 amino acids was determined by microsequencing using the Edman degradation technique on the intact molecule and on fragments produced by various enzymatic and chemical cleavages. The COOH-terminal end could not be sequenced however.

A synthetic gene encoding 155 of the residues of HuTNF-β was constructed for expression in *E. coli* (6). This construction for the gene reflected the assumption that the additional undetermined COOH-terminal residues were not necessary for bioactivity. However extracts purified from *E. coli* cultures containing an expression plasmid lacking the unknown COOH-terminal region were not active in the L929 bioassay suggesting that the missing COOH-terminal residues were indeed necessary for the cytotoxic activity of HuTNF-β.

Fragments of the synthetic gene were used as probes to isolate the HuTNF-β cDNA sequence (6). Messenger RNA was isolated from cultures of nonadherent human peripheral blood lymphocytes stimulated with PMA, thymosin-α1 and staphylococcal enterotoxin B. Oligo(dT)-primed poly(A^+)RNA was used to prepare a cDNA library in vector λgt10. About 10,000 clones were screened under conditions of low stringency with a probe prepared from the NH_2-terminal coding (116 bp in length) region of the synthetic HuTNF-β gene. Two clones that hybridized with the ^{32}P-labeled probe were plaque purified. These two cDNA clones also strongly hybridized with labeled HuTNF-β probes prepared from two additional segments of the HuTNF-β synthetic gene. The longest cDNA clone encoded the entire amino acid sequence of HuTNF-β (see Fig. 1). Recombinant TNF-β was determined to be 171 residues in length with a M_r of approximately 18,660. An N-linked glycosylation site at residue 62 probably accounted for the increased size (M_r 25,000) described for natural TNF-β.

Sixteen COOH-terminal amino acid residues not identified by protein sequencing were encoded by the HuTNF-β cDNA sequence. A hybrid expression plasmid was prepared by splicing onto the inactive synthetic plasmid coding sequences for the 16 additional amino acid residues. Extracts from *E. coli* cultures containing this hybrid expression plasmid contained significant L929 bioactivity. The absence of carbohydrate residues on rHuTNF-β does not appear to affect its in vitro cytotoxic activity because the specific activity of rHuTNF-β on L929 cells approximates that of the natural HuTNF-β ($2.5–13 \times 10^7$ versus 4×10^7 U/mg, respectively) (6,33).

The 20,000 M_r form of HuTNF-β lacks 23 NH_2-terminal residues when compared with the 25,000 M_r form. A wide range of sizes for HuTNF-β have been reported from 15,000 to over 150,000 M_r. However this probably does not indicate a family of related HuTNF-β proteins, because polyclonal and monoclonal antibodies raised against natural or rHuTNF-β neutralize all the L929 bioactivity from the RPMI-1788 B-lymphoblastoid cells and from stimulated nonadherent lymphocyte cultures. In addition, hybridization studies indicate that HuTNF-β is encoded by a single gene on chromosome 6 (34). This size heterogeneity is probably due to protein aggregation or degradation, or both.

HOMOLOGIES AMONG HUMAN TUMOR NECROSIS FACTOR-α, MURINE TUMOR NECROSIS FACTOR-α, AND HUMAN TUMOR NECROSIS FACTOR-β

The comparison of the amino acid sequences of HuTNF-α and HuTNF-β indicates that these two proteins share 35% identity and 51% homology when conservative substitutions are considered. The hydrophobic COOH-terminal amino acids in particular are significantly conserved which may indicate this region is important for certain biological activities of the two proteins. While HuTNF-β contains no cysteine residues both HuTNF-α and MuTNF-α contain two cysteine residues at position 69 and 101 that are involved in a single intramolecular disulfide bond (B. Aggarwal, personal communication). In contrast to HuTNF-α, which lacks potential *N*-glycosylation sites, HuTNF-β contains a glycosylation site at residue 62. Further, an amino acid comparison between HuTNF-α and MuTNF-α reveals an overall homology of approximately 79%. The MuTNF-α contains one potential *N*-glycosylation site at Asp-7 which agrees with previous reports describing the glycoprotein nature of partially purified native murine TNF (14). A complete presentation of the amino acid homologies among HuTNF-α, MuTNF-α, and HuTNF-β is illustrated in Fig. 1. It is interesting that a recently purified cytokine from the murine macrophage cell line J774.1 (necrosin) may be identical to MuTNF-α (35).

BIOLOGICAL PROPERTIES

In Vivo Biological Activities of Recombinant Human Tumor Necrosis Factors α and β

The tumor necrosis activity of rHuTNF-α and rHuTNF-β has been measured by the classic in vivo assay using methylcholanthrene-induced BALB/c Meth A sarcoma (13). The assay is as follows: female CB6F1 mice bearing an approximately 0.75-cm average diameter intradermal Meth A sarcoma (7–10 days after tumor injection) were injected intravenously with various doses of either rHuTNF-α or rHuTNF-β. Control mice were injected with phosphate-buffered saline. Twenty-four hours after the intravenous injections, the tumors were scored visually for hemorrhagic necrosis. A comparison of the necrosis activities of rHuTNF-α and rHuTNF-β is presented in Table 1. Both rHuTNF-α and rHuTNF-β induced similar degrees of necrosis at all the doses tested. In addition, necrosis could be induced by either TNF after intramuscular, intraperitoneal, and intralesional administration (6,7).

Table 1 Necrosis of Meth A Sarcoma after Intravenous Injection of rHuTNF-α and rHuTNF-β

Treatment	No. of animals	Mean necrosis ± SD[a]
PBS[b]	49	0.08 ± 0.24
rHuTNF-α		
50 μg	19	2.7 ± 0.6
15 μg	20	2.6 ± 0.6
5 μg	19	2.6 ± 0.8
2.5 μg	28	2.1 ± 1
1 μg	20	1.5 ± 0.9
rHuTNF-β		
50 μg	20	2.4 ± 1
15 μg	20	2.7 ± 0.8
5 μg	29	2.2 ± 1
1 μg	30	1.4 ± 0.9

In the maximum response, denoted by 3, 50–75% of the tumor mass is markedly necrotic; 2 denotes a moderate response that is 25–50% hemorrhagic necrosis; 1 denotes a minimal response of 25% hemorrhagic necrosis; and 0 denotes no visible necrosis.

[a]P values of all groups compared with PBS controls were <.001 as determined by Student's *t* test. Results were obtained from three independent experiments.

[b]Phosphate-buffered saline.

In Vitro Biological Properties of Recombinant Human Tumor Necrosis Factors α and β

Sugarman et al. have conducted an extensive in vitro screen on a panel of 23 human tumors (Table 2) and 12 murine tumor cell lines (Table 3) (36). Of the 35 cell lines screened, rHuTNF-α was active (i.e., induced greater than 25% reduction in cell viability as determined by crystal violet staining after a 72-hr incubation) on 36% of the cell lines. Two aspects of the in vitro studies need further discussion. First, rHuTNF-α enhanced the growth of five normal human fibroblast cell lines but none of the transformed cell lines. This property of rHuTNF-α was previously unreported but clearly demonstrates the possible role for HuTNF-α in the regulation of normal cell functions (36). Second, the synergistic antitumor effect(s) of TNFs and IFNs (36-38) is of considerable interest because it may provide a way to substantially enhance the sensitivity of cancer cells to the cytotoxic/cytostatic effects of the TNFs. Recently, it was shown that rHuIFN-γ increases the total number of rHuTNF-α receptors on human cervical carcinoma cells (ME-180) two- to threefold without substantially changing the affinity constant (39,68,69). This increase in receptor number may be one explanation for the synergistic antitumor effect observed between rHuTNF-α and rHuIFN-γ (36). However changes in the receptor number cannot explain the synergistic antitumor activities observed between particular chemotherapeutic agents and rHuTNF-α (40).

A major biological activity of both TNFs is their ability to influence a variety of human neutrophil functions in vitro (41,42,63). Further, the treatment of neutrophils with a combination of rHuIFN-γ and rHuTNF-β resulted in an activation greater than that observed by either agent alone (41,42). In addition, the stimulation of neutrophil adherence to endothelial cells by rHuTNF-α has been reported (43). The importance of these findings is further emphasized considering the neutrophil's involvement in host defense against microbial infections, inflammatory responses, tumor surveillance, and immune regulatory mechanisms (44-46).

Of greater importance perhaps is the finding that neutrophils can mediate endothelial injury in vitro (47). It is tempting to speculate a possible association between the antitumor and the neutrophil-activating abilities of the TNFs. Thus it is important to determine whether or not TNF-activated neutrophils can modify vascular integrity, and thereby play

Table 2 Summary of Responses of Human Cell Lines to rHuTNF-α In Vitro

Cell line		In vitro sensitivity
A549	Lung carcinoma	–
BT-20	Breast carcinoma	+
BT-475	Breast carcinoma	+
Calu-3	Lung carcinoma	–
G-361	Melanoma	–
Hela	Cervical carcinoma	–
HT-1080	Fibrosarcoma	–
HT-29	Colon carcinoma	–
KB	Oral epidermoid carcinoma	–
LS174T	Colon carcinoma	–
MCF-7	Breast carcinoma	+
ME-180	Cervical carcinoma	+
RD	Rhabdosarcoma	–
Saos-2	Osteogenic sarcoma	–
SK-Co-1	Colon carcinoma	–
SK-Lu-1	Lung carcinoma	–
SK-MEL-109	Melanoma	+
SK-OV-3	Ovarian carcinoma	–
SK-OV-4	Ovarian carcinoma	+
SK-UT-1	Uterine carcinoma	–
T24	Bladder carcinoma	–
WIDR	Colon carcinoma	+
W-38-VA13	SV40-transformed WI38	–

(–) Represents $<25\%$ cytostasis/cytotoxicity.
(+) Represents $\geq 25\%$ cytostasis/cytotoxicity.
Sensitivity to rHuTNF-α was determined by the crystal violet-staining procedure as previously outlined (33).
Source: taken with permission from Ref. 36.

Table 3 Summary of Responses of Murine Cell Lines to rHuTNF-α In Vitro

Cell line		In vitro sensitivity
B6MS2	Chemically induced sarcoma	+
B6MS5	Chemically induced sarcoma	+
B16F10	Melanoma	–
CMS4	Chemically induced sarcoma	+
CMS16	Chemically induced sarcoma	+
CMT-93	Rectal carcinoma	–
L-929	Fibroblast	+
Meth A	Chemically induced sarcoma	+
MMT	Breast carcinoma	+
SAC	Malony transformed 3T3	+
S49	Lymphoma	–
WEHI-164	Sarcoma	+

(–) Represents < 25% cytostasis/cytotoxicity.
(+) Represents ⩾ 25% cytostasis/cytotoxicity.
Sensitivity to rHuTNF-α was determined by the crystal violet staining procedure as previously outlined (33).
Source: taken with permission from Ref. 36.

a role in the induction of tumor necrosis in vivo. Collectively, the data reported to date demonstrate that TNFs exert antitumor effects in vitro and in vivo and immunomodulatory activities on human neutrophil functions in vitro. These facts may be of help in the evaluation of tumor responses in patients treated with TNF and in the elucidation of TNF regulation of immune functions associated with tumor growth inhibition.

Many of the in vitro biological properties of rHuTNF-α and rHuTNF-β have been characterized only within the last 3 years as a result of the availability of these recombinant proteins in a form free of contaminating lymphokines and/or endotoxin. We have included Table 4 to describe some recently characterized activities of TNF-α and TNF-β.

Nomenclature of Human Tumor Necrosis Factors α and β

As discussed in the foregoing sections HuTNF-α and HuTNF-β are products predominantly of distinct cell types (macrophages and lymphocytes, respectively)

Table 4 Biological Activities of Tumor Necrosis Factors

Activity	Ref.
Induces hemorrhagic necrosis of tumors	6,7
Induces IL-1 production	51,58
Activates neutrophil functions	41–43
Suppresses lipoprotein lipase activity in adipocytes	51,59
Induces cachexia in animals	52
Induces cytotoxic/cytostatic effects on tumor cell lines	36
Synergizes with interferon-gamma to enhance antitumor activities	36
Enhances proliferation of normal diploid fibroblasts	36
Stimulates bone resorption	53
Inhibits proliferation of hematopoietic progenitor cells	54
Alters cell cycle progression of tumors	55
Enhances efficacy of certain chemotherapeutic drugs	40
Involved in endotoxin-induced shock	56
Antiviral activity	60–62
Stimulates cartilage degradation	70
Modulates endothelial cell functions	43,64,65
Stimulates HLA, B, and HLA-DR expression	57,66,67

and are antigenically distinct polypeptides that share significant amino acid homology (see Fig. 1). In addition to manifesting similar in vitro and in vivo biological activities (discussed in the two previous sections), it has been shown that these two molecules share a common receptor on human cervical carcinoma cells ME-180 (39). Furthermore, the genes that encode both proteins are structurally similar and are closely linked on human chromosome 6 as reported recently (34,48).

It can be reasoned that the nomenclature issue for HuTNF-α and HuTNF-β is analogous to that of the three types of interferons (α, β, and γ). The interferons are also products of different cell types and are antigenically distinct but share many biological functions besides antiviral activity. The term *interferon* reflects a major function shared by all three proteins. The greek letter designations serve to distinguish their specific physical and biological properties. The nomenclature TNF-β, rather than *lymphotoxin*, is in harmony with this concept.

In addition, the term lymphotoxin does not accurately reflect possibly the most important known property of the molecule, i.e., tumor necrosis activity. Alternatively TNF-β is the more appropriate term because it is descriptive of the tumor necrosis activity, it implies the structural homology with TNF-α, and it maintains the distinct entity of the molecule. Others have discussed the possible presence of a family of antitumor effector molecules and that materials being used as lymphotoxin could be related to TNF (49). To avoid possibly confusing terminology in this area we recommend the use of this new nomenclature. A more detailed explanation for the basis of the new nomenclature has been published (27).

SUMMARY

Discoveries of a tumor necrosis substance in serum of experimental mice and of cytotoxic factor(s) in cultures of stimulated lymphoid cells have triggered intense research efforts that have culminated in the production of recombinant materials purified to homogeneity of two distinct human tumor necrosis factors namely alpha and beta. The two molecules are encoded by two genes on chromosome 6, show significant amino acid homology, and are efficacious in mice. Apart from their shared tumor necrosis abilities, HuTNF-α and HuTNF-β have a number of similar biological activities that they can manifest alone or in concert with IFN-γ. The wide spectrum of biological activities exhibited by tumor necrosis factors may be an indication of their importance in immunological and homeostatic phenomena.

ACKNOWLEDGMENTS

The authors wish to thank Dr. David V. Goeddel for his helpful suggestions in the preparation of this manuscript.

REFERENCES

1. Gray, P. W., Leung, D. W., Pennica, D., Yelverton, E., Najarian, I., Simonsen, C. C., Derynck, R., Sherwood, P. J., Wallace, P. M., Berger, S. L., Levinson, A. D., and Goeddel, D. V. (1982). *Nature 295*:503.
2. Taniguchi, T., Matsui, H., Fujita, T., Takaoka, C., Kashima, N., Yoshimoto, R., and Hamuro, J. (1983). *Nature 302*:305.
3. Gray, P. W. and Goeddel, D. V. (1983). *Proc. Natl. Acad. Sci. 80*:5842.

4. March, C. J., Mosley, B., Larsen, A., Cerretti, D. P., Braedt, G., Price, V., Gillis, S., Henney, C. S., Kronheim, S. R., Grabstein, K., Conlon, P. J., Hopp, T. P., and Cosman, D. (1985). *Nature 315*:641.
5. Auron, P. E., Webb, A. C., Rosenwasser, L. J., Mucci, S. F., Rich, A., Wolff, S. M., and Dinarello, C. A. (1984). *Proc. Natl. Acad. Sci. 81*: 7907.
6. Gray, P. W., Aggarwal, B. B., Benton, C. V., Bringman, T. S., Henzel, W. J., Jarrett, J. A., Leung, D. W., Moffat, B., Ng, P., Svedersky, L. P., Palladino, M. A., and Nedwin, G. E. (1984). *Nature 312*:721.
7. Pennica, D., Nedwin, G. E., Hayflick, J. S., Seeburg, P. H., Derynck, R., Palladino, M. A., Kohr, W. J., Aggarwal, B. B., and Goeddel, D. V. (1984). *Nature 312*:724.
8. Bruns, P. (1888). *Bertr Z. Klin. Chir. 3*:433.
9. Coley, W. B. (1891). *Ann. Surg. 14*:199.
10. Gratia, A. and Linz, R. (1931). *C.R. Soc. Biol. (Paris) 108*:427.
11. Shear, M. J., Turner, F. C., Perrault, A., and Shovelton, T. (1943). *J. Natl. Cancer Inst. 4*:81.
12. Algire, G. H., Legallais, F. Y., and Anderson, B. F. (1952). *J. Natl. Cancer Inst. 12*:1279.
13. Carswell, E. A., Old, L. J., Kassel, R. L., Green, S., Fiore, N., and Williamson, B. (1975). *Proc. Natl. Acad. Sci. USA 72*:3666.
14. Green, S., Dobrjansky, A., Carswell, E. A., Kassel, R. L., Old, L. J., Fiore, N., and Schwartz, M. K. (1976). *Proc. Natl. Acad. Sci. USA 73*:381.
15. Helson, L., Green, S., Carswell, E. A., and Old, L. J. (1975). *Nature 258*:731.
16. Matthews, N. and Watkins, J. F. (1978). *Br. J. Cancer 38*:302.
17. Matthews, N. (1981). *Immunology 44*:135.
18. Ruff, M. R. and Gifford, G. E. (1981). In *Lymphokines.* Edited by E. Pick. Academic Press, New York, p. 235.
19. Williamson, B. D., Carswell, E. A., Rubin, B. Y., Prendergast, J. S., and Old, L. J. (1983). *Proc. Natl. Acad. Sci. 80*:5397.
20. Rubin, B. Y., Anderson, S. L., Sullivan, S. A., Williamson, B. D., Carswell, E. A., and Old, L. J. (1985). *J. Exp. Med. 162*:1099.
21. Govaerts, A. (1960). *J. Immunol. 85*:516.
22. Rosenau, W. and Moon, H. D. (1961). *J. Natl. Cancer Inst. 27*:471.
23. Ruddle, N. H. and Waksman, B. H. (1968). *J. Exp. Med. 128*:1267.
24. Granger, G. A. and Williams, T. W. (1968). *Nature 218*:1253.
25. Rosenau, W. (1968). *Fed. Proc. 27*:34.
26. Granger, G. A. and Kolls, W. P. (1968). *J. Immunol. 101*:111.
27. Shalaby, M. R., Aggarwal, B. B., Rinderknecht, E., Svedersky, L. P., Finkle, B. S., and Palladino, M. A. Jr. (1986). *J. Immunol. 136*:2335.

28. Hoffman, M. K., Oettgen, H. F., Old, L. J., Mettler, R. S., and Hammerling, U. (1978). *J. Reticuloendothel. Soc. 23*:307.
29. Mannel, D. H., Moore, R. N., and Mergenhagen, S. E. (1980). *Infect. Immun. 30*:523.
30. Ruff, M. R. and Gifford, G. E. (1981). *Infect. Immun. 31*:380.
31. Aggarwal, B. B., Kohr, W. J., Hass, P. E., Moffat, B., Spencer, S. A., Henzel, W. J., Bringman, T. S., Nedwin, G. E., Goeddel, D. V., and Harkins, R. N. (1985). *J. Biol. Chem. 260*:2345.
32. Pennica, D., Hayflick, J. S., Bergman, T. S., Palladino, M. A., and Goeddel, D. V. (1985). *Proc. Natl. Acad. Sci. 82*:6060.
33. Aggarwal, B. B., Moffat, B., and Harkins, R. N. (1984). *J. Biol. Chem. 259*:686.
34. Nedwin, G. E., Nylor, S. L., Sakaguchi, A. Y., Smith, D., Jarret-Nedwin, J., Pennica, D., Goeddel, D. V., and Gray, P. W. (1985). *Nucl. Acids Res. 13*:6361.
35. Kull, F. C. Jr. and Cuatrecasas, P. (1984). *Proc. Natl. Acad. Sci. 81*: 7932.
36. Sugarman, B. J., Aggarwal, B. B., Haas, P. E., Figari, I. S., Palladino, M. A., and Shepard, H. M. (1985). *Science 230*:943.
37. Stone-Wolf, D. H., Yip, Y. K., Keller, H. C., Le, J., Destefano, D. H., Rubin, B. Y., Rinderknecht, E., Aggarwal, B. B., and Vilcek, J. (1985). *J. Exp. Med. 159*:828.
38. Lee, S. H., Aggarwal, B. B., Rinderknecht, E., Assisi, F., and Chiu, H. (1984). *J. Immunol. 133*:1083.
39. Aggarwal, B. B., Eessalu, T. E., and Haas, P. E. (1985). *Nature 318*:665.
40. Palladino, M. A. and Figari, I. S. (1986). (in preparation).
41. Shalaby, M. R., Aggarwal, B. B., Rinderknecht, E., Svedersky, L. P., Finkle, B. S., and Palladino, M. A. (1985). *J. Immunol. 135*:2069.
42. Shalaby, M. R., Assisi, F. C., Aggarwal, B. B., Svedersky, L. P., and Palladino, M. A. (1984). *Fed. Proc. 43*:1924.
43. Gamble, J. R., Harlan, J. M., Klebanoff, S. J., Lopez, A. F., and Vadas, M. A. (1985). *Proc. Natl. Acad. Sci. 82*:8667.
44. Weiss, S. and LoBuglio, A. (1983). In *Advances in Inflammation Research.* Edited by G. Weissmann. *5*:107.
45. Babior, B. M. (1978). *N. Engl. J. Med. 298*:659.
46. Kay, H. D. and Smith, D. L. (1983). *J. Immunol. 130*:475.
47. Harlan, J. M., Killen, P. D., Harker, L. A., Stricker, G. E., and Wright, D. G. (1981). *J. Clin. Invest. 68*:1394.
48. Pennica, D. and Goeddel, D. V. (1986). In *Gene Cloning in Lymphokine Research.* Edited by D. Webb and D. V. Goeddel. (in press).
49. Granger, G. A., Orr, S. L., and Yamamoto, R. S. (1985). *J. Clin. Immunol. 5*:217.

50. Dinarello, C. A., Cannon, J. G., Wolff, S. M., Bernheim, H. A., Beutler, B., Cerami, A., Figari, I. S., Palladino, M. A., and O'Connor, J. V. (1986). *J. Exp. Med. 163*:1433.
51. Torti, F. M., Dreckmann, B., Beutler, B., Cerami, A., and Ringold, G. M. (1985). *Science 229*:867.
52. Beutler, B. A., Milsark, I. W., and Cerami, A. (1985). *J. Immunol. 135*: 3972.
53. Bertolini, D. R., Nedwin, G. E., Bringman, T. S., and Mundy, G. R. (1986). *Nature 319*:516.
54. Degliantoni, G., Murphy, M., Kobayashi, M., Francis, M. K., Perussia, B., and Trinchieri, G. (1985). *J. Exp. Med. 162*:1512.
55. Darzynkeiwicz, Z., Carter, S. P., and Old, L. J. (1987). *J. Cell Physiol.* (in press).
56. Beutler, B., Milsark, I. W., and Cerami, A. C. (1985). *Science 229*:869.
57. Collins, T., Papierre, L. A., Fiers, W., Strominger, U. L., and Pober, J. S. (1986). *Proc. Natl. Acad. Sci. USA 83*:446.
58. Nawroth, P. P., Banks, I., Handley, D., Cassiemeris, J., Chess, L., and Stern, D. (1986). *J. Exp. Med. 163*:1433.
59. Patton, J. S., Shepard, M. S., Wilking, H., Lewis, G., Aggarwal, B. B., Eessalu, T. E., Gavin, L. A., and Grunfield, C. (1986). *Proc. Natl. Acad. Sci. USA 83*:8313.
60. Kohase, M., Henricksen-DeStefano, D., May, L. T., Vilcek, J., and Sehgal, P. B. (1986). *Cell 45*:659.
61. Mestan, J., Digal, W., Mittnacht, S., Hillen, H., Blohm, D., Moller, A., Jacobsen, H. M., and Kirchner, H. (1986). *Nature 323*:816.
62. Wong, G. H. W. and Goeddel, D. V. (1986). *Nature 323*:819.
63. Klebanoff, S. J., Vadas, M. A., Harlan, J. M., Sparks, L. H., Gamble, J. R., Agosti, J. M., and Waltersdorph, A. M. (1986). *J. Immunol. 136*: 4229.
64. Pober, J. S., Bevilacqua, M. P., Mendvick, D. L., Lapierre, L. A., and Fiers, W. (1986). *J. Immunol. 136*:1680.
65. Nawroth, P. P. and Stern, D. M. (1986). *J. Exp. Med. 163*:740.
66. Chang, R. J. and Lee, S. H. (1986). *J. Immunol. 137*:2853.
67. Pfizenmaier, K., Schevrich, P., Schluter, C., and Kronke, M. (1987). *J. Immunol. 138*:975.
68. Tsumimoto, M., Yip, Y. K., and Vilcek, J. (1986). *J. Immunol. 136*: 2441.
69. Ruggiero, V., Tavernier, J., Fiers, W., and Baglioni, C. (1986). *J. Immunol. 136*:2445.
70. Saklatvala, J. (1986). *Nature 322*:547.

Index